Art that Tells the Truth

Creative Methods are a shortcut to what we didn't know we knew. In working from a student's or client's own imagination and psychological material, a person discovers who they are and what they need to expand and move forward.

This enriching and inspiring book on creative methods demonstrates the power and effectiveness of the creative approach in guidance and counselling settings. The twenty chapters in this volume focus on the importance and joys of play, creative expression, and imagination in effective learning: as we develop, observe, and interact with our own creations we can arrive at fresh insights by tapping into the wisdom of the unconscious mind. Creative methods often provide a new perspective on difficult emotions and allow us to perceive what they're trying to tell us. Chapter topics include the following: Embodied Theatre Ecology; the Use of Poetry with Clients Recovering from Anorexia; Retirement Life Writing; the Value of Metaphors in Grieving; the Construction of New Narrative Identities in Careers; Dance Movement Psychotherapy as an Approach to Depression; Psychodrama and Philosophy in Learning Self-care by Encountering the "Unknown Other"; Artistic Tools for Psychotherapeutic Work with Children and Youth; Temporal Chair Work; Identity Learning through Paintings; and the ways in which Poetry Can Help us Bridge Cultural Divides and Inform Career Learning Practices.

This volume will be of value and interest to students, researchers, teachers, professionals, and practitioners of psychology, behavioural sciences, mental health, counselling, and education. The chapters in this book were originally published as special issues in the *British Journal of Guidance & Counselling.*

Reinekke Lengelle is Associate Professor of Interdisciplinary Studies at Athabasca University, Canada, and a researcher at The Hague University, the Netherlands. Her book *Writing the Self in Bereavement: A Story of Love, Spousal Loss, and Resilience* won the Best Book Award for Ethnography in 2021 and the International Qualitative Inquiry Book Award in 2022.

Deirdre Hughes is Associate Professor at the University of Warwick's Institute for Employment Research (IER), Coventry, UK. She is an international careers practitioner researcher and senior policy adviser. She led and co-edited an international series of Special Issue Journals on behalf of the *British Journal for Guidance & Counselling.* In 2012, she was awarded a Queen's Honorary Medal (2012) for her services to lifelong guidance.

Liane Hambly is an international career coach, supervisor, and educator of career development professionals. She is the co-author of the best-selling book *Creative Career Coaching: Theory into Practice* (2019) and works with organisations worldwide to strengthen the confidence and skills of their practitioners.

Art that Tells the Truth

Art that Tells the Truth

Creative Methods in Guidance and Counselling

Edited by
Reinekke Lengelle, Deirdre Hughes & Liane Hambly

Routledge
Taylor & Francis Group
LONDON AND NEW YORK

First published 2024
by Routledge
4 Park Square, Milton Park, Abingdon, Oxon, OX14 4RN

and by Routledge
605 Third Avenue, New York, NY 10158

Routledge is an imprint of the Taylor & Francis Group, an informa business

British Library Cataloguing-in-Publication Data
A catalogue record for this book is available from the British Library

ISBN13: 978-1-032-62957-5 (hbk)
ISBN13: 978-1-032-62962-9 (pbk)
ISBN13: 978-1-032-62965-0 (ebk)

DOI: 10.4324/9781032629650

Typeset in Myriad Pro
by codeMantra

Publisher's Note
The publisher accepts responsibility for any inconsistencies that may have arisen during the conversion of this book from journal articles to book chapters, namely the inclusion of journal terminology.

Disclaimer
Every effort has been made to contact copyright holders for their permission to reprint material in this book. The publishers would be grateful to hear from any copyright holder who is not here acknowledged and will undertake to rectify any errors or omissions in future editions of this book.

To my mother Maria Hiske, my daughters Sophia Aurora and Maya Vita, and my son-in-law Caleb Bert who are all artists and know that art is both luxury and necessity.

— Reinekke Lengelle

To my grandchildren Felicity, Rose, Bertie and Shay may your future lives be filled with creativity and kindness.

— Deirdre Hughes

To my students and colleagues who make such a difference to people's lives.

— Liane Hambly

Contents

Citation Information

The following chapters were originally published in the *British Journal of Guidance & Counselling*, volume 46, issue 3 (2018) and volume 48, issue 1 (2020). When citing this material, please use the original page numbering for each article, as follows:

Chapter 1

Embodied Theater Ecology: illuminating the gap through bridging depth psychology's encounter with performative inquiry
Kirsten Frantzich and Lynn Fels
British Journal of Guidance & Counselling, volume 46, issue 3 (2018), pp. 272–281

Chapter 2

Is poetry therapy an appropriate intervention for clients recovering from anorexia? A critical review of the literature and client report
Christine E. Ramsey-Wade and Ellen Devine
British Journal of Guidance & Counselling, volume 46, issue 3 (2018), pp. 282–292

Chapter 3

The warm bathwater of working life slowly ebbing away: retirement stories and writing for therapeutic purposes
Jeannie K. Wright
British Journal of Guidance & Counselling, volume 46, issue 3 (2018), pp. 293–303

Chapter 4

Enter centre stage, the case study…
Deborah A. Lee
British Journal of Guidance & Counselling, volume 46, issue 3 (2018), pp. 304–314

Chapter 5

Walking in a fairy tale forest in search of a second primitivity with the help of Little Red Riding Hood
Michiel de Ronde
British Journal of Guidance & Counselling, volume 46, issue 3 (2018), pp. 315–325

Chapter 6

Cures for the heart: a poetic approach to healing after loss
Patricia A. McClocklin and Reinekke Lengelle
British Journal of Guidance & Counselling, volume 46, issue 3 (2018), pp. 326–339

Chapter 7

Construction of narrative identity based on paintings
Katarzyna Garwolińska, Piotr K. Oleś and Anna Gricman
British Journal of Guidance & Counselling, volume 46, issue 3 (2018), pp. 340–348

Chapter 8

Art dialogue methods: phronèsis and its potential for restoring an embodied moral authority in local communities
Heidi S. C. A. Muijen and René Brohm
British Journal of Guidance & Counselling, volume 46, issue 3 (2018), pp. 349–364

Chapter 9

Arts for the blues – a new creative psychological therapy for depression
Ailsa Parsons, Joanna Omylinska-Thurston, Julianne Harlow, Shelly Haslam, Jessica Hobson, Kerry Nair, Linda Dubrow-Marshall, Scott Thurston, Julia Griffin and Vicky Karkou
British Journal of Guidance & Counselling, volume 48, issue 1 (2020), pp. 5–20

Chapter 10

Towards a deeper integration of creative methods in counselling: some thoughts about frameworks for practice
Valerie Thomas
British Journal of Guidance & Counselling, volume 48, issue 1 (2020), pp. 21–29

Chapter 11

Inter-professional learning: initial observations of the art psychotherapy tools used in the post-qualifying postgraduate training in counselling children and young people
Blanka Hubena and Judith Mulcahy
British Journal of Guidance & Counselling, volume 48, issue 1 (2020), pp. 30–39

Chapter 12

Career assessment and creativity: potential complementarity or a contradiction in terms?
Mark Watson and Mary McMahon
British Journal of Guidance & Counselling, volume 48, issue 1 (2020), pp. 40–51

Chapter 13

The vocational ID – connecting life design counselling and personality systems interaction theory
Marc Schreiber, Adrian Gschwend and Marie-Louise Susanne Iller
British Journal of Guidance & Counselling, volume 48, issue 1 (2020), pp. 52–65

Chapter 14

Use of narratives and collage in the exploration of the self and the meaning of a career
Anne Chant
British Journal of Guidance & Counselling, volume 48, issue 1 (2020), pp. 66–77

Chapter 15
Bridging cultural divides with the power of poetry: an educator's reflection
Caylee Kreller
British Journal of Guidance & Counselling, volume 48, issue 1 (2020), pp. 78–88

Chapter 16
Dialogical Temporal Chair Technique
Małgorzata Łysiak
British Journal of Guidance & Counselling, volume 48, issue 1 (2020), pp. 89–97

Chapter 17
Innovative career construction counselling for a creative adolescent
Jacobus Gideon Maree
British Journal of Guidance & Counselling, volume 48, issue 1 (2020), pp. 98–113

Chapter 18
The philosophy of self-care, individuation and psychodrama: exploring creative means to encountering the "unknown other" in self
Barbara A. Schellhammer
British Journal of Guidance & Counselling, volume 48, issue 1 (2020), pp. 114–124

Chapter 19
Standards of performance and aesthetics in counselling and beyond
Morten Nissen
British Journal of Guidance & Counselling, volume 48, issue 1 (2020), pp. 125–136

Chapter 20
Transforming career stories through poetry: a group-based career counselling intervention
Esther Wafula
British Journal of Guidance & Counselling, volume 48, issue 1 (2020), pp. 137–151

Notes on Contributors

René Brohm, De Nieuwe Kleren van de Wolf, Zwolle, the Netherlands.

Anne Chant, Centre for Career and Personal Development, Canterbury Christ Church University, UK.

Ellen Devine, Expert by Experience, Bristol, UK

Linda Dubrow-Marshall, School of Health & Society, University of Salford, UK.

Lynn Fels, Arts Education, Faculty of Education, Simon Fraser University, Vancouver, Canada.

Kirsten Frantzich, PhD, Licensed Psychologist and Independent Scholar, Los Angeles, USA.

Katarzyna Garwolińska, Kontekst Foundation, Warsaw, Poland.

Anna Gricman, Institute of Psychology, John Paul II Catholic University of Lublin, Poland.

Julia Griffin, Voidance Company, Manchester, UK.

Adrian Gschwend, Career Counselor and Consultant, St. Gallen, Switzerland.

Liane Hambly, Career Development, International Career Coach, Supervisor, and Educator, UK.

Julianne Harlow, Faculty of Health and Social Care, Edge Hill University, UK.

Shelly Haslam, Faculty of Health and Social Care, Edge Hill University, UK.

Jessica Hobson, Lancashire Fire and Rescue Service, UK.

Blanka Hubena, Therapeutic Studies, School of Psychology and Therapeutic Studies, University of South Wales, Newport, UK.

Deirdre Hughes, Institute for Employment Research, University of Warwick, Coventry, UK.

Marie-Louise Susanne Iller, IAP Institute of Applied Psychology, Zurich University of Applied Sciences (ZHAW), Switzerland.

Vicky Karkou, Professor of Arts and Wellbeing, Director of the Research Centre for Arts and Wellbeing, Faculty of Health, Social Care and Medicine, Edge Hill University, UK.

Caylee Kreller, Ontario Institute for Studies in Education, University of Toronto, Ontario, Canada.

Deborah A. Lee, Department of Professional Psychology, School of Psychology, University of the West of England, Bristol, UK.

Reinekke Lengelle, Faculty of Humanities and Social Sciences, Athabasca University, Canada.

Małgorzata Łysiak, Institute of Psychology, John Paul II Catholic University of Lublin, Poland.

Jacobus Gideon Maree, Department of Psychology, University of Pretoria, South Africa.

Patricia A. McClocklin, Faculty of Humanities and Social Sciences, Athabasca University, Canada.

Mary McMahon, School of Education, The University of Queensland, Brisbane, Australia.

Heidi S. C. A. Muijen, Centre for Philosophical Counselling, Thymia, Weesp, the Netherlands.

Judith Mulcahy, Independent Consultant, Newport, UK.

Kerry Nair, The Christie NHS Foundation Trust, Manchester, UK.

Morten Nissen, School of Education, Aarhus University, Copenhagen, Denmark.

Piotr K. Oleś, Institute of Psychology, John Paul II Catholic University of Lublin, Poland.

Joanna Omylinska-Thurston, School of Health & Society, University of Salford, UK and Greater Manchester Mental Health NHS Foundation Trust, UK.

Ailsa Parsons, School of Health & Society, University of Salford, UK.

Christine E. Ramsey-Wade, Centre for Appearance Research, University of the West of England, Bristol, UK.

Michiel de Ronde, Institute for Applied Social Sciences, University Applied Sciences Rotterdam, the Netherlands.

Barbara A. Schellhammer, Munich School of Philosophy SJ, Germany.

Marc Schreiber, IAP Institute of Applied Psychology, Zurich University of Applied Sciences (ZHAW), Switzerland.

Valerie Thomas, Independent Scholar, UK.

Scott Thurston, School of Arts, Media and Creative Technology, University of Salford, UK.

Esther Wafula, School of Human and Social Sciences, Department of Psychology and Counselling, Daystar University, Nairobi, Kenya.

Mark Watson, Department of Psychology, Nelson Mandela University, Port Elizabeth, South Africa.

Jeannie K. Wright, Department of Counselling, University of Malta, Malta.

Acknowledgements

We would like to thank all the authors who participated in the creation of the "Creative Methods" Special Issues that have become this book and who have expressed their enthusiastic support for the project. We also thank the reviewers, patient co-editors, and production editors at the *British Journal of Guidance & Counselling*. We also thank our Routledge editor Anveshi Gupta and Editorial Assistant Ria Goyal for making this book project a reality.

Introduction—Art that Tells the Truth: Creative Methods in Guidance and Counselling

Reinekke Lengelle, Deirdre Hughes and Liane Hambly

Painter Pablo Picasso is known for this evocative statement, *"We all know that Art is not truth. Art is a lie that makes us realise truth, at least the truth that is given us to understand"*. What he seems to be pointing to is a fundamental principle of human development: we learn through play, through imagination, and through make-believe, and as we observe and interact with our own creations, we come to understand ourselves better. This collection of twenty chapters on *Creative Methods* in guidance and counselling settings aims to demonstrate the power and effectiveness of introducing creative approaches. We engaged with this project because we saw and believed that Creative Methods can give us a new perspective on difficult emotions and life events and allow us to perceive what we might learn. Working creatively can be a shortcut to the unconscious, drawing from the student's or client's own imagination and psychological material, allowing new life-giving perspectives to emerge.

When Reinekke first began working in the field of Writing for Wellbeing 25 years ago (Den Elzen & Lengelle, 2023), she noticed that her students often experienced miraculous insights through exercises that stimulated them to play. She was much less likely to see this unfolding when she asked them to answer more rational-sounding questions. In her work in Career Writing (Lengelle & Meijers, 2015), when she stimulated people to think about their career aspirations, it was much more useful to ask them to "write down what you childhood hero would say to you now about the question you posed at the start of this workshop…" and have them write a dialogue with Spiderman or Pippy Longstocking than if she asked them to "please write out what you think you would like to be doing in five years".

Likewise, in working in career counselling, Liane found that clients engaged at a deeper level when using multi-sensory methods – they were more likely to arrive at "lightbulb" moments and regard the process as powerful whereby images and metaphors encouraged them to explore the constructs they held about their selves and opportunities. Using the body in activities such as chair work (Cardoso & Duarte, 2020) enabled them to discover their more confident and self-compassionate self; physically standing back to view the situation gained critical distance and unearthed their ability to answer their own questions. When used in shorter sessions and with a lighter touch, clients of all ages often found the sessions more meaningful and engaging.

Deirdre grew up in Northern Ireland in the 1970s during "The Troubles". She witnessed first-hand the psychological damage to individuals' confidence and self-esteem that often came from divided communities and overtly formal ways of working with young people and adults, particularly with those most vulnerable. She understood the importance of dignity, tolerance, and respect and noticed how easily these could disappear when left unattended. This is where Creative Methods applied skilfully in guidance and counselling can make a positive difference to individuals' lives regardless of circumstance, age, gender, race, religion, or sexuality. For some, unavoidable suffering is difficult to escape though this does not have to define one's life forever as our well-being hinges greatly on the perspectives we may take (Frankl, 1955). Her clients taught her that reshaping those perspectives was possible through creative approaches, noting the importance as well of having a safe "places and spaces" to tell their stories and to create a livelihood and/or meaningful life – that is, to fundamentally nurture people as described in this book.

Our experiences and awareness of the potential of Creative Methods in guidance and counselling led us to work on this topic, and the chapters you see here were originally articles published as Parts I and II of the Creative Methods symposium issues with the *British Journal of Guidance and Counselling* published in 2018 and 2020.

THE CHAPTERS

Part I

Creative Methods are intended to inform and support researchers, practitioners, educators, and those they serve. As artist and writer William Blake might have said, one needs "a firm persuasion" (cited in Whyte, 2001, p. 3) to gain wisdom and insights into life, and in the process of expanding the evidence base for Creative Methods in guidance and counselling we are affirmed that this is both essential and rewarding.

In our original call for papers, we identified several reasons that Creative Methods are essential to guidance and counselling; for instance, they reintroduce playfulness, which is an often-undervalued capacity of humans that can help create space to respond to serious questions. Creative Methods allow us to be less resistant to the so-called "negative" feelings and they let us break rank with the rational linear thinking, planning, efficiency, and goal orientation that has dominated policy and some practice discourses. In essence, this has suppressed the creative, sensory, and feeling side of human needs and behaviours. Indeed, a common theme that appeared in all the chapters is the importance of making room for the affective before connecting that with more cognitive articulations and solutions.

It is only by embodying feelings and putting words to what happens that people can make use of what they learn about themselves and others. Fundamentally creative work bridges a gap we experience between a sense of being both an "I" and a "me" and helps us make meaning out of experience – in particular when we perceive things to be discordant in our relationships with ourselves, others, and the wider world.

The methods described in the following chapters may sound new to some, but this is likely because educational practice is still frequently associated with reproductive modes of working and knowing. As counsellors, guidance professionals, educators, and students in the field of human development, there is still a tendency to focus on "information provision" and "knowledge transfer" and "skill building" as if by default. The invitation that creative methods offer is to work differently – to shift to more personalised and meaning-oriented modes of learning. This requires reflexive practice, tuning in, and being both associative and structured in our responses. Ultimately, people will access and construct personal wisdom by listening in, hearing the body speak, following their passions, and creative urges (or nurturing the tiny first whisperings of such urges). In this way, people have the opportunity to develop a stronger inner voice or clear whatever is in the way.

This book begins with the creative method, Embodied Theatre Ecology, where authors Frantzich and Fels show the importance of the somatic in psychotherapy and provide a variety of activities that a counsellor can do within therapy when words fall short. This method intends to "bridge the gap between lived experience and the words we have to express that lived experience". Snippets of "Nell's" (a client) story are told and how a person might use "body as an ear" or work with "evocative objects".

In the second chapter in this collection, Ramsey-Wade and Devine explore the potential of using poetry therapy to work with those with anorexia. The authors provide a thorough description of the poetry-therapy field and research in the area of writing for personal development, both which have developed extensively over the last 50 years. The chapter includes the personal story of one of the authors, showing how poetry helped her put words to feelings that she experienced as bodily discomfort, where bodily sensations and emotions felt like weapons and not resources.

Wright's chapter is third and addresses the world of work, in particular leaving the "warm bathwater" of paid work. What does this mean for someone's sense of self and their personal story? Here writing for therapeutic purposes is the methodology and the reader will see how "Images in creative writing can help individuals to connect with feelings that they are not consciously aware of, connect with themselves and with others".

This chapter is followed by Lee's work which makes use of a playwriting format to get across the idea that one of the risks of using case studies is that it reduces clients to their problems and therapists to a summation of their credentials and professional experience. Lee helps us instead to become aware of a "co-existence criterion" and does this in dialogue with "Kate" who is in therapy. Lee speaks about a warmth in the work they do together and she ends with the question, does what I'm doing "permit me to go into dialogue?" inviting others to consider this as well.

Next is a consideration of the ideas of author and educator De Ronde who takes his coaches into the woods for a walk and a talk and initiates an embodied conversation process with prompts from Little Red Riding Hood. He proposes that the danger of reflection is that we see ourselves as objects we can reflect upon and this creates a division "between human and nature, and between the person and him – or herself" which can "be a source of alienation and depression, because it fractures a more primitive connection between the self and nature". His remedy is this unique coaching approach, which involves a "combination of the sensation of *participation mystique* with the ability to reflexively find one's own path of life".

McClocklin and Lengelle's chapter follows with an exploration of grieving and how poetry can become an important way of expressing pain and making sense of loss. Here the authors also examine how grieving is repressed and complicated in our society and how poetry allows for its expression. Three specific types of metaphors are explored here as well and how they might bring meaning and solace. In this chapter, McClocklin speaks specifically of the loss of her husband and how poetry became a way to express and make sense of his death and how the urge to write erupted inside her. At the time the authors wrote the original article, Lengelle did not know that she herself would be facing widowhood but the writing here set the tone for her own poetic expression when her spouse Frans Meijers was also diagnosed with cancer as McClocklin's husband had been. Such synchronicities frequently mark the work of those involved with creative methods, and we can draw strength from the timing of events, as Lengelle did.

Garwolińska, Oles, and Gricman present a narrative-based creative method where images of paintings are used to explore the story of self. The material used in working with clients is a set of 100 colour copies of paintings. A person is asked to choose a number of these pictures and tell his or her life story based on the images. Like some of the other methods, the ability to speak of one's self often works better by using indirect means, whether that is a movement the body makes, a poem that emerges in the face of grief or illness, or telling one's stories in response to specific objects and images.

The final chapter in this Part I collection is the work of Muijen and Brohm and it looks at "healing organizational rifts" through an Art-Dialogue method. It explains how art invokes the senses in sense-making. The authors also make a strong case for becoming "conscious, critical, cosmopolitan citizens" and breaking out of our comforting routines to take a stand in our troubled times. They advocate the development of a moral compass through a game that includes symbolic pictures, paintings, music, and dialogue. As their work is more focused on what we can all do to improve life in a broader societal context, we chose to put their chapter as a capstone piece of the first issue of the journal where this piece was first published. After all, the creative methods that we are presenting here aim to heal and inspire the individual and are ultimately intended to serve the greater whole.

Part II

"Life isn't a support system for art. It's the other way around". Stephen King

In the year since the publication of the first *Creative Methods Special Issue (Part I above)*, Reinekke Lengelle lost her work and life partner, Dr Frans Meijers, to cancer. During his illness, Reinekke wrote a series of poems that she shared with Frans to help them talk about his conscious journey towards death. She also began writing a book on grieving that was eventually published under the title "Writing the Self in Bereavement" (Routledge, 2021). It was not lost on us when we wrote the editorial for Issue II (Part II here) that engaging with a creative method had helped Reinekke to make meaning of this loss. Creative, expressive, and reflective writing allows people who engage this way to stay close to feelings, to actively and consciously grieve, to perhaps share the process (and therefore stay connected with others), and ultimately to craft a story of resilience and reverence, instead of one of depression or victimhood. Indeed, it should not be surprising that creative methods can be profoundly useful in guidance and counselling policies and practices.

Part II of this volume on Creative Methods engages with a diversity of contexts, locations, and arts forms – including dialogue, therapies, poetry, and psychometrics – and brings together theoretical and practice-based perspectives on the question of what creativity can bring to guidance and counselling practices in individual and social contexts. From an interdisciplinary viewpoint, Lechevalier and Laugier (2019) have argued that the complexity and uniqueness of different situations mean that we cannot reduce or predict the outcome or result of human activities. Instead, such difficulties require creative and tailormade responses and the contributions here feature ways in which to work and think about those responses.

The reflexive approaches presented in section include methods and concepts for working in hybrid contemporary form, particularly at a time when theories and models of identity and human behaviour from all disciplines of the social sciences are evolving. In considering the importance of cultural influences, Arthur (2018) has indicated that insufficient attention has been paid to the alignment between the client's cultural worldview and the cultural worldview of the counsellor, as expressed through selected theoretical preferences. The scholars and practitioners within this series set out the value of different creative and methodological approaches in guidance and counselling within differing (and culturally varied) client groups.

Despite growing evidence that creative methods have much to offer guidance and counselling practice, there are abiding assumptions about what "art" is and who it might serve. There are two stereotypes that surround the arts that may block people from readily considering creative methods as viable approaches in this context. The first assumption is that one must be wildly creative to engage with arts and the second is that artists are a separate breed, doing their separate thing which seems unconnected with the realities of daily living. The article turned chapter in this and the previous special issue on this topic (Lengelle, Hambly, & Hughes, 2018), however, convincingly show that these stereotypes are false: engaging with the arts is not just the purview of the talented or the quirky and the arts are proving increasingly vital as an avenue for healing.

In a newsletter review of the book "Creative Calling" by Chase Jarvis, Von Stackelberg (2019) writes, "… the big realization that's coming over the next decade is how important creative expression is for health, and that everyone should do some sort of creative work as close to daily as possible" (p. 1). When writing the editorial, "Connecting to the Muses" for Part I of this Special Issue on Creative Methods (Lengelle, Hambly, & Hughes, 2018), we mentioned the importance of art and creativity in engaging the emotions and restoring playfulness to educational practice. In the second issue (Part II of this book) we show similar themes but are impressed by the research methodologies used, the ability of these methods to breakthrough aforementioned assumptions, and the clear applications here for practitioners.

The first chapter in this section in this collection by Parsons et al. shows creative and methodological rigour as the authors determine which elements of existing therapies for depression are truly helpful and apply these to the development of their practice. They do so in order to further develop and examine the potential reasons for the efficacy of Dance Movement Therapy (DMP). They identify seven vital elements of useful treatment in the context of depression through a Thematic Synthesis approach.

Thomas advocates for a deeper integration of creative methods within counselling and proposes that one way forward would be to develop more inclusive frameworks for this practice. To this end, she considers some of the ways clinicians and theorists, particularly from the creative/expressive arts therapies, have sought to develop integrative approaches for imagination-based therapeutic practices. This overview also pays attention to attempts within talking therapies to develop more descriptive/functional models for the use of mental imagery that allow an integration across theoretical orientations.

This is followed by Hubena and Mulcahy's chapter who focus on the advantages of using creative methods in counselling and in the training of those working in Child and Young People counselling. They indicate that in using creative methods, counsellors in training often reflected on the strength of these experiences and were surprised by how these arts-based techniques resulted in impacts not experienced before, such as cutting through layers of resistance and bringing up powerful personal insights.

Watson and McMahon combine quantitative career testing (i.e. matching-based psychometric methods) with narrative career counselling (i.e. the storytelling method) as a means of allowing clients to emotionally respond to test scores as well as to take a more holistic perspective of what those scores could mean within the context of their present lives. The Integrative Structured Interview is presented here as a creative and theoretically inspired method. They address the question about the potential complementarity of quantitative and creative approaches and conclude that creativity adds richness to the scores generated using more instrumental tests.

Schreiber et al. introduce the Vocational ID which integrates linguistic and visual representations of a career counselling client's self. They present a theoretical framework and its practical applications, including a case study as an illustration. Whilst this serves primarily to facilitate career counselling from a Life Design perspective, it also readily connects with many other cited theoretical approaches and counselling methods.

Chant draws on her own career questions and outlines how she developed ways of working with collage with her clients. She argues that although social constructivist theories infuse writing on career counselling practice, this doesn't mean practical methods are being implemented. Chant concludes that the collage approach can identify what narrative career researcher and counsellor, Savickas (2011) calls "preoccupations" (i.e. the life issues, born of pain) which inform career choice or occupations (i.e. choice of career).

Kreller, in the next chapter, looks for ways in which poetry can help heal cultural divides. As social injustice becomes increasingly apparent and eurocentric education remains ubiquitous around the world, in this chapter Kreller shows how those teaching must be willing to examine their internalised stereotypes. She makes use of Hermans's (1996) Dialogical Self Theory (DST) in order to describe and explore identity and the writing of poetry as an exploration of self.

Łysiak describes how problems might be responded to by having a temporal dialogue with our past, present, and/or future self, using a Dialogical Temporal Chair Technique. Her method combines DST with Gestalt and cognitive behavioural techniques. In essence, the idea here is that we are not only multi-voiced and able to dialogue with various I-selves but that we can glean vital insights and create useful tensions within ourselves by doing so. This creative form of "time travel" might, for instance, lead some to evaluate what they might learn from the past and what future self they might aspire to becoming.

Maree focuses on innovative career construction counselling for a creative adolescent. He adopts a case-study approach, drawing on a career construction counselling intervention that includes assessment and (meta-) reflective dialogue to investigate the participant's career-life story. Evidence shows that this approach can assist in helping to celebrate and draw on the client's sense of creativity. He argues that multiple case and quantitative studies are needed on the topic including more longitudinal research.

This is followed by Schellhammer who produces a compelling argument using the philosophical concept of "self care" to assert that we cannot truly meet another if we are not willing to look at our own inner workings first. She discusses the use of psychodrama and inner team methods as practical ways to enact her ideas on fostering "self care" as foundational to social well-being. Schellhammer argues for the need to develop "alien-ability" (Fremdheitsfähigkeit) by encountering our own discomfort and fear and engaging with the stranger within us before we can ultimately engage with the stranger out there in a multicultural society.

Nissen discusses standards in relation to Danish experiments with transforming drug counselling through aesthetic documentation: a hybrid of art with narrative practice. He contends that this can also have a wider application to youth work and social work. Concepts of performance and standards are discussed, followed by a critique of ways to customise counselling through formalised feedback. Prototypes are considered as a means of helping to overcome stigmatisation, and linkages made to trans-disciplinary knowledge which differ from traditional dominant scientific forms.

Kenyan researcher Wafula explains the potential use of writing poetry for career reflection. She presents a design for a career-learning intervention made for college students in order to respond to the transition from school-to-work that is often rife with insecurity. Using the work of various career construction scholars, she designs a group modality that uses poetry reading and writing tasks to allow students to create more empowering narratives from disempowering ones. Based on her integration of the various existing narrative-based methods and theories, she concludes that although few in Kenya are familiar with poetry therapy, it may be a valuable avenue for fostering career-learning in her country.

Conclusions

We hope practitioners and students learning how to design research or creative projects will use this book, as well as scholars looking to be inspired to learn and try new methods. However, complex policy issues surround these scholarly and practical activities, inviting new questions.

- How can professionals make the case for greater investment in creative methods in guidance and counselling?
- Which options are the most likely to have an impact and should be encouraged?
- What kind of research methods are best suited to examine the effects of creative methods?
- What is the best way to build a consideration of creative methods in guidance and counselling into existing or forthcoming government policies?
- Some approaches may benefit only those most able to pay for such services; therefore, what are the ethical implications in this regard for both clients and professionals?

Human civilisation is facing profound cultural and environmental challenges (Wallace-Wells, 2019) and with those challenges come existential questions about survival and meaning. Individuals also face uncertain economic and environmental futures and increasingly precarious work conditions (Blustein, Kenny, Di Fabio, & Guichard, 2019). Fundamentally, we want to give both scholars and practitioners from across disciplines a space to reflect upon and draw out exactly how they develop and apply creative methods and to address how methods crossover and/or transform service design and delivery over the next quarter of a century.

References

Arthur, N. (2018). *Counselling in cultural contexts: Identities and social justice*. Cham: Springer. 2 (1): 37. [Crossref], [Google Scholar]

Blustein, D. L., Kenny, M. E., Di Fabio, A., & Guichard, J. (2019). Expanding the impact of the psychology of working: Engaging psychology in the struggle for decent work and human rights. *Journal of Career Assessment, 27*, 3–28. https://doi.org/10.1177/1069072718774002 [Crossref], [Web of Science ®], [Google Scholar]

Cardoso, P. M., & Duarte, M. E. (2020). Two-chair dialogue: An emotion-focused technique applied to career counselling. *British Journal of Guidance & Counselling, 49*(2), 177–186. https://doi.org/10.1080/03069885.2020.1782833.

Den Elzen, K. & Lengelle, R. (Eds) (2023). *Writing-for-wellbeing: Theory, research, and practice*. New York: Routledge.

Frankl, V. (1955). The *doctor and the* soul (originally titled *Ärztliche Seelsorge*). NewYork: Random House.

Hermans, H. J. M. (1996). Voicing the self: From information processing to dialogical interchange. *Psychological Bulletin, 119*, 31–50. https://doi.org/10.1037/0033-2909.119.1.31 [Crossref], [Web of Science ®], [Google Scholar]

Lechevalier, S., & Laugier, S. (2019). Innovation beyond technology: Introduction. In S. Lechevalier (Ed.), *Innovation beyond technology: Science for society and interdisciplinary approaches*. London: Springer. 1(1):1–21. [Crossref], [Google Scholar]

Lengelle, R. (2021). Writing the self in bereavement: *A* story of love, spousal loss, and resilience. Routledge. https://doi.org/10.4324/9781003124009.

Lengelle, R., & Meijers, F. (2015). Career writing: Creative, expressive, and reflective approaches to narrative career learning and guidance. *The Canadian Journal of Career Development, 14*, 19–31.

Lengelle, R., Hambly, L., & Hughes, D. (2018). Connecting to the muses. *British Journal of Guidance & Counselling, 46*, 269–271. https://doi.org/10.1080/03069885.2018.1442917 [Taylor & Francis Online], [Web of Science ®], [Google Scholar]

Picasso, P. (1923, May). Picasso speaks. *The Arts, New York*, pp. 315–326. Retrieved from www.learn.columbia.edu/monographs/picmon/pdf/art_hum_reading_49.pdf [Google Scholar]

Savickas, M. L. (2011). *Career counselling*. Washington, DC: American Psychological Association. [Google Scholar]

Von Stackelberg, H. (2019, November 27). Wednesday musings. *Newsletter*. [Google Scholar]

Wallace-Wells, D. (2019). *The uninhabitable earth: A story of the future*. London: Penguin Random House. [Google Scholar]

Whyte, D. (2001). *Crossing the unknown sea: Work as a pilgrimage of identity*. New York: Riverhead Books. [Google Scholar]

Embodied Theater Ecology: illuminating the gap through bridging depth psychology's encounter with performative inquiry

Kirsten Frantzich and Lynn Fels

ABSTRACT

This article presents a new approach to psychological practice that dwells within the somatic, expressive, imaginal, poetic, narrative, and performative. Embodied Theater Ecology (ETE) as a form of Performative Inquiry is introduced and presented. This approach involves the performative unfolding of unlanguaged stories that lie at the heart of our clients' experiences of themselves and their worlds. The origins of this creative method are offered along with six principles and practices: Body as Ear; Undoing; Image & Central Metaphor; Living Artifacts & Evocative Objects; The Natural World; and Witnessing as Attending. The authors end with a call for practitioners to engage in the principles and practices of ETE as a means of calling into presence the hidden, the forgotten, the yet-to-be known stories embodied within us.

A young woman, Nell[1], sits voiceless across from me, she no longer has words. Minutes earlier, she had reported that she was 'in transition' at her workplace, in her primary relationship, and most recently, with friends. She then stops mid-sentence. We sit in silence for a long time. The silence is broken. Her voice weary, 'Words,' she says, 'Why is it all we have are words? Words, words, words. I feel so much more. Words aren't enough.' 'Words are not enough,' I reflect.

As a psychotherapist and fellow human being, I resonate with this young woman who finds herself lost in translation. We all have moments where words are insufficient and we all work with individuals who struggle to articulate what they feel, what they want to say. Despite the challenge of articulating significant human experiences, Nell, like each of us, has a story, multiple stories, often only partly known, sensed, waiting to be shared. To share our stories we must first discover our language and, in discovering it, we must live with the bittersweet knowledge that there may always be a gap between the fullness of our experience and the limitations of the communicative forms we have to express it (Frantzich, 2013; Romanyshyn, 2007).

Although it is often so difficult to express our most poignant stories, 'coming to a sense of fulfilment in life has a great deal to do with the capacity for self expression' (Frantzich, 2013; Rock, 1990, p. 57). The pain of language lost is echoed by philosopher Gaston Bachelard in his call and response, 'Where is our first suffering? … The hours when we have hoarded within us things left unsaid' (1942/1983, p. 195). Nell was giving voice to this same kind of first suffering, a suffering that many who come to us also feel.

This article introduces Embodied Theater Ecology (ETE), as a way to help individuals identify their most poignant untold stories and traverse the gap between saying (language) and being (Heidegger,

1947/1977), between lived experience and the ability to know it and convey it. ETE invokes possibilities for embodied expression of profound experiences that language, as such, is unable to touch.

Foundations for embodied theater ecology

Being a Juilliard trained actor with a PhD in depth psychology, I (Kirsten Frantzich) have long been interested in the interstices of psychology and performance. As a professional woman in the field, I questioned the nearly exclusive reliance on linear, verbal processes of communication that often had not reached those unspoken dimensions of human experience that I longed to touch and found so vivid and satisfying as an actor. Although Freud knew words have a kind of magical power, he too acknowledged, citing Goethe, that 'in the beginning there was the deed, action' ('Im Anfang war die Tat.' Cited in Freud, 1926/1959, p. 188). My conviction about the value of embodied expression and inquiry was further strengthened and affirmed by the work of theatre director Mary Zimmerman and scholar-artist Lynn Fels.

I remember being moved by a particular scene in Zimmerman's 2002 Broadway hit *Metamorphoses* and her pivotal character Alcyone who made her mythic way, eventually transforming, through love and loss. While producing *Metamorphoses,* Zimmerman was enduring a traumatic separation from her partner of 17 years and said 'something is born out of these places' (Moyers, 2002). Working on her play was 'a poetic bridge between myth and modernism,' (Garwood, 2003) essentially traversing the gap between lived experience and personal expression. Alcyone's story uncannily mirrored themes secreted in the heart of my own family of origin's unexpressed traumatic experience. These primordial family events lay in my being, appearing unexpectedly as fragments, broken pieces, or vaguely sensed lost memories disconnected from my own consciously told life story. They gathered only gradually, bricolage-like, as they do for so many with whom we work, long before any organised conscious awareness. Zimmerman's own personal story and play affirmed the possibility of finding ways to bring the orphaned, voiceless, fragments of unlanguaged experience into vital, embodied, theatrical performance.

My dream of uniting theatre and psychology by tapping the transformational power of life stories was reinforced when introduced to Fels' Performative Inquiry (PI) in the field of arts education. PI focuses on ways lived experiences resonate through performance and become individually and universally recognisable and revelatory. PI invites individuals to consider performance as an 'action site of learning' (1999, p. 46) and inquiry, recognising that engagement through form and through the interruption of form leads to new possible action (Fels & Stothers, 1996). PI investigates through embodied explorations the individual and communal scripts we perform, how individuals are performed by their environments, the interplay between our bodies, imagination, and memories, in relationship with others, and how performance as an action site of inquiry, learning, and reflection can lead to new understanding, new ways of being awakened. Encountering Fels' work, not to mention the person herself, led me to wonder anew in what ways the theatrical stage might provide fresh opportunities for individuals to discover and tell their own unlanguaged embodied stories. To be even more precise, how might the theatrical stage provide a radically open space and time for individuals' stories to tell themselves, to allow their orphaned stories to speak for themselves?

My response to these questions was to explore and eventually arrive at an organic, new approach to psychological practice called Embodied Theater Ecology. ETE began as a heuristic, personal inquiry within the performative arts that later found justification and support in psychological theory and research. Psychologically speaking, ETE is grounded in the thought and practice of depth psychology, particularly in its more imaginal and archetypal versions. Artistically speaking, it was infused with and inspired early on by contemporaries of both Freud and Jung such as vocal researcher and psychotherapist Alfred Wolfsohn and visual artist Joan Miró. Further inspiration came from Peter Brook, Jerzy Grotowski, and Wolfsohn's protégé, Roy Hart. More recent performative influences include Anne Bogart, Pina Bausch, and Enrique Pardo's [with Linda Wise] Pantheatre. The approach shares crucial values, purposes, and practices with somatic and expressive therapies and imaginal, poetic, and narrative inquiries, all of which are also grounded in depth psychological theory and practice. Other kindred therapeutic approaches include psychodrama, therapeutic enactment, body/mind psychotherapy, expressive arts therapy, and most notably, Comprehensive Resource Model (CRM).

ETE is an organic, spontaneous, embodied, non-linear process that moves away from anything programmatic, predetermined, scripted, or analyzed. ETE emphasises personal, moment by moment awakening and revelation in which the client is surrendered to and moved by spontaneously emerging images, affects, and sensory experiences. Thus, one might think of ETE not only as an approach to counselling and psychotherapy but also as a catalyst for theatrical creation. I will introduce ETE and then identify and discuss central premises and actions that educators, counsellors, and psychotherapists might find applicable in their own work.

Minding the gap between experience and language

Embodied theater ecology pursues the ways embodied theatrical language bridges the gap between our lived experience and the words we have to express that experience. ETE invites individuals to experience and become absorbed by the unknown through acts of creative availability, awakening, and embodied languaging. ETE recognises that we each carry stories that are hidden, forgotten, and often unrecognised within us and that given time, attention, and attunement these stories find ways, through the availability of the individual, to tell themselves. ETE investigates what it means to *un-do* rather than do, inviting the individual into sensory receptivity and availability.

ETE trusts the work will come, will illuminate, and will assert itself through the individual's spontaneously emerging experience of their orphaned story as it is embodied in elusive fragments: unexpected memories and feelings, images, felt-sensations, impulses, metaphors, sounds, all coming in moments that startle (Fels, 2012). ETE engages an embodied phenomenology of being that attends to the imaginal, metaphorical, relational, contextual, breath and impetus of an embodied moment. ETE invites and taps into the hidden stories, gaps of understanding, silences, and revelations that speak to us through surrender, through being moved, that, as van Manen (2007) writes:

> reside or resonate in the body, in our relations with others, in the things of our world, and in our very actions [and undoing]. These are the kinds of knowledge that cannot necessarily be translated back or captured in conceptualizations and theoretical representations. In other words, there are modes of knowing that inhere so immediately in our lived practices – in our body, in our relations, and in the things around us – that they seem invisible. (p. 22)

The distinctiveness of ETE may be seen in six key principles and practices: Body as Ear; Undoing; Image and Central Metaphor; Living Artifacts and Evocative Objects; The Natural World; and Witnessing as Attending.

Body as ear: listening with one's whole being

As Nell is sitting with me, I encourage her to move onto the floor mat in the open area of my office. An empty space, a metaphorical stage, I invite her to listen to her body, to attend to feelings emanating through her bones, her skin, her flesh, from toes, up through her thighs, hips, along the long reach of her spine … as she feels into her being, the first 'tug' comes.[2]

Here, rather than working from a script or structured improvisational techniques (such as what one might find in drama therapy or psychodrama), I invite her to use her body as an ear, listening to what is but remains invisible, unknown, and unspoken. The essence of this process is akin to the creative attitude and philosophy of Joan Miró. Miró's painting, *The Policeman* (1925), hangs in the Art Institute of Chicago. The title card accompanying it reads:

> Soon after Joan Miró moved to Paris in 1920, he met a new group of painters and writers united in merging the unconscious world with the rational world in order to produce the new language of Surrealism. To release images

> of this higher realm he embraced *automatism,* a spontaneous working method much like free association . . . .'Rather than setting out to paint something,' he said, 'I begin painting and . . . the picture begins to assert itself, or suggest itself under my brush. . . . Even a few casual wipes in cleaning my brush may suggest the beginning of a picture.' (Sweeney, 1948, p. 112)

Miró was adept at automatic drawing. Although his approach was similar to Surrealism, he was unwilling to align himself with any movement. Instead, he had a curiosity and passion for the furthering of what he called his *symbolic language* through art (Erben & Duchting, 2004). As in ETE, Miró emphasised symbolic language that 'promotes universal communication among people, no matter where they come from or where they are going' (p. 235). Like Miró's automatic drawing, in ETE, embodied images spontaneously assert themselves from themselves rather than from theatrical technique or method.

Undoing as embodied process

Whereas performative inquiry is rooted in *action* such as knowing, doing, being, creating, and *reflecting* (Fels, 1995, 1999, 2010), embodied theater ecology is rooted in *receptivity,* that is, being, undoing, and not-knowing (Frantzich, 2013, p. 323). Engaging ETE, with its direct turn to the body as a form of active imagination, deliberately deferring will and intention, an individual is surrendered to the story hidden within as it spontaneously unfolds, impulse by impulse, movement by movement, sound by sound, and, at some point, word by word. Yoga therapist Cobb (2008) captures the process in this way:

> The individual is called into a willingness to receive information in whatever way it wants to come – as a feeling, a sensation, a thought, an image, a memory, a color, a sound, a smell or a taste – followed by a letting go of censoring, editing or otherwise cleaning up what comes. (p. 144)

In her undoing, Nell hears a tug that awakens and opens her to receive whatever happens next. She feels a slowly surging sensation rising up through her body. She feels her interior being, offering, emptying, expanding outward far beyond herself. A window of awareness opens to her story and also to the universe. This universality feels so immense she panics and shuts it down, waiting until she has the capacity – perhaps the container or grounded-ness – to hold whatever this moment might reveal. Her experience is felt, not yet articulatable. No words.

Through ETE, the unspoken story moves the individual through embodied automatism. The individual is not atop a chair imagining sitting in a chair; instead there is nothing between the individual and the source, nothing between the body and the chair. The individual is with the chair and the chair is with the individual; embodied active imagination, automatism, re-membering, not-knowing, and knowing. Miró with his asserting canvas, and a splash of red, a canvas moving to become.

Dancer, poet and scholar Celeste Snowber writes that what we cannot yet articulate dwells deep within the body as embodied knowing (2017). She observes that conventional ways of articulating what we know abandon us, and what is as yet unknown only may be accessed through the body – 'Embodied inquiry as a place of opening' (Snowber, 2014, p. 119). As writer Hélène Cixous acknowledges, 'writing is not arriving; most of the time it's not arriving. One must go on foot, with the body' (1994, p. 203). Thus we are called, into inarticulateness, to awaken the cells of our body, within which the untold stories dwell. The initial awakening to our human plight becomes possible through a performative embodied inquiry that moves an individual through darkness into light, absence into presence, inarticulateness to embodied being.

Image as emergent central metaphor

Nell enthusiastically returns a week later. She is grinning. I grin back saying, 'Looks like you have something to share?' 'I have it!' she responds. 'Have what?' I ask. 'Remember the feeling I was trying to translate, a kind of levity? I thought of so many things: circus arts, speeding bicycles, nothing seemed right. Last night, frustrated, I was sprawled face up on my bed looking at the ceiling, stumped. Then, I fell asleep. This morning, I woke with the most amazing dream! A female figure in the dream was speaking to me. She would approach, retreat, come close, and then move away. I realised she was on a swing. A swing! A swing feels perfect. How's that for levity?'

As an individual continues to work in an inquiring, resolute openness with the unknown, he/she will often stumble upon an image evoking a central metaphor on which his/her orphaned story hinges. This image may appear in dreams, desires, myths, and through other lived and artistic influences. Image emerges 'as a kind of shared language, forming a collective imaginal space' that increases the complexity of mutual exploration (Marks-Tarlow, 2012, p. 174). Psychologist and artist Terry Marks-Tarlow goes on to describe the body's use of 'metaphor to bridge disconnected experience, create somatic templates, and weave the illusion of constancy during continual change' (p. 154). Through this preverbal aspect of emergent, imagistic availability the individual may be swept along by his/her experience discovering in the process the potentiality of trusting the unknown. Within ETE, that which is moved becomes the movement not representation or pantomime; the image needs no interpretation. Through embodied being the individual becomes the image from unknown origins and that is where the meaning is found. Through metaphoric possibility experience is transformed, value is marked, and relationship illuminated. Individuals are able to hold the metaphoric mirror up to themselves, seeing afresh, as long as those involved 'can refrain from becoming impatient and attempting to irritate the image into meaning' (Romanyshyn, 2007, p.149). There is a wisdom and awareness offered by the unknown that the everyday world does not possess. As an individual is moved by and with images, there is 'a fair chance of finding what we seek in vain in the conscious world' (Fidyk, 2010, p. 4; Frantzich, 2013, p. 312), beyond linear human understanding stories transmute into a form humans may feel body to body.

Living artifacts and evocative objects

Nell arrives for her appointment. 'What do we have here?' I inquire. 'Suitcases,' she replies, holding the handle of one large, marble cream case and another matching boxy overnight bag. 'They were my aunt's. 1950s. Cool, huh?' 'Wow, amazing,' I reply. 'They were returned to our family after her death. I had them in my apartment.' 'Good, let's let them play with you today and see what happens. Find a place that feels right for them in the room.' Nell puts the suitcases in the centre. I invite her to find a comfortable place near them. She choses to sit cross-legged on the floor, her back against the larger suitcase. She sits in silent attention. 'Let's begin by breathing. As you breath more deeply allow your abdomen to rise and fall with the breath. Bring your attention to your body. Feel your sit bones on the floor, the back of your legs, the felt sense of your ankles against the mat, the tight bend of your knees, your back, touching your suitcase. Now, let the suitcase feel into you and you into it. Listen with body as ear. Open yourself to experiencing the suitcase, being with it, and simultaneously moved by it.' I turn on instrumental music. She breathes deeply. No words.

Living artifacts are meaningful original items that are directly linked to an individual's story. Living artifacts differ from Winnicott's transitional objects as their aim is not to ease a developmental step toward self actualisation, rather, they are valued for the metaphorical or emotional meaning they possess due to their direct relationship to a person, place, or event. Their inherent legacy aids the individual's re-membering through embodied performative connection to the individual's stories and the central metaphor that guides them on their artistic, therapeutic way: A swing lifts an individual to the heavens, revealing a potentiation, a levity and promise; while a suitcase may pull the same individual to the earth, grounding, heavy, the weight, perhaps, of responsibility. Living artifacts differ from evocative objects, yet they are complimentary exploratory items.

Items an individual is drawn to that capture a symbolic element of their lived experience yet do not have direct involvement in the individual's story are called *evocative objects*. Evocative objects evoke affect without words. They are gathered while the individual lives life being receptive to what arrives when not knowing what he/she is looking for. Examples of evocative objects include: a doll discovered in a thrift shop, an old coat from a garage sale, pennies collected on the sidewalk, a plastic bathtub found in a junk yard. One of the wonderful surprises of being moved by and with a living artifact or evocative object is that they are rarely engaged with by the individual in their traditional sense. They often surprise with their imaginative potentiality and varied applications and uses, metaphorical and imaginal.

After closing her eyes, feeling into the moment, Nell begins to slowly move back and forth in contact with the suitcase. She moves methodically, windshield wiper-like, swiping the case clean with her back. The movement becomes extended, fluid, sweeping, and then more vigorous, like a bear scratching its back on a tree. I put my foot against the base of the suitcase providing support against her movement. Tentatively she begins to move her fingers as her hands fall off of her lap and braille-like, dust the floor finding the edges of the suitcase. Her chest arches out, her arms back behind her clutch the large marble case. She lets out an immense sigh. 'Notice where you are led, what arises, allow your senses to respond to the encounter,' I invite. Time passes, she continues, drawn by the living artifact into further exploration and movement. Eventually, she sits on top of the suitcase like a rider on a horse, then slides down it to the floor, the case eventually toppling onto its side. She wraps herself around it like a question mark. She remains still, then slowly comes back to sitting. She pries the suitcase open like a big mouth, chomping, then leaves it open like a silent scream. By the end of our session she has climbed inside the suitcase and closed it on herself. There she remains breathing, quiet, animal-like until it is time to leave.

Living artifacts are as varied as our lived experiences. Artifacts welcomed into ETE sessions include: shoes, clothing, furniture, jewellry, household items, music boxes, even the remains of a door. Working without intension or expectation with body as ear, listening acutely to the artifact or object while keeping a keen awareness of the longings, feelings, and images within, requires awake-ness and letting-be-ness. An individual may experience somatic sensations, memory flashes, pronounced breathing and sighs; emit sounds and vocalizations recognisably human and other-than-human; word fragments and phrases; all of these holding the potential revelation of the yet to be known, perhaps even leading to a full, performative text.[3]

When living artifacts and evocative objects are used simply, offering just enough insight yet not too much information, those who witness the work may experience it as a Rorschach inkblot, a gateway into their own re-membering. Living artifacts and evocative objects used during an individual's sessions offer a layering, a fleshing out of the central metaphor, increased 'releasement toward things' (gelassenheit), literally, the 'gathering-of-letting-be-ness' (Heidegger, 1959/1966, pp. 54–55). This releasement into being is also encouraged through encounters with the natural world.

Natural worlding: re-wilding the work

I watch a turkey feather spin between Nell's fingers, brushing her thighs. She shares a meaningful experience that took place the first day she arrived at her new apartment. The duplex was located on a city street yet the back yard flowed into protected parkland. Upon her arrival, deposit and first month's rent in hand, she headed down a stone path that wrapped around the duplex into her new back yard. 'This,' she exclaims, 'is when I was stopped in my tracks.' 'Really? Why?' I ask. 'Turkeys! Honestly, I was astounded!' 'Turkeys? How curious.' She continues, 'I began to count them, ten! Completely blocking any possibility of getting to my back door. Wisely, I gave them the right of way,' she laughs, then elaborates. 'I waited a few minutes, dumbfounded, and eventually went all the way around the other side of the duplex to get inside.' 'What an unexpected surprise,' I respond. Nell continues, 'This was only the beginning, this band of turkeys has been there ever since that first day and they are full of surprises. Last week walking through the parkland, I stumbled on this feather. It felt like a perfect item to bring into our work together. An offering from the turkeys.'

Engaging the natural world as a way of being with oneself and experiencing the other-than-human is a critical component of ETE. The natural world often evokes a softening of human defenses, awakening receptivity. An individual may experience an increased availability to him/herself, others, and other-than-human beings. There is often increased openness and less need to self protect as an individual stands gazing at the expanse of the ocean, looks up the powerful stone face of Half Dome or lays on a bed of autumn leaves watching the clouds' incremental movement. Human receptivity is awakened, rigidity becomes more pliable. The body is felt in new ways, there is an experience of one's humanness, one's grass-ness, one's tree-ness, one's sky-ness (Frantzich, 2013).

Swedish poet and psychologist, Tranströmer (1987), writes poetry to thread together experience beyond words. His poetry speaks to the natural world's profound ability to language experience through the act of existing:

> Tired of all who come with words, words but no language I went to the snow-covered island. The wild does not have words. The unwritten pages spread themselves out in all directions! I come across the marks of a roe-deer's hooves in the snow. Language, but no words. (pp. 158–159)

The natural world invites humans to remember their most primordial source, oneness with and regard for beings as a whole. For an individual with whom the natural world offers a sense of belonging to something larger, within it there is often a releasement towards and beyond being-ness, drawing him/her into the humbling recognition of belonging to and within the expansive web of life.[4]

Inviting the natural world and its ancient ecology into human explorations encourages us as practitioners to ask these questions: What might we understand about our

> human wholeness once we liberate psychotherapy, coaching, education, and religion from indoor consulting rooms, classrooms, and churches? What happens when we rewild our techniques and practices for facilitating human development – not by merely getting them out the door and onto the land or waters, but, much more significantly, by fashioning approaches in which our encounters with the other-than-human world are the central feature? (Plotkin, 2013, p. 7)

What is rehabilitated in our various practices when nature becomes a vital centre and humanity is allowed its wildness (Plotkin, 2013)? What might arise as other-than-human encounters are embraced as central to the experience of being human?

Although most practitioners meet individuals in their offices, the natural world can still be engaged with during sessions. Individuals are encouraged to spend designated time alone in nature: walk through the woods, lay in a meadow, build a small stone cairn, dance or journal by the warmth of a fire. They are invited to bring back discoveries, images, objects, awarenesses, and creations that arrive during their other-than-human encounters. Their discoveries may be integrated within their sessions potentially illuminating their stories, as well as their process of personal awakening, wellbeing, and experience of aliveness.

Witnessing: a way of attending

Nell and I are here in the space together. The burden that is her untold, unknown story is unfolding in my presence, within our presence, a reciprocal offering, receiving, through which movement, image, voice, text, living and evocative artifacts expose a being-ness that reveals the story yearning to be released. Here, with the swing as levity, the turkey feather, the suitcases waiting in the empty space, bodies are listening as ear, gathering, re-membering – moving what she and I do not yet know. Within embodied presence and release, her story will arrive between the lines, in the pauses, within the flourish of looped letters, on bended knee in reverence, through listening and receiving, beholding together what is revealed, and not yet revealed. Until, in breath, in body, in voice, she arrives and in her arriving, I am drawn, too, into my own awakening.

Theatre director Peter Brook once wrote that for theatre to exist all one needs is an empty space, a person walking across, and someone to witness the action

> I can take any empty space and call it a bare stage. A man walks across this empty space whilst someone else is watching him, and this is all that is needed for an act of theatre to be engaged. (1968, p. 7)

There are multiple understandings of the role of *witness* in theatre, somatic practices, and life, yet here in the intimacy of embodied performative revelation and the birthing of an inarticulate story, bearing witness, it is vital that practitioners engage without intent or desire for a result. Meaning is not sought, nor are we invited to interpret. Instead, it is our task as practitioners to 'be with' those we serve as 'a radical selfless activity' (Craig, 2000, p. 268), receiving and attending to the subtleties of their unique embodied language. This invitation is not a stepping away from oneself, but a coming into oneself. It invites an at oneness with oneself that makes it possible to 'transcend that self in order to be with-and-for the other' (p. 270). Rather than doing, practitioners are called into undoing and it is our undoing that shares an affinity with Eastern thought and midwifery. As practitioners we attend to an emptiness of being while easing the passage of what is birthed through each individual we serve. By way of profound presencing there is an exchange, an eventual participatory sharing, in which 'not only is the theatre [empty space] about the audience [practitioner] seeing, it is where the audience [practitioner] witnesses the actor [individual] seeing. ... The drama [moment] is a drama [moment] of unfolding sight' (Bogart, 2007, p. 81).

As practitioners we become embodied containers for the experience of the other, embracing our own experience of body as ear. In listening to the other we experience and know ourselves, and the other again, in return. Neuropsychologist Allen Schore and psychoanalyst Bromberg (2011) refer to this process as 'right brain to right brain state sharing' (p. xxvii). During the process we experience gaps, silences, and absences in ourselves and in the other where once invisible realities can dare to appear. If we can manage to keep our linear, ambitious, efficient selves out of the way we may experience the wisdom of poet Leonard Cohen's words 'forget your perfect offering ... there is a crack in everything/that's how the light gets in' (1993, p. 373). Thus, understanding can unfold 'within and out of presence ... with a witness who is present to presence' (Romanyshyn, 2007, p. 221).

ETE for practitioners: work with selves

As I sit with Nell, I prepare myself to receive, to hold the space. I empty myself, simultaneously, drawing breath in through my chest, abdomen, and into my pelvis. I feel my body root deeply into the mat, floor, the pylons of the building, beyond the concrete, through layers of time-worn earth, arriving at the liquid core of my/our Being. Aware of my own letting-be-ness, void of intent, prejudgments, expectations, I wait. Ready to attend to her first flicker of light.

Practitioners interested in exploring ETE with clients are strongly encouraged to experience it for themselves. The majority of us have been trained in traditional, cognitive, verbal modes of therapeutic languaging. Regardless of our conventional training, which is not to be discounted, few have had the opportunity to experience for ourselves modalities emphasising embodied forms of inquiry, expression, and communication. We now know through recent infant, affect, and neuroscience research that our most primordial modes of expression, communication, and connection are not verbal but somatic and emotional. ETE invites practitioners to become aware of psychological barriers, biases, assumptions, prejudices, and personal limitations not only through emotional and cognitive awareness but also through the mysteries that only the body knows and can speak.

Embodied theater ecology: an embodied reclamation of language

Throughout this introduction to embodied theater ecology we have done our best to give voice and language to an approach involving processes that originate and operate largely prior to verbal language. Clearly our words alone are not enough to help practitioners bridge the gap between this written introduction and the actual experience of ETE. We are convinced the gaps that are inherent in our effort can be reconciled, at least in part, by aspiring embodied practitioners' own engagement with the kinds of involvements we have described: by experiencing one's body as ear; by undoing as embodied process; by attending to images and metaphor as they appear in the peripheries of awareness; by paying attention to, gathering and dwelling with evocative fragments, artifacts, and objects; by being in nature in new, radically open ways; by witnessing attention to the flow of embodied experience. What mattered for Nell, beyond the languaging of her story, was its awakened, enlivened, embodied release into the world.

Allowing the body to articulate orphaned stories can bring one into a way of being in which old habits of engagement become visible, hidden fears and defenses are revealed, forsaken hopes are reawakened and re-membered. We think of this as the essential promise of what Hannah Arendt called natality (1958), where some of the most basic questions of human existence can be asked. Who are you? What has been forgotten? What needs reclamation? What untold stories lie dormant in our being? What languages are not-yet-imagined? ETE aspires to evoke experiences relevant to these questions. Spiralling through embodied layers of time – past, present, future, transgenerational – is a re-turning to what has been personally, ancestrally, communally, culturally forgotten. And in the re-turning, re-membering, encountering ghosts, secreted stories, haunted forgettings, illuminating the embodied articulateness of the moment, here and now, we encounter ourselves anew, as if for the first time.

Notes

1. The character Nell is a composite of several clients that would represent a clinical process of ETE.
2. Fels (2012) uses the metaphor 'tug on one's sleeve' as a signalling of those moments that call us to attention.
3. In one version of ETE, time is taken to be enveloped in, embody, and create a full theatrical piece with an invited audience. The performance takes place where those who attend enter the process through the natural world and move into being participant-witnesses with/of the performance.
4. It is important to acknowledge that there are those unfamiliar with the out of doors and who do not feel at home in the natural world. This too is respected valuable information. Their discomfort and dis-ease is one place to begin in joint exploration and in gentle introduction.

Disclosure statement

No potential conflict of interest was reported by the authors.

References

Arendt, H. (1958). *The human condition*. Chicago, IL: University of Chicago Press.

Bachelard, G. (1983). *Water and dreams: An essay on the imagination of movement* (E. Farrell, Trans.). Dallas, TX: Dallas Institute Publications, Dallas Institute of Humanities and Culture. (Original work published 1942).

Bogart, A. (2007). *And then you act*. New York, NY: Routledge.

Bromberg, P. (2011). *The shadow of the tsunami: And the growth of the relational mind*. New York, NY: Routledge.

Brook, P. (1968). *The empty space*. New York, NY: Antheneum.

Cixous, H. (1994). *The Helene Cixous reader* (S. Sellers, Ed.). New York, NY: Routledge.

Cobb, E. (2008). *The forgotten body: A way of knowing and understanding self*. Hadwick, MA: Satya House.

Cohen, L. (1993). *Stranger music: Collected poems and songs*. Toronto, ONT: McClelland & Stewart.

Craig, P. E. (2000). Sanctuary and presence: An existential view of the therapist's contribution. *The Humanistic Psychologist, 28*(1-3), 267–274. doi:10.1080/08873267.2000.9976996

Erben, W., & Duchting, H. (2004). *Miró (Taschen 25th Anniversary)*. Koln, Germany: Taschen.

Fels, L. (1995). In dialogue with Grumet: Erasing the line. *Educational Insights*. Retrieved from http://ccfi.educ.ubc.ca/publication/insights/archives/v03n01/fels.html

Fels, L. (1999). *In the wind clothes dance on a line: Performative inquiry as methodology* (*Unpublished doctoral dissertation*). University of British Columbia, Vancouver, British Columbia, Canada.

Fels, L. (2010). Coming into presence: The unfolding of a moment. *Journal of Educational Controversy, 5*(1), 1–15.

Fels, L. (2012). Collecting data through performative inquiry: A tug on the sleeve. *Youth Theatre Journal, 26*(1), 50–60. doi:10.1080/08929092.2012.678209

Fels, L., & Stothers, S. (1996). Academic performance: Between theory and praxis. In J. O'Toole & K. Donelan (Eds.), *Drama, culture and education* (pp. 255–261). Brisbane, AUS: IDEAS.

Fidyk, A. (2010). Hermaphrodite as healing image: Connecting a mythic imagination to education. *Journal of Jungian Scholarly Studies, 6*(1), 1–32.

Frantzich (a.k.a. Allen), K. (2013). *Theater of the psyche: The emergence of embodied theater ecology and the stage as home (be)coming* (*Doctoral dissertation*). Pacifica Graduate Institute, Carpinteria, CA.

Freud, S. (1959). The question of lay analysis. In J. Strachey (Ed. & Trans.). *The standard addition of the complete psychological works of Sigmund Freud* (Vol. 20, pp. 177–258). London: Hogarth Press. (Original work published 1926).

Garwood, D. (2003, January). Myth as public dream: The metamorphosis of Mary Zimmerman's *Metamorphoses*. *PAJ: A Journal of Performance and Art, 25*(1), 69–78.

Heidegger, M. (1966). *Discourse on thinking*. New York, NY: Harper & Row. (Original work published 1959).

Heidegger, M. (1977). Letter on humanism. In F. A. Capuzzi & J. G. Gray (Trans.) *Basic writings* (pp. 193–242). New York, NY: Harper & Row. (Original work published 1947).

Marks-Tarlow, T. (2012). *Clinical intuition in psychotherapy: The neurobiology of embodied response*. New York, NY: W.W. Norton & Company.

Moyers, B. (2002, March 22). Bill Moyers interviews Mary Zimmerman [Transcript]. NOW with Bill Moyers. Retrieved from http://www.pbs.org/now/transcript/transcript_zimmerman.html

Plotkin, B. (2013). *Wild mind*. Novato, CA: New World Library.

Rock, W. P. (1990). *Performing inside out*. Chicago, IL: Between Two Worlds Press.

Romanyshyn, R. D. (2007). *The wounded researcher: Research with soul in mind*. New Orleans, LA: Spring.

Snowber, C. (2014). Dancing on the breath of limbs: Embodied inquiry as a place of opening. In A. Williamson, G. Batson, S. Whatley, & R. Weber (Eds.), *Dance, somatics, and spiritualities: Contemporary sacred narratives* (pp. 115–130). Bristol, UK: Intellect Books.

Snowber, C. (2017). *Embodied inquiry*. Rotterdam, NL: Sense.

Sweeney, J. J. (1948, February). Joan Miró: Comment and interview. *Partisan Review, XV*(2), 206–212.

Tranströmer, T. (1987). *Tomas Tranströmer: Selected poems, 1954–1986*. R. Bly (Ed.). New York, NY: Ecco Press.

van Manen, M. (2007). Phenomenology of practice. *Phenomenology & Practice, 1*(1), 11–30.

Is poetry therapy an appropriate intervention for clients recovering from anorexia? A critical review of the literature and client report

Christine E. Ramsey-Wade and Ellen Devine

ABSTRACT
Poetry therapy is an arts-based psychotherapeutic intervention, often delivered in groups. This paper argues that the process and benefits of poetry therapy may be particularly suited to clients recovering from anorexia, as an adjunct to other treatments. Poetry therapy and its history are described briefly, and the relevance of poetry therapy for clients recovering from anorexia is outlined. After one client contributes her experience of this treatment for illustration, the paper offers a review of the evidence base for poetry therapy for eating disorders, and argues that, while research is limited, further research is warranted. Finally, a description of one form of clinical application is offered, to enable replication.

Poetry therapy

What is poetry therapy?

Poetry therapy is 'the intentional use of poetry and related forms of literature and creative writing for personal growth and healing' (McCulliss, 2011b, p. 94). It can be distinguished from reading bibliotherapy or self-help, where a client may read a text at home or on prescription from a librarian, with no therapist to assist the client to process the material for therapeutic ends (Mazza, 2003). While poetry and therapy are both largely language based and concerned with communication, insight and authenticity (Hedges, 2005), poetry therapy can be distinguished from creative writing in general, as the focus here is on the process of writing and its therapeutic benefits rather than the finished product (Alschuler, 2006). It therefore overlaps and yet remains distinct from the fields of narrative therapy and expressive writing (Mazza, 2003).

Mazza created a multidimensional clinical model of poetry therapy, which was then tested via therapist surveys to verify its accurate representation of current practice (Mazza & Hayton, 2013). This flexible model is known as the RES model (Mazza, 2003), as shown in Figure 1, and sets out the range of techniques poetry therapists may use. The Receptive – Prescriptive mode describes interventions where a published piece of writing is read with a client, and reactions are used to develop a therapeutic exploration or dialogue. The Expressive-Creative mode captures the therapeutic use of creative writing, journaling or letter writing, either within or outside the counselling session. Finally, the Symbolic – Ceremonial mode encapsulates the therapeutic benefits of performance and recitation, through ritual or storytelling, and the cultivation of metaphorical thinking.

A brief history

Poetry therapy is now an established profession in the US. It arose in the late 1960s and 1970s in hospital clinics and libraries (Gorelick, 2005), leading to the establishment of accredited and certified training routes in the US, the National Association of Poetry Therapy, and the peer-reviewed *Journal of Poetry Therapy*. The National Coalition of Creative Arts Therapies Associations in the US now lists some of the goals of poetry therapy as:

- Developing an understanding of oneself and others through poetry and other forms of literature
- Promoting creativity, self-expression, and greater self-esteem
- Strengthening interpersonal and communication skills
- Expressing overwhelming emotions and releasing tension
- Promoting change and increasing coping skills and adaptive functions (Gorelick, 2005, p. 119)

Process, characteristics and benefits

Like other expressive or arts-based therapies, poetry therapy is characterised by the use of the imagination, imagery and metaphor (Hedges, 2005; Malchiodi, 2005). By enhancing self-expression, poetry therapy can also enable independence from therapy (Alschuler, 2006), which is an important aim in more chronic presentations. Importantly, poetry therapy is presented 'as a tool, not a school' (Gorelick, 2005, p. 124), in that it can be practiced by a range of professionals across a spectrum of psychotherapeutic models. For example, poetry therapy in psychodynamic practice may focus on catharsis and unconscious processes (Perlin, 2009) or the written word as a transitional object (Steinberg, 2004), whereas poetry therapy in existential practice may focus on giving voice to unfolding experience, clarifying and magnifying being (Furman, 2003), or maintaining vitality in the face of the givens of existence (Gorelick, 2005). It can also be a culturally-sensitive practice, particularly where poetry, lyrics and language form a strong part of a client's cultural heritage (Mohammadian et al., 2011; Reynaga-Abiko, 2008). It can be a developmentally-sensitive practice as well, as

Receptive-Prescriptive mode – introducing published work into sessions for therapeutic ends

Expressive-Creative mode – encouraging client expression through writing

Symbolic-Ceremonial mode – the therapeutic use of performance and recitation

Figure 1. Mazza's (2003) RES model of poetry therapy.

adolescents may already be using poetry and lyrics to identify, articulate and communicate their feelings (Reynaga-Abiko, 2008).

There is a rich literature documenting how different clinicians have incorporated poetry into their therapeutic work (Nylund, 2002; Speedy, 2004). Alschuler (2006) stated that poetry therapy is usually offered as a group-based intervention, and many other practitioners attest to the therapeutic power of poetry in group work (Bolton, 1999). McLoughlin (2000) presented an excellent case study describing a poetry therapy group offered from a psychodynamic perspective in a hospice. He has described how the group functioned as a transitional space, after Winnicott (1971), while offering consolation and a space for growth and development during a time of change. In this sense, poetry therapy can be particularly suited to ward-based work, with some authors describing how poetry therapy can enhance bonds between patients (Golden, 1995; Leedy, 2006). However, this intervention can be difficult to access for clients with learning disabilities such as dyslexia or clients who have had difficult experiences of schooling. Treatment targets the ability to symbolise, by supporting clients to access metaphor and imagery (Bolton & Latham, 2004). So, while clients who lack imaginal capacity can be difficult to engage, the intervention targets this deficit in its attempts to repair the bridge between the body and experience.

Many writers agree that poetry therapy is most effective as an adjunct to therapy (Heimes, 2011; Mazza, 2003; McCulliss, 2012; Perlin, 2009), in part to support clients with the painful process of accessing difficult emotions and experiences (Esterling, L'Abate, Murray, & Pennebaker, 1999). This strengthens the case for this intervention to be offered as part of a package of care, such as in psychiatric hospitals, where poetry therapy can encourage expression, peer interaction and engagement in groups through the use of an expressive, 'strength-based technique' (Kerner & Fitzpatrick, 2007, p. 333) that can potentially be less confrontational or threatening than other groups (Alschuler, 2006).

Anorexia nervosa – the need for innovative treatments

Anorexia is often a complex presentation, where new, accessible and cost-effective (i.e. group-based) treatments are needed (NICE, 2004; Reynaga-Abiko, 2008). As East, Startup, Roberts, and Schmidt (2010) have pointed out, anorexia nervosa lags behind other psychiatric disorders in terms of evidence and treatment. Writing is already used in many treatment programmes for anorexia, by perhaps writing letters to anorexia my enemy and anorexia my friend as a motivational intervention, or encouraging clients to externalise anorexia as a bully through their writing from a narrative perspective (Schmidt, Bone, Hems, Lessem, & Treasure, 2002; Treasure & Alexander, 2013). Clients recovering from anorexia often voice their dissatisfaction with traditional treatments, which can be experienced as reductionist, with staff appearing to focus primarily on weight gain (Robbins & Pehrsson, 2009). There is a need to create space for clients' ambivalence around recovery, which is why poetry therapy is being explored as a particularly appropriate and creative intervention for anorexia (Kaplan, 2002; Robbins & Pehrsson, 2009). Developing new treatments for anorexia can be difficult, however, due to the high levels of avoidance that are a part of the presentation (Schmidt et al., 2002). There is a need therefore for new and effective treatments which specifically target avoidance (Frayne & Wade, 2006).

Poetry therapy and anorexia

Is there a case for considering arts-based psychotherapeutic interventions using creative writing, literature and poetry as particularly suitable for clients recovering from anorexia? East et al. (2010) have argued that writing-based treatments can target experiential avoidance through exposure to feelings and thoughts, thus improving psychological flexibility. They cite Pennebaker's (1997) work as they contend that these interventions also target the difficulties expressing emotions commonly seen in anorexia, through a 'disinhibitory' effect (East et al., 2010, p. 181). They also suggest that engagement with emotional experience is key to recovery from anorexia, which is why treatments which focus more on cognitive control over their environment (i.e. CBT) are less effective with this presentation. Hornyak and Baker (1989) also observed that clients recovering from eating disorders can present as very cut off from themselves, emotionally and cognitively, and that experiential and arts-based therapies can help to re-build that bridge. Schmidt et al. (2002), Howlett (2004) and Treasure and Whitney (2010) have all described writing-based treatments that can be used as 'a way in' to facilitate emotional expression and processing in order to address or challenge misattributions – which can then increase support and understanding between families and clients, reducing isolation and stigmatisation (Schmidt et al., 2002). Importantly, Alschuler (2006) and Boone and Castillo (2008) also have written that poetry therapy may be particularly useful with 'resistant' or highly defended clients, as the intervention is explorative and works indirectly, enabling reflection and revelation. Writing poetry is cathartic, and so can help to express feelings, increase confidence through risk-taking, enhance insight, and reduce anxiety (Alschuler, 2006).

Alexithymia is commonly experienced by clients affected by anorexia and many other mental health presentations, and has been shown to have debilitating effects, even after controlling for other factors (Stockdale, 2011). Treatment, as in therapeutic creative writing, becomes about expression (Howlett, 2004; L'Abate & Sweeney, 2011). Poetry therapy may be able to assist alexithymic clients to identify and experience emotions as opposed to somatising them or acting them out (Alschuler, 2006; Stockdale, 2011). Research into the use of expressive writing in particular indicates the benefits of integrating and organising experience by translating it into a narrative, which creates distance from the events, improves perspective and increases a sense of control (Treasure & Whitney, 2010). Further, East et al. (2010) have reasoned that perspective-taking could be among the mechanisms by which writing can target the theory of mind deficits which are often observed in clients recovering from anorexia.

Where anorexia cannot be managed in the community, there is a need for psychiatric group interventions for day patients or inpatients which can encourage engagement in group therapy. Alschuler (2006) has made the case that poetry therapy, like other art therapies, is particularly suitable here, as it can encourage expression and peer interaction in a less confrontational or threatening way than a more intense group psychotherapy. Poetry therapy also has the potential to be an empowering intervention for clients recovering from anorexia. As it is focused on meaning and expression, and not solely on weight gain, it can give voice to clients' experiences, and help to shift any sense of blame from the self to the disorder (Robbins & Pehrsson, 2009), using narrative and other approaches to encourage the externalisation of the anorexic 'bully' (Treasure & Alexander, 2013).

Woodall and Andersen (1989) provided an excellent psychodynamic conceptualisation of the experience of anorexia which makes plain the appropriateness of poetry therapy for clients in recovery. Expression and communication are important, they maintain, as silence can be a feature of an anorexic presentation; a refusal to speak can be a component of the ambivalence toward treatment and recovery. Poetry therapy works with meaning, like poetry and psychotherapy, and its precise use of metaphor offers a way to reconnect with emotions. It can be less threatening to initially connect with a non-present poet through their writing, circumventing defences, and identification with poems can bring relief and strength. Writing poetry becomes a way of communicating personal meaning, and brings pleasure in accomplishment. Poetry therapy therefore provides indirect access to therapy and facilitates expression, and as it reduces self-censoring or reticence, it increases clients' sense of effectiveness and assertiveness, 'providing a means of transforming into words what is communicated physically through the symptoms of anorexia nervosa' (Woodall & Andersen, 1989, p. 205).

Client report

The first author contacted the second author, a former client, while drafting this paper, and invited her to contribute a written report of her experience of attending a poetry therapy group as part of her treatment. The second author kindly agreed, and, with permission, what follows is in her own words.

My truth

I took part in a poetry therapy group when I was an inpatient in an eating disorders unit. Prior to going into hospital, I had not received any treatment for anorexia. I was at the beginning of a long process, and during my time as a hospital inpatient and day patient, I took part in a variety of therapy groups. Today, six years after I was discharged from hospital, it is the poetry group that stands out in mind as the group in which I could be at my most honest, my most creative, and my most open to possibilities, with multiple truths existing alongside each other.

For me, anorexia has often been an attempt to be perfect, when inside I have always believed myself to be bad. The feeling of badness is not, entirely, rooted in fact or reason, but more a physical sensation. I am intelligent, can apply logical thinking and be incredibly rational. I sometimes feel that there are two brains inside my head: a rational brain which is fully in agreement with all the people, therapists, family and friends around me who repeatedly point out the blindingly obvious – I'm not fat, it's ok to eat, I am a good person – and a second brain which does not use words and does not respond to them, but instead uses emotions, sensations, and bodily urges as its weapon. For a long time, I have hated this sensation brain and have tried to cut myself off from everything it demands. Anorexia is my way of coping with the bodily sensations that have no words. Anorexia numbs that pain and takes you to a place where everything is constant and predictable, where everything is level and reassuring; like a fixed metre poem using rhyming couplets, it feels safe.

Therapy sessions like CBT appeal to the rational brain. The problem with CBT is that my sensation brain cannot connect with the words or the logical arguments that CBT presents, and so, when the session is over, the rational brain tries its hardest to stay in control, but ultimately the sensation brain is stronger and wins out. I remain anorexic.

The poetry group takes a different approach. During the group we read poems, such as the series by Gross (1998) about his daughter's anorexia, which describe the reality of how it feels to have anorexia. The poems put the unbearable chaos inside of me into something external, something fixed and on a page. The poems did not attempt to explain anorexia in its entirety and, most importantly, they did not always attempt to challenge the thoughts and behaviours associated with the illness. Instead, the poetry group gave me a space to start to recognise the sensations that for so long I had tried to cut off from and, slowly, to learn that those sensations are valid. Learning to accept and tolerate emotions, sensations and desires is a major part of my ongoing recovery, and I still read and write poems as a way to engage with myself on a level that is rational. Moreover, I read poems when I am in distress, as the rhythm and sound of them soothes the part of me that is hurting, perhaps like a lullaby soothes a child.

During the poetry therapy group, writing poems with other members of the group was also incredibly powerful. Anorexia can be a very isolating illness; you cut yourself off from your own feelings, and that results in an inability to properly connect with other people around you. By writing a poem with the other group members, we were able to create something together that validated our experiences as a group. We created a book of all the poems we made which was kept in the lounge on the ward. When new patients were admitted, I would watch them open the book and read the poems. I hoped, and believe, that the poems offered them comfort as they helped them recognise their own struggles and their own hopes through the words of others.

I do not think that poetry therapy is a replacement for all other therapies and believe that CBT is a much needed strategy for learning to make changes to behaviours, but I do think that poetry therapy offers something that talking therapies do not. As the person reads a poem, they are given the opportunity to engage in that poet's world and in the poet's feelings, which often seems safer than diving straight into your own messy mix of sensations. Poetry therapy allowed me to reach the intangible, the nameless sensations, the silent noise, the core of my illness and the key to my recovery.

The evidence base

For this paper, a literature review was conducted using the terms 'poetry therapy,' 'bibliotherapy' and 'therapeutic writing' in the indexes *PsychInfo* and *Google Scholar*, so that research from all related fields which may indicate the potential of poetry therapy could be examined. The majority of these publications were descriptive and employed no standardised research method. A small number of relevant quantitative and qualitative research papers were found, which mainly showed support for poetry therapy as an intervention, with some caveats. Firstly, research from the related area of expressive writing will be outlined, followed by a review of quantitative and qualitative studies of the use of poetry and creative writing for therapeutic purposes.

Expressive writing

There is a sizable amount of research on the therapeutic benefits of the related area of expressive writing, stemming from Pennebaker's (1997) work. Esterling et al. (1999) summarised well this extensive literature, which shows expressive writing to be as effective or nearly as effective as a short-term psychotherapy intervention, based on self-report outcome measures, for clients with minor issues. Esterling et al. (1999) summarised other research which shows that expressive writing is associated with less doctor visits, less days off sick, and improved liver and immune function. Interestingly, some further work has examined change processes, exploring the roles of cognitive change, levels of disclosure and confrontation of events (Esterling et al., 1999). However, the majority of this research has been conducted with healthy university students and over a few sessions only. Greenhallgh (1999), for example, was sceptical of the value of such expressive writing studies, arguing that they overstate the case, are badly designed, and largely miss the point, in that writing therapy is much more of an art than a science.

Most research to date regarding writing and eating disorders has examined interventions which apply expressive writing in the Pennebaker (1997) paradigm in some way to eating disorder symptomatology in non-clinical samples. For example, East et al. (2010) have reported a preliminary trial of expressive writing tasks on features linked to eating disorders in a student sample. The study reported positive results, but employed very small numbers. Earnhardt, Martz, Ballard, and Curtin (2002) also applied an expressive writing task to students, using an inclusion criterion of negative body image markers. Both the control group and the expressive writing group showed improvements, however. The authors offered many ideas as to why this may be, such as the placebo effect, a social desirability effect or pre-test sensitisation. As both the control and the experimental groups were invited to do some writing in this design, another explanation for these results, however, may lie in the effectiveness of writing in general, rather than any particular paradigm of writing intervention. Similarly, Frayne and Wade (2006) compared the effects of a written emotional expression task and a planning task control on bulimic symptoms. Again, both groups showed improvements, which the authors took to indicate a need for further research. Likewise, Johnston, Startup, Lavender, Godfrey, and Schmidt (2010) did not find that an expressive writing intervention offered via email made any significant difference in reducing bulimic symptoms in a non-clinical group, when compared with a control distraction task. The authors argue for more research using qualitative methods to examine the nature of the therapeutic process.

All of these studies also point to the need for more research with clinical samples. Robinson and Serfaty (2008) presented the results from a pilot randomised controlled trial of email therapy for bulimia nervosa and binge eating disorder. Interestingly, they found only a non-significant difference between an unsupported self-directed expressive writing task and therapist administered email therapy for bulimia, which could also indicate that writing in general can be a helpful intervention for clients recovering from eating disorders.

Poetry therapy

Quantitative research

The majority of the limited numbers of research studies on the effectiveness of poetry as an art therapy intervention follow a broadly quantitative research design, but with very limited subject numbers. Boone and Castillo (2008) used an experimental design to examine the effect of an online poetry therapy intervention for counsellors experiencing secondary PTSD symptoms. The experimental group, which was invited to respond to poetry, experienced more clinical benefit than the controls who were not, as measured by the Impact of Events Scale. Echoing the case material presented earlier, Mazza (2003) documented experimental research by himself and Golden (1995) showing that poetry therapy interventions, and the collaborative creative writing exercise in particular, facilitate important group processes such as advancing group cohesion compared to controls – a factor cited by Yalom (2005) as key to effective group therapy. Lowe (2006) recorded biological evidence of the effectiveness of writing emotional poetry or reading positive poems by measuring levels of an antibody which defends against infection before and after writing and reading. Antibody levels rose after writing emotional poems but not after writing more neutral poems, nor did they rise in the control group who wrote no poetry. Antibody levels also rose after reading positive poems, and not after reading negative or neutral poems. The sample sizes in this study were again small however, and no control group is mentioned in the reading study.

Mohammadian et al. (2011) reported a small scale evaluation of a group poetry therapy intervention which involved reading poetry for therapeutic purposes. The poetry therapy group showed significant decreases in their scores on depression, anxiety and stress on the Depression Anxiety Stress Scale compared to the control. In Tegner, Fox, Philipp, and Thorne's (2009) study, a poetry therapy group in which clients wrote individually during the session, shared their work with each other, and responded to each other's writing, was offered to clients being treated for cancer. Their research documents the intervention's ability to reduce anger and the need to control emotions in this client group, but the study again only involved small numbers of participants. Finally, Heimes conducted a systematic review of the evidence for poetry therapy in 2011. Unsurprisingly, he found that existing work, while highlighting both the cost-effectiveness and efficacy of poetry therapy, only fit low levels of evidence as determined by the University of Oxford's Centre for Evidence Based Medicine (CEBM), due to their designs and low participant numbers. He also found that the majority of the existing research was conducted in the US, and that more was needed from elsewhere in the world.

Qualitative research

Heimes (2011) also acknowledged the lack of fit between a systematic review using the CEBM's standards for levels of evidence, and poetry therapy, which may be more suited to qualitative research methods that explore meaning and expression. There have been some qualitative investigations of poetry therapy. Jensen and Blair (1997), for example, explored the tensions between writing for therapeutic purposes and creative writing practice in a community-based writing group for ex-mental health service users. Mazza (2003) summarised historical research, including case studies and qualitative surveys of staff and patients at hospitals where poetry therapy was offered, which indicate good up-take of the intervention, advancements in group cohesion, particular benefits for withdrawn patients, and that the intervention was less beneficial for those with limited cognitive functioning. Kidd, Zauszniewski, and Morris (2011) presented an interesting piece of qualitative research using grounded theory to analyse interview data collected from carers of people with dementia about their experiences of writing poetry. Emerging themes around the possible experienced benefits included self-affirmation, catharsis of negative emotions and the validation of positive emotions, a sense of achievement, increased acceptance, greater empathy, the opportunity to reflect, greater self-awareness, fun, positive challenge, and an increased energy for helping others, some of which can also be seen in the earlier client report. More recently, Petrescru, MacFarlane, and Ranzijn (2014) collected feedback from four participants after a poetry writing group intervention for clients with early stage dementia. Client feedback on the poetry workshops was overwhelmingly positive, but this exploratory study did not analyse any of this data rigorously.

Naturally, research on poetry therapy and eating disorders is even more limited, perhaps in part due to the difficulty of evaluating interventions in eating disorder treatment programmes with many components (Kaplan, 2002). However, Robbins and Pehrsson (2009) set out a moving case report of an anorexic client responding to published poems in therapy, to good effect.

The need for more research

The chorus of voices in the literature calling for more research on the effectiveness of poetry therapy is overwhelming (Gorelick, 2005; Heimes, 2011; Hornyak & Baker, 1989; Johnston et al., 2010; L'Abate & Sweeney, 2011; McArdle & Byrt, 2001; McCulliss, 2011a, 2012; Schmidt et al., 2002), particularly in regards to poetry or arts-based therapies for anorexia (Kaplan, 2002; Robbins & Pehrsson, 2009). Jensen and Blair (1997) point out that most papers in this area are based on clinical opinion unsubstantiated by evidence. In other words, they present many theories about how this intervention creates its benefits written by enthusiastic advocates, in the face of a dearth of actual research, qualitative or quantitative. Wright and Chung (2001) concurred, and contrasted well the literature produced by artists and writers against those by psychotherapists or other health professionals, in terms of their different emphases, tone and subjects. However, they contended that publications from both are needed, and they note with interest that work from both groups seems to be reaching similar conclusions. Mazza (1993) proposed a research agenda which prioritises qualitative and quantitative process and outcome research examining the effects of poetry therapy on specific groups, and the experiences and perceptions of those who engage in creative writing for therapeutic purposes. Mazza (2003) went on to articulate the ethical imperative for upgrading research on poetry therapy and arts therapies in general, in the service of ensuring that clients have access to most appropriate treatments for their presentations. Nicholls (2009) has gone further, and has criticised the emphasis in the literature on health psychological research and publications on expressive writing, as compared to research on poetry therapy or therapeutic creative writing. Like Heimes (2011) and Johnston et al. (2010), she recommends the use of more appropriate research methods in this work as well, such as phenomenological research methods and other designs that capture the experience of writing. Writing itself could also be used as a research tool or process as part of this work (Nicholls, 2009).

Jensen and Blair (1997) set out one primary problem, in that most published papers do not define their terms well. As they could therefore be discussing different interventions, there is a real need for clarity in the field. Mazza (1993, 2003) also emphasised the importance of setting out the detail of the intervention under study, its context, and the presentations to which it is being applied, so that research is transparent and replicable. While there is debate in the field regarding the relative weight of therapist effects and relational factors (Wampold & Imel, 2015) versus standardised interventions tested in controlled trails (Roth & Fonagy, 2005), further quantitative research employing a standardised protocol could bring this intervention to the attention of a wider audience, such as commissioners and service managers.

A replicable model

Mazza (2003) offered a group poetry therapy procedure which incorporates all three modes of the RES model and which could be applied to a wide variety of client groups and presentations.

In each session, after a brief opening round, the poem written by the group at the last session is circulated. Group members are invited to read this to themselves in silence, before a volunteer is sought to read the piece aloud in the room, to allow for a different kind of processing of the piece and the therapeutic benefits of reading poetry aloud. Group members are then invited to share their gut reactions to a part of or the whole poem, perhaps in terms of what grabs their attention, what feelings are now arising, what they dislike about the poem or what they would like to change. Their responses are linked by the facilitator to the difficult experiences they are facing, leading to a group exploration of the meaning of change or the lived experience of recovery. At intervals, the group leader or any group member can offer a further piece of published poetry, writing or song lyrics in the same manner, to enable the recognition of their experiences in others, a deeper examination of these, and an application of these insights to their journey (McCulliss, 2011a).

Towards the end of the session, the group leader facilitates a collaborative creative writing exercise, to support the group to collectively write a poem summarising their overall reflections from the session or their relationship to a particular theme which arose, often using an image or metaphor that naturally emerged during the discussion. In typing up this collaborative poem and selecting published poems based on their discussion for next week's session, the group facilitator demonstrates to group members that they are being held in mind collectively and individually in between appointments.

Mazza (2003) has offered guidance on poem selection, useful poems, questions to prompt reflections and self-supervision tools in the core text *Poetry Therapy: Research and Practice*.

Conclusion

Poetry therapy is a promising arts-based therapeutic intervention with clear applications for clients recovering from anorexia. More qualitative research examining rigorously what clients experience as helpful and the process of change is needed. Further quantitative research examining the efficacy and effectiveness of poetry therapy is also needed to evidence whether this approach should be more widely available, and to impact future practice. One interesting body of research involves the use of software, such as Pennebaker's Linguistic Inquiry and Word Count programme or NVivo, to document types of language used and changes in language over time (Esterling et al., 1999; Santarpia, Tellène, & Carrier, 2013). For example, Santarpia, Dudoit, and Paul (2015a, 2015b) analysed a poetry therapy intervention using interviews, published haiku, and the creative writing of haiku using the Tropes semantic analysis software programme, and showed changes in language over the course of the intervention that indicated therapeutic change. Finally, a wider, more systematic literature review specifically investigating whether poetry therapy could improve outcomes for clients diagnosed with anorexia nervosa, incorporating more search terms and more databases, could guide future practice, commissioning and research.

Disclosure statement

No potential conflict of interest was reported by the authors.

ORCID

Christine E. Ramsey-Wade http://orcid.org/0000-0003-4318-0286

References

Alschuler, M. (2006). Poetry, the healing pen. In S. Brooke (Ed.), *Creative therapies manual* (pp. 253–262). Springfield, IL: Charles C Thomas Publisher Ltd.

Bolton, G. (1999). *The therapeutic potential of creative writing: Writing myself.* London: Jessica Kingsley Publishers.

Bolton, G., & Latham, J. (2004). 'Every poem breaks a silence that had to be overcome': The therapeutic role of poetry writing. In G. Bolton, S. Howlett, C. L. Lago, & J. K. Wright (Eds.), *Writing cures: An introductory handbook of writing in counselling and therapy* (pp. 106–122). Hove: Routledge.

Boone, B. C., & Castillo, L. G. (2008). The use of poetry therapy with domestic violence counselors experiencing secondary posttraumatic stress disorder symptoms. *Journal of Poetry Therapy, 21*(1), 3–14. doi:10.1080/08893670801886865

Earnhardt, J. L., Martz, D. M., Ballard, M. E., & Curtin, L. (2002). A writing intervention for negative body image: Pennebaker fails to surpass the placebo. *Journal of College Student Psychotherapy, 17*(1), 19–35. doi:10.1300/J035v17n01_04

East, P., Startup, H., Roberts, C., & Schmidt, U. (2010). Expressive writing and eating disorder features: A preliminary trial in a student sample of the impact of three writing tasks on eating disorder symptoms and associated cognitive, affective and interpersonal factors. *European Eating Disorders Review, 18*(3), 180–196. doi:10.1002/erv.978

Esterling, B. A., L'Abate, L., Murray, E. J., & Pennebaker, J. W. (1999). Empirical foundations for writing in prevention and psychotherapy: Mental and physical health outcomes. *Clinical Psychology Review, 19*(1), 79–96. doi:10.1016/S0272-7358(98)00015-4

Frayne, A., & Wade, T. D. (2006). A comparison of written emotional expression and planning with respect to bulimic symptoms and associated psychopathology. *European Eating Disorders Review, 14*(5), 329–340. doi:10.1002/erv.731

Furman, R. (2003). Poetry therapy and existential practice. *The Arts in Psychotherapy, 30,* 195–200. doi:10.1016/S0197-4556(03)00052-2

Golden, K. M. (1995). The effect of collaborative writing on cohesion in poetry therapy groups (Doctoral dissertation, The American University). *Dissertation Abstracts International Section A: Humanities and Social Sciences,* 56(3), ProQuest Information & Learning, US.

Gorelick, K. (2005). Poetry therapy. In C.A. Malchiodi (Ed.), *Expressive therapies* (pp. 117–140). New York: The Guilford Press.

Greenhallgh, T. (1999). Writing as therapy. *British Medical Journal, 319*(7205), 270–271. doi:10.1136/bmj.319.7205.270

Gross, P. (1998). *The wasting game.* London: Bloodaxe Books Ltd.

Hedges, D. (2005). *Poetry, therapy and emotional life.* Abingdon: Radcliffe.

Heimes, S. (2011). State of poetry therapy research (review). *The Arts in Psychotherapy, 38*(1), 1–8. Retrieved February 26, 2014. doi:10.1016/j.aip.2010.09.006

Hornyak, L. M., & Baker, E. K. (1989). Introduction. In L. M. Hornyak & E. K. Baker (Eds.), *Experiential therapies for eating disorders* (pp. 1–7). New York, NY: Guilford Press.

Howlett, S. (2004). Writing the link between body and mind: The use of writing with clients suffering from chronic stress-related medical disorders. In G. Bolton, S. Howlett, C. L. Lago, & J. K. Wright (Eds.), *Writing cures: An introductory handbook of writing in counselling and therapy* (pp. 85–94). Hove: Routledge.

Jensen, C. M., & Blair, S. E. E. (1997). Rhyme and reason: The relationship between creative writing and mental wellbeing. *British Journal of Occupational Therapy, 60*(12), 525–530. doi:10.1177/030802269706001205

Johnston, O., Startup, H., Lavender, A., Godfrey, E., & Schmidt, U. (2010). Therapeutic writing as an intervention for symptoms of bulimia nervosa: Effects and mechanism of change. *International Journal of Eating Disorders, 43*(5), 405–419.

Kaplan, A. S. (2002). Psychological treatments for anorexia nervosa: A review of published studies and promising new directions. *The Canadian Journal of Psychiatry, 47*(3), 235–242. doi:10.1177/070674370204700303

Kerner, E. A., & Fitzpatrick, M. R. (2007). Integrating writing into psychotherapy practice: A matrix of change processes and structural dimensions. *Psychotherapy: Theory, Research, Practice, Training, 44*(3), 333–346. doi:10.1037/0033-3204.44.3.333

Kidd, L. I., Zauszniewski, J. A., & Morris, D. L. (2011). Benefits of poetry writing intervention for family caregivers of elders with dementia. *Issues in Mental Health Nursing, 32,* 598–604. doi:10.3109/01612840.2011.576801

L'Abate, L., & Sweeney, L. G. (2011). *Research on writing approaches in mental health.* Bingley: Emerald Group Publishing.

Leedy, N. (2006). The therapeutic value of poetry. In S. Brooke (Ed.), *Creative therapies manual* (pp. 263–268). Springfield, IL: Charles C Thomas Publisher Ltd.

Lowe, G. (2006). Health-related effects of creative and expressive writing. *Health Education, 106*(1), 60–70. Retrieved February 26, 2014. doi:10.1108/09654280610637201

Malchiodi, C. A. (2005). Expressive therapies: History, theory and practice. In C. A. Malchiodi (Ed.), *Expressive therapies* (pp. 1–15). New York: The Guilford Press.

Mazza, N., & Hayton, C. (2013). Poetry therapy: An investigation of a multidimensional clinical model. *The Arts in Psychotherapy, 40*(1), 53–60. doi:10.1016/j.aip.2012.10.002

Mazza, N. (1993). Poetry therapy: Toward a research agenda for the 1990s. *The Arts in Psychotherapy, 20*(1), 51–59. doi:10.1016/0197-4556(93)90031-V

Mazza, N. (2003). *Poetry therapy: Research and practice.* New York: Brunner-Routledge.

McArdle, S., & Byrt, R. (2001). Fiction, poetry and mental health: Expressive and therapeutic uses of literature. *Journal of Psychiatric and Mental Health Nursing, 8*(6), 517–524. Retrieved February 26, 2014. doi:10.1046/j.1351-0126.2001.00428.x

McCulliss, D. (2011a). Bibliotherapy. In L. L'Abate & L. G. Sweeney (Eds.), *Research on writing approaches in mental health* (pp. 67–83). Bingley: Emerald Group Publishing.

McCulliss, D. (2011b). Poetry therapy. In L. L'Abate & L. G. Sweeney (Eds.), *Research on writing approaches in mental health* (pp. 93–114). Bingley: Emerald Group Publishing.

McCulliss, D. (2012). Bibliotherapy: Historical and research perspectives. *Journal of Poetry Therapy, 25*(1), 23–38. doi:10.1080/08893675.2012.654944

McLoughlin, D. (2000). Transition, transformation and the art of losing: Some uses of poetry in hospice care for the terminally ill. *Psychodynamic Counselling, 6*(2), 215–234. doi:10.1080/135333300407558

Mohammadian, Y., Shahidi, S., Mahaki, B., Mohammadi, A. Z., Baghban, A. A., & Zayeri, F. (2011). Evaluating the use of poetry to reduce signs of depression, anxiety and stress in Iranian female students. *The Arts in Psychotherapy, 38*(1), 59–63. Retrieved February 26, 2014. doi:10.1016/j.aip.2010.12.002

National Institute for Health and Clinical Excellence. (2004). *NICE clinical guideline 9: Eating disorders.* Retrieved from www.nice.org.uk/cg9

Nicholls, S. (2009). Beyond expressive writing: Evolving models of developmental creative writing. *Journal of Health Psychology, 14*(2), 171–180. Retrieved February 26, 2014. doi:10.1177/1359105308100201

Nylund, D. (2002). Poetic means to anti-anorexic ends. *Journal of Systemic Therapies, 21*(4), 18–34. doi:10.1521/jsyt.21.4.18.23323

Pennebaker, J. W. (1997). Writing about emotional experiences as a therapeutic process. *Psychological Science, 8*(3), 162–166. doi:10.1111/j.1467-9280.1997.tb00403.x

Perlin, E. (2009). *Breaking addictions with biblio/poetry therapy.* Bloomington, IN: AuthorHouse.

Petrescru, I., MacFarlane, K., & Ranzijn, R. (2014). Psychological effects of poetry workshops with people with early stage dementia: An exploratory study. *Dementia, 13*(2), 207–215. doi:10.1177/1471301212456279

Reynaga-Abiko, G. (2008). Culturally competent group therapy with Latina adolescents and young adults with eating disturbance: The use of poetry and music. In S. Brooke (Ed.), *The creative therapies and eating disorders* (pp. 159–172). Springfield, IL: Charles C Thomas Publisher Ltd.

Robbins, J. M., & Pehrsson, D. (2009). Anorexia nervosa: A synthesis of poetic and narrative therapies in the outpatient treatment of young adult women. *Journal of Creativity in Mental Health, 4*(1), 42–56. doi:10.1080/15401380802708775

Robinson, P., & Serfaty, M. (2008). Getting better byte by byte: A pilot randomised controlled trial of email therapy for bulimia nervosa and binge eating disorder. *European Eating Disorders Review, 16*(2), 84–93. doi:10.1002/erv.818

Roth, A., & Fonagy, P. (2005). *What works for whom? A critical review of psychotherapy research.* London: Guilford Press.

Santarpia, A., Dudoit, E., & Paul, M. (2015a). The discursive effects of the haiku-based SADUPA poetry technique in palliative care. *Journal of Poetry Therapy, 28*(3), 179–194. doi:10.1080/08893675.2015.1051288

Santarpia, A., Paul, M., & Dudoit, E. (2015b). L'usage de la poésie haïku en psycho-oncologie[The use of the Haiku poetry in psycho-oncology]. *Psycho-Oncologie, 9*, 127–134. doi:10.1007/s11839-015-0523-5

Santarpia, A., Tellène, J., & Carrier, M. (2013). Les effets d'un protocole d'écriture poétique SANTEL sur l'image érotique du corps dans le traitement du cancer féminin : étude pilote[The effects of poetry-writing SANTEL on erotic body image in remission of cancer in women: A pilot study]. *Psycho-Oncologie, 7*(3), 156–162. doi:10.1007/s11839-013-0426-2

Schmidt, U., Bone, G., Hems, S., Lessem, J., & Treasure, J. (2002). Structured therapeutic writing tasks as an adjunct to treatment in eating disorders. *European Eating Disorders Review, 10*(5), 299–315. doi:10.1002/erv.465

Speedy, J. (2004). The contribution of narrative ideas and writing practices in therapy. In G. Bolton, S. Howlett, C. L. Lago, & J. K. Wright (Eds.), *Writing cures: An introductory handbook of writing in counselling and therapy* (pp. 25–34). Hove: Routledge.

Steinberg, D. (2004). From archetype to impressions: The magic of words. In G. Bolton, S. Howlett, C. L. Lago, & J. K. Wright (Eds.), *Writing cures: An introductory handbook of writing in counselling and therapy* (pp. 44–55). Hove: Routledge.

Stockdale, B. (2011). Writing in physical and concomitant mental illness: Biological underpinnings and applications for practice. In L. L'Abate, & L.G. Sweeney (Eds.), *Research on writing approaches in mental health* (pp. 23–35). Bingley: Emerald Group Publishing.

Tegner, I., Fox, J., Philipp, R., & Thorne, P. (2009). Evaluating the use of poetry to improve well-being and emotional resilience in cancer patients. *Journal of Poetry Therapy, 22*(3), 121–131. doi:10.1080/08893670903198383

Treasure, J., & Alexander, J. (2013). *Anorexia nervosa: A recovery guide for sufferers, families and friends.* London: Routledge.

Treasure, J., & Whitney, J. (2010). Writing as a tool for developing reflective capacity and emotional processing. In J. Treasure, U. Schmidt, & P. Macdonald (Eds.), *The clinician's guide to collaborative caring in eating disorders: The new Maudsley method* (pp. 150–166). London: Routledge.

Wampold, B. E., & Imel, Z. E. (2015). *The great psychotherapy debate: The research evidence for what works in psychotherapy* (2nd ed.). New York, NY: Routledge.

Winnicott, D. W. (1971). *Playing and reality.* London: Routledge.

Woodall, C., & Andersen, A. E. (1989). The use of metaphor and poetry therapy in the treatment of the reticent subgroup of anorectic patients. In L. M. Hornyak, & E. K. Baker (Eds.), [online] (pp. 191–206). New York, NY: Guilford Press.

Wright, J., & Chung, M. C. (2001). Mastery or mystery? Therapeutic writing: A review of the literature. *British Journal of Guidance & Counselling, 29*(3), 277–291. doi:10.1080/03069880120073003

Yalom, I. D. (2005). *The theory and practice of group psychotherapy.* New York: Basic Books.

The warm bathwater of working life slowly ebbing away: retirement stories and writing for therapeutic purposes

Jeannie K. Wright

ABSTRACT
"What am I without paid work?" Some would say, "A non-person." Others might say, "Free!" The experience of retirement is explored using creative writing for therapeutic purposes. Written from the perspective of fictional British retirees from different workplaces, the paper offers a view of how expressive and reflective writing can be both therapy and research at times of transition. Little in the literature on retirement in the UK uses the "experience near" approaches of writing as inquiry. This paper will point out some of the benefits of research methods that are "up close and personal", culturally embedded and embodied. Encouraging the use of playful, creative writing in individual counselling and in groups is one of the aims of this paper.

Introduction

This article is about retirement. I can often write what I can't say – started young and have developed the habit. Some of the material for this article is therefore drawn from my personal writing; "journalling" is not quite right, although there is now a substantial literature about regular expressive writing as a therapeutic tool (Bolton, 2011; Thompson & Adams, 2015). I started with a list, that simplest and least threatening form of writing. The list was in answer to a question: What would I miss if I retired? *"Identity, the printer, working with some of the students, status, some of my colleagues, structure, IT Services, some of the students, talking about ideas, a sense of purpose and routine, an income. Did I mention the printer?"* The metaphor in the title, "the warm bathwater of working life" is an example of showing, not telling. One purpose of this article is to draw attention to the value of creative writing tools as part of helping strategies for those who struggle with the move out of paid work, and all that that implies. Images in creative writing can help us to connect with feelings that we are not consciously aware of, connect with ourselves and with others. I wasn't fully aware of how important – and at times comforting – paid work has been in my life until that metaphor of the warm bathwater emerged.

Of course choosing to leave paid work is a privilege. For Tony, the taxi driver in the dialogue below, choice has been very limited. Dialogue is a more extended form of creative writing and in this example introduces some of the tensions for people who are ageing and dealing with externally imposed upheavals in their working lives:

Tony, now a taxi driver (who was an engineer) asks me, "What do you do?"
He waits while I struggle with the seatbelt with arthritic fingers, an older male driving an older female. He has picked me up from a UK University residence with a suitcase, so he knows I have some connection with the University. There's a pause. I decide on, "I teach."

We move on to the fog forecast and then, watching the hard hats and steel –toe- capped builders arrive at the site across from where I live. There's another pause. I forego silence.
"This place employs a lot of people," I say and he's off.
He was "retired" from production engineering after a takeover.
Tony: "This town used to be everything engineering, now the University must be the biggest employer, or maybe the hospital. Can't imagine a more pathetic job than driving. The one good thing about it is I go home when I like, get up when I like."
The light is red. We turn into the one scenic drive in this battered and historically carpet-bombed city. The road is suddenly tree-lined and curves down to the station.
Me: "With your qualifications and experience, it seems a waste. You could be passing on your knowledge." Am I being deliberately provocative?
The back of his neck straightens,
Tony: "Well, of course I applied for technician jobs. I thought they'd have my name written on them. No response from any of them. Even when I stopped putting my date of birth on applications. The only reason I got on to this was through an argument. Down at the dole, they started saying I'd got to take shelf stacking. I snatched the card up from the desk, 'Right, I'll go for this!' And it was training to drive taxis, if you can call it training. There's no holiday pay and of course, when you don't have a company car, sick pay, pension- that's when you realise what you had."
He's angry and I estimate I may be another five minutes sitting in the back of this car. Tony carries on talking about what he misses from his previous engineering life, and how he only has a year to go before retirement proper, that is collecting his pension.
We're now in a bowl of fog, then up and out into the sun outside the station.
Tony: "Do you want a receipt?"
I imagine the invoice, 20 min counselling, or is it biographical or ethnographic research? He has told his story and been heard. He may feel valued, or may not. Other passengers may have taken the other seat, telling their stories, not listening to the driver's.

Writing activities

Self writing takes many forms, starting with lists (Bolton, Field, & Thompson, 2011; Field, Bolton, & Thompson, 2006). Many people carry the old shame of school, and being told they can't write, but everyone writes lists. Some clients have brought examples of their writing to our work and we've used them together. For example:

- Unsent letters/emails
- Song lyrics
- Poems on stones then thrown as far as you can
- Dream journals
- Dialogues with other people or with parts of yourself.

There is a long tradition of using creative writing in career, health and therapeutic settings and an increasing research literature (Lengelle & Meijers, 2014; Williamson & Wright, in press).

Using fictional characters, such as Tony and Leslie, who will appear in this article is a way of distancing, and allows more freedom of expression, especially if there is traumatic memory (Etherington, 2003). Tony and Leslie are fictional in the sense that they have emerged from my imagination but also reflect my experience and relationships, of course. This is an ethical as well as creative decision. No story is ever about only one person, the writer (Tullis, 2013). The ethics of personal and fictional writing as published narrative research, similar to those of writing autoethnographies are fraught and will be returned to (Josselson, 2007; Wyatt & Adams, 2014).

Unsent letters/emails

The unsent letter, now more likely to be an email or tweet, is a familiar therapeutic writing tool. It's crucial that the writer chooses whether to press send, or not.

> Dear students and colleagues,
>
> I'm taking my mono-functional equipment (a clock) and leaving you to it.
> Updating the yellowing handouts? Yes, I can see the need for that, but becoming part of an entertainment industry on social media? No.
> Updating Twitter every time I turn round because Marketing says so? No.
> Hot desking? Good luck with that.
> All the best
> Leslie – the grey-haired one who used to teach you … .(Enter a subject as desired)

Leslie's rant, to former students and colleagues, expresses hurt. For some, leaving paid work is forced; they would prefer to stay in the workplace, possibly even to die in harness. Leslie is ambivalent. She writes in a journal entry:

"I'm very tired and fed up. The work just irritates me now. I don't really want to do it any more. It pays though, and sometimes does that thing of distracting: work as anaesthesia. I suppose I'll have to find other painkillers."

In the UK, at last count, three quarters of people aged over 50 are still in work and 1 in 8 people aged over 65 are still in the paid work force. Encouraged by governmental policies, staying in paid work for people between the ages of 50 and 74 is a growing area of opportunity (Office for National Statistics https://www.gov.uk/government/news/employment-minister-calls-on-businesses-to-create-more-opportunities-for-older-workers).

Encouraging written expression is very much part of my practice, mostly in writing groups rather than with individuals (Wright, 2012). There is solidarity in groups. I wrote this paragraph about retirement in a supportive writing group over three years ago:

> Wherever *or whatever you've been able to hang this life around, you're suddenly, like your Skoda in the works car park, the oldest on the corridor. The departmental mug shots show rows of youthful and middle aged faces. You're elderly, a crone and a half. And there's not much of the "elder" in terms of respect when reflecting on feeling elderly in this particular workplace. Shaming is the organisational leverage that pushes many out.*

Based on experience of retirees and those about to leave paid work in wealthier parts of the world, I'm conscious of how gender and social class impact on retirement stories. Economically, the current historical period in the UK and other parts of the "global north" is rare in that retirement is cushioned by pensions – for some. Even fifty years ago, although still linked with ageing, retirement was not a viable, financial option; now for some it means index-linked pensions and potentially a more leisured and desirable life-style (Blake, 2006). So why is Leslie so resistant to the idea of more leisure time?

> "It's the day of the leaving do. I have specifically asked not to have one, and feel relieved that it's partly diluted by two others moving on from this workplace. It's outside too – not in some cramped corridor, with bought cakes and some colleagues looking anxiously at their phones in case they're missing an email/Tweet/Facebook post. The genial Head of Department makes jokes and refers to me as 'retiring'. That's not what I'm about to do. However, he seems unable to accept that I'm going to get another job, and definitely not about to set off on a Saga cruise. 'All the best, Leslie,' he says. We all smile, drink the warm wine and go back to work."

One of the major strengths of the kind of creative writing illustrated here is the freedom to express thoughts and feelings openly, anywhere and with any kind of equipment, from the pencil and back of anything that's write-able on, to the tablet/phone/laptop. The privacy of this first write is essential. There is no audience, no judge, no critic (Wright & Bolton, 2012).

Autoethnography, writing as inquiry and ethics

The creative traditions and colours of writing for therapeutic purposes run into approaches to research where writing about personal experience is honoured, such as in autoethnography and writing as inquiry (Richardson & St Pierre, 2005). One of the differences is that the "product" of the writing is more dominant, rather than the writing process. For example, during transitions between jobs and between countries, for me, personal writing is anchoring and the reflection it affords in re-reading full of insight (Wright, 2009). The jump from personal and therapeutic (this writing is for my eyes only) to producing writing within a cultural and political envelope for publication has hazy boundaries: it helps me to understand the experience from a wider angle; it may also connect with others' experience and it raises complex ethical issues.

"Autoethnography is a way of caring for the self." (Adams, Holman Jones, & Ellis, 2015, p. 62).

Is it? There is a kind of protection in writing, and paradoxically, deciding to publish that intimate, autoethnographic writing is also a risky way to share vulnerabilities (Wright, 2003). Once the given audience is invited in, there's no way of taking back the invitation, and the occasional need to "speak" to a wider audience leaves me feeling exposed, and not just about me, but also about the other people who are inevitably woven into the parts of my life I choose to write about. Most of my writing goes into cupboards or in bags under beds. Ethically, that is a much safer option. Those writings have done their job as a kind of therapy; they have no need to go anywhere else – it's a private outpouring and not for anyone else's eyes.

Do the unique and emotionally powerful insights of autoethnographic accounts make it worth the anguish of risking publication? Sometimes. As an approach to research, this is contested ground. Essentially, as some of the leaders in the field argue, it's worth it because of the possible connections with other people; that personal story might do some "good in the world". Certainly finding autoethnographer Ron Pelias' evocative writing about the indecision facing him at the end of an academic career made me smile (Pelias, 2015). Hanging on, or letting go – I felt he understood my dilemma as I read about his.

As Tony Adams says in a recent film by Kitrina Douglas about autoethnography, "I can write about homophobia in my life in ways that no interviewer could ever capture" (Douglas & Carless, 2016) https://www.youtube.com/watch?v=7nTX3BkUrmA. Accessed 20.9.16.

Autoethnography is a useful part of the repertoire of social science research but is not for the faint-hearted. Your personal thoughts and feelings, once in print, cannot be changed or taken back (Holman Jones, Adams, & Ellis, 2013; Wyatt & Adams, 2014).

Writing poetry

Poetry is a "hotline to the heart" in poet Andrew Motion's image. Perhaps that is why people tend to turn to poetry in difficult times. Also, there's potentially more freedom to be private and to under-share than in unsent letters or journal entries. Symbolic language and metaphor have a power that allows us to attend to that which is left out, and is perhaps unthinkable (Cixous & Calle-Gruber, 1994/1997). Some of the tools of poetic writing, for example, rhythm (try reading aloud), metaphor and a quality of conciseness are illustrated in the fragments of poetry below:

If she were male

If she were male
She'd be monstrous
Napoleonic
Swaggering, bullying
Power loving.

She's a strong red wine
Fine tannins with black cherries
Lively acidity and a
Chocolaty complexion.
Belligerent, beating
The competition

(And even those not competing).
Swearing, smoking, shouting:
"I nearly made him cry"
Agitating, aggressive,
"I don't back down".

And when they asked us
When she retired
To evaluate her management style
We said:
"We love her but
She works too hard."

Borrowing from journal entries and from fragments of poetry that tend to record the negatives, this article might have denied the positives of leaving paid work.

Retired as a purring cat

The days when I stay in bed for a bit.
Grey, cold days when
Scraping ice off the windscreen would have meant an even
Darker, earlier start.
So, with a book or radio and cup of tea,
I lie there.
Retired as a purring cat.
For some, retirement can't come soon enough and is anticipated with joy.

Celebration

Getting away from some of the horrors of working lives is a good reason to retire. Choosing to spend time on cherished hobbies and with family, there may be many causes for celebration in plans for the future without paid work:

Leaving that job with an early retirement package was the happiest day of my life.

Given luxuries, like enough money to pay the bills, some retirees luxuriate in the time "to stand and stare". In earlier centuries the leisured classes would have been permanent retirees; now there is a pensioned way out of toil for some working people – they have the space for creativity and the money to pay: daytime classes – singing, Pilates, circle dancing, bowls, foreign holidays, more time with the water-colour painting and other creative hobbies. Their new identity is cause for celebration, away from the toxicities of some work places. Life without paid work, of course, is very different for those without good pensions, who struggle to pay bills, who need to sort through the reduced vegetables in the supermarket.

Others move into more than full-time volunteering. The pressures and pleasures of running the local Oxfam branch or the University of the Third Age (U3A) feel familiar and reassuring. It's like a job without a pay packet. The empty days in the diary are all filled up and there's a feeling of usefulness that is worth a lot in terms of social capital.

Advertisements for the wealthy over – 60s feature: cruises, gated retirement communities with swimming pools, Quality Riser Recliners, stair lifts, incontinence pads, machinery and ramps for getting pets in and out of cars. Aimed at a particular and monocultural demographic (a recent article about the writer Alan Bennett in a UK newspaper featured ads for all of the above) I object to the stereotyping. Most advertisements targeted at this group feature images of smiling, white-haired couples celebrating on a tropical beach hand in hand (the couples are usually heterosexual); or sitting by the log burner, along with the pedigree Labrador (the kennels will pamper him when they finish that expensive wine and decide on another spa-break). After all, privileged and blessed with no mortgage and big pensions, some of my peer group would argue that retirement is their due: One long holiday.

A recent series in a UK newspaper, *the Guardian*, debated the new "flexible" retirement age, gender and retirement and argued for 5 pillars of successful ageing/leaving paid work. The economic divide for those looking to retire happily is clear: https://www.theguardian.com/membership/ng-interactive/2017/jan/16/the-new-retirement-catch-up-with-this-series.

Fear and shame

The landscape of growing old is not pretty – for some. The decline of taken-for-granted health – the physicality of ageing, curved spines, arthritis, hair-loss, high blood-pressure and the consequent losses of vanity, mobility and independence – can be full of fear. Asking for help may not be easy and shame seems to be part of the package.

Retirement from paid work is the anteroom to death, after all, and if we take a pessimistic view, that's all there is to it: Dementia, stroke, chronic illnesses await. The fears underlying the decision to move out of that warm water of working life, to let it ebb away, or have the plug pulled abruptly, can be paralysing.

The incompetence and inadequacy I'm drenched in, when faced with the technological speedway that living and working now presents, brings out the Luddite. Let me out of here. Like Maya Angelou, in her poem, "The last decision," the question arises of what to give up next, but life itself:

Angelou bemoans print being too small and not being able to read because of the 'wavering black things on the page'. As eyesight fails with age, the distress of giving up even the quiet enjoyment of reading is distressing, even humiliating.

Writing can be less exposing, less shaming in managing those feelings than face-to-face conversations – even, perhaps especially, with counsellors. Shame is connected to loss of identity as part of the work-force and connected to leaving part of a younger stage of life. Shame is felt, as well, with the various physical indicators of declining years: can't hear – poor old thing; can't see – scrabbling about in the bag for the glasses; and worse. We won't approach incontinence – yet.

Telling stories to ourselves in writing is a way of reclaiming ourselves before risking saying the words out loud (Etherington, 2003).

Leslie writes an unsent email to a friend. Leslie is the reader/audience, she "hears" her own story:

> Dear B,
> It started with buying the tartan shopping trolley, one of those 'old woman' trollies. It sat outside the shop with its wheels, slowly rusting. I was struggling to carry stuff and didn't want to use the car any more. My grown-up (should know better) kids took the Michael out of me. They loved playing around with it – its clever sets of wheels going up and down steps. So, I bought it. Even if it were purple, as in that famous Jenny Joseph poem, it wouldn't be cool. Is this it now, pushing a shopping trolley with the other bent heads? I can hear you laugh, 'I pull mine'.
>
> What it means to me is: no strength, weak back, no car. Then I see a typically cheery Edward Bond play, all about dead soldiers, women in war, dead babies and there it is! Part of the very cool stage set. I wheel it up and down steps – those wheels really are clever – it takes the bottles and tins and, what John Shuttleworth calls big box powders that used to go in the boot of the car in the supermarket car-park. That detail of a theatre designer's imagination is now part of my life. Is this it now?

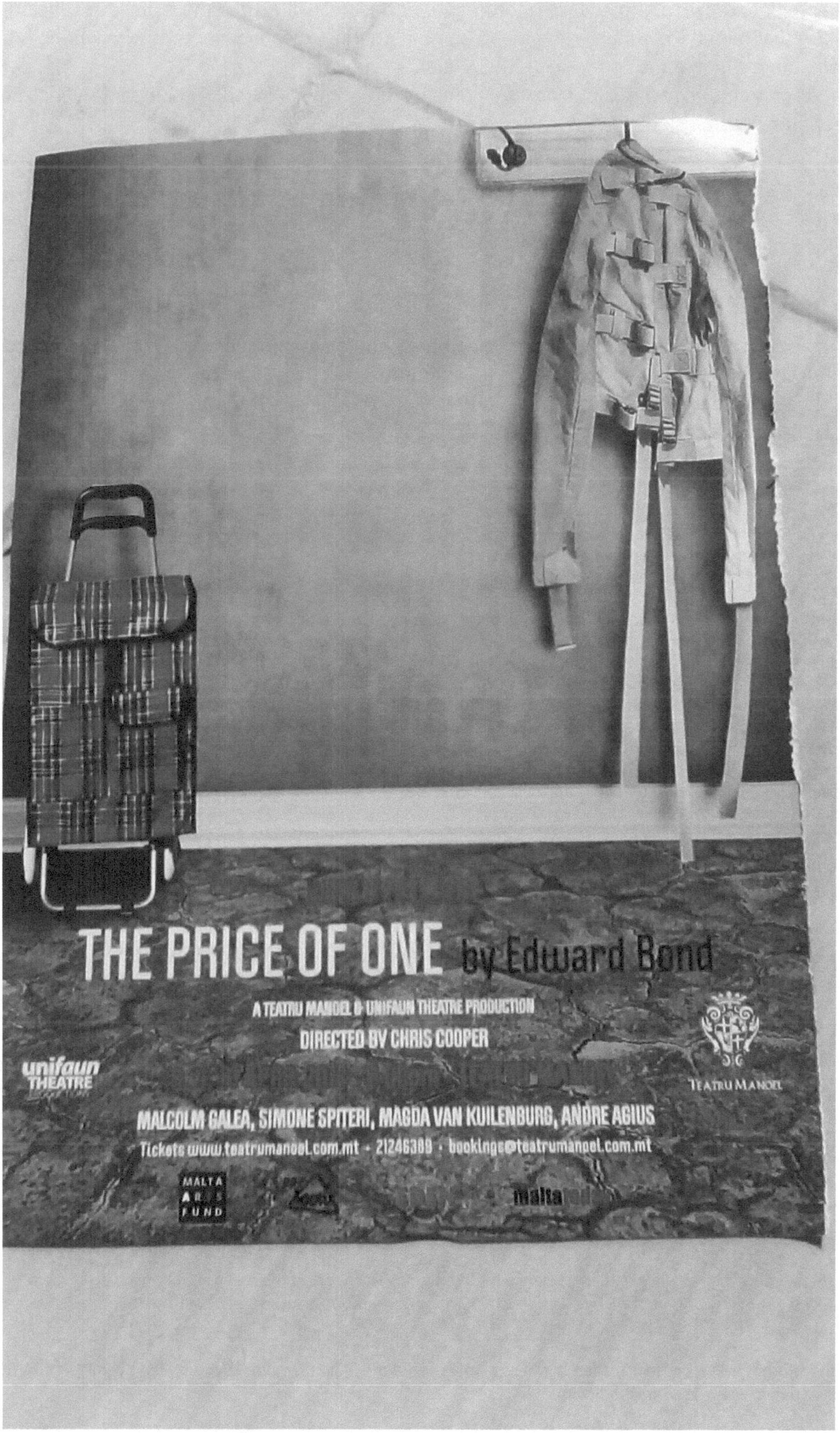
THE PRICE OF ONE by Edward Bond
A TEATRU MANOEL & UNIFAUN THEATRE PRODUCTION
DIRECTED BY CHRIS COOPER
unifaun THEATRE
TEATRU MANOEL
MALCOLM GALEA, SIMONE SPITERI, MAGDA VAN KUILENBURG, ANDRE AGIUS
Tickets www.teatrumanoel.com.mt - 21246389 - bookings@teatrumanoel.com.mt
MALTA ARTS FUND
malta

Some prefer to draw, to sing, to take photographs as their way of expressing themselves, including the feelings that might accompany retirement. Combining these creative methods with writing is fun, and again, more fun in a group (Rogers, 1993/2000).

The risks of boredom and isolation are overcome by replacing paid work with unpaid – yet … Even volunteering carries a risk of shame:

Didn't think there'd be an interview. I looked at the job description and thought: I could do that. It's an entry-level job - that's how I got into the voluntary sector 40 years ago! Now they are shortlisting and interviewing, and it's all unpaid. Imagine if I didn't get it !

Resistance

Certainly, although not the focus of this article, retirement is a gendered story. Leslie, the reluctant retiree (RR) chooses to write a dialogue with an optimistic and cheery part of herself about the differences between her and her happily retired partner, Gordon. She calls this upbeat part of her, "the life begins at 60" or LBA.

The reluctant retiree (RR):
I'm bored.
The Life Begins At 60 retiree (LBA):
Well, go out then – 10,000 steps a day remember.
RR: It's cold and I'd rather listen to the radio, but I can't work this new digital one. Anyway, it'll be dark by 3 and it's half past 2 now.
LBA: You need a time-table – go on – schedule all those Pilates classes, picking up the grandchildren every other day, canvassing for the Green Party, volunteering at the library, walking the dog, University of the Third Age foreign film group, choir, Latin dancing, oil-painting for beginners …
RR: I need a job. I'm bored. When I think of that lot, I'm tired and bored.
LBA: Gordon's not bored. He's out early every day, using his bus pass to get down at the boat yard. He meets his mates, has a brew-up – he's never been so happy. "Should have done it years ago," is what he's saying about retiring. He's always asking you to go with him, help with the cleaning, get together with the other wives.
RR: Why do you think I want to go back to work? Sitting around some freezing cold club room on a damp canal tow-path, talking about cleaning fluids – no thank you. Work was a much better distraction.
LBA: Don't get grumpy. People don't like grumpy.

Even the status and potential cushioning of voluntary responsibilities can't prevent the undermining behaviour experienced from younger people. Leslie says of a nurse: "She is treating me like a little old woman."

Some little old women are happy grandmothers and some are not. Leslie writes:

'Sitting in parks in the drizzle, scraping dog-shit off kids' shoes, boring afternoons when the grandchildren have gone and nobody to talk to except Gordon … this is no life.

The privacy of writing is key. Gordon won't read this. Leslie writes online, password protected, and sometimes even deletes what she's written. Leslie uses writing to resist being poured into the moulds waiting for her to settle into now she's no longer "out at work".

Jane Speedy's very alive, illustrated book about life after a stroke in her late fifties is made up of layers of fragmented poetic text and full-colour images (Speedy, 2015). It is not a stroke memoir; neither is its major focus the leaving of a professional career although changes in working life and identity are central. It's about resistance:

'This is my embodied/visceral/textual resistance to narrative coherence and my means of bringing experience to life … I am giving an account of this life as an act of homage or gratitude. I am so glad that I am not dead. (Speedy, 2015, p. 14)

'Grounded' from her work as an academic, Speedy writes about the fear of certain nurses, shared by the "confused elderly women" she was in hospital with.

Having known these women, however, I now no longer fear old age. (Speedy, 2015, p. 15)

Jane Speedy finds ways of layering visual images, stores, academic words, poetic fragments that build up and expand with the reading.

One way to resist has always been to join with others. The creation of writing groups for those who are thinking of retiring or have finally left the paid job is a rich alternative to one-to-one counselling. Such groups, whether facilitated by therapists, creative writers, neither or both are illustrated by some of the writing by members of Lapidus, an international words for wellbeing association. The organisation publishes a journal, holds conferences and advertises groups and workshops mostly in the UK (www.lapidus.org.uk).

Writing groups

"The process felt both powerful and liberating. Being able to answer as my 'other person' in the dialogue activity was surprising; in fact, the answer was not what I expected at all, even though I wrote it myself. "(Feedback from a UK self-writing group participant).

The setting: The room, a corporate and rather too carpeted space is changed when the coloured paper, pens, pencils, pastels, and music arrives. We are due to spend three hours together and have some materials online and in paper form as support.

Posters around the room say: "Gag the inner critic!" "Spelling and grammar don't matter." "Forget school rules." It is made clear in the "ground-rules" that we are here not to produce works of art, poems or prose to be judged and evaluated. This writing is different and is "for your eyes only until and if you choose to share it."

Tony is one of 16 people in the group. He has been asked to think about a recent experience when he felt a strong emotion, noticing how feelings work in the body. Tony's struggle with writing seems to be freed up:

"If I can't say what's been happening out loud to another human being and I can't write it down what can I do? What do I like doing, they ask.

Dancing.

Lately I haven't been dancing much, but the wedding at the weekend was great. One of the bands was a combination of Irish jigs and reels plus – I couldn't stop myself dancing. It's a tonic to move around to music in a group of other people. I stood watching for a while, too hot to carry on.

What happened to the playful me?"

Tony uses a written dialogue with different parts of himself, as in Matt Haig's writing through depression which a friend has loaned him (Haig, 2015):

DANCER:	you don't do this often enough. The music has a real impact on you, right through your feet to the top of your head – and the dancing even more so. What stops you dancing more?
WORK ETHIC:	it's all right for you. You haven't got bills at the back of your mind all the time, and people pressurising you.
DANCER:	all work and no play ….. anyway, you're going to leave all that behind in another month. Retirement – yay!
ANXIOUS:	I was worried all the way there thinking you wouldn't be able to find your way there to that wedding. And then you had to drive back and I knew you'd get lost.
FROZEN ONE:	Silence
DANCER:	You did get there and you got home okay. And you felt better
ANXIOUS:	Yes, I did – for a while. I was worried you'd feel tired all day after all that dancing though, and you did.

Memoir writing, creative writing classes, retirement and transition writing groups are all part of the same process. They involve writing (and reading) close to life. The Irish writer, Nuala O'Faolin writes in her memoir:

There is an idea current in the prevailing culture that writing about something that pains you heals the pain. I was not, when I began writing my life story, and am not now, healed of my mother. But you do gain a small distance from anything by keeping it in suspension in your mind while you work at finding the words to fit it. The process is so slow and incremental that you don't notice its effect, but the point is that it is a process… (O'Faolain, 2003, p. 36)

Yes, it is a process of, and perhaps it can only be understood by trying it out.

Endings

Not all choose to retire, to end their paid career, or find the decision easy, even if the choice is theirs. Tools from creative writing, and especially writing in groups, eases the isolation and allows emotional expression. Feedback from writing groups includes, "it's like reading my own mind", and, "It seems to be all in, body, mind, spirit."

This article has focused on a transition; the metaphor about the warm bathwater of working life slowly ebbing away might capture the experience for some. Others might resonate more with a feeling of the bath plug being yanked and a cold shower turned on. The grey pound may well be powerful, but life without work is a challenge – even more so if there aren't enough pounds in the pension to cover the cost of living. For others, retirement means enjoying all that work got in the way of, hobbies, family, holidays and all – none the less, this shift represents a transition which can be challenging.

A dilemma with autoethnographic and writing as inquiry intended for publication is how to manage the ethical tensions, but for those who use therapeutic writing for their own private purposes, publication is not the point.

Writing creatively, and particularly in groups, can be a way to connect with self, others and sometimes a wider audience during times of transition. This kind of writing is about imagination and intuition, with rational thinking and intellect taking a back seat, as with most forms of creativity. The tools of creative writing are simple, need no special equipment – and can be adapted for self-help, group work and as an adjunct to the therapeutic relationship. Writing can be "life-support", throughout the life stages (Williamson, 2015).

Disclosure statement

No potential conflict of interest was reported by the author.

References

Adams, T. E., Holman Jones, S., & Ellis, C. (2015). *Autoethnography: Understanding qualitative research*. New York: Oxford University Press.

Angelou, M. (1986). *And still I rise*. London: Virago Press.

Blake, D. (2006). *Pension economics*. London: John Wiley & Sons.

Bolton, G. (2011). *Write yourself: Creative writing and personal development*. London: Jessica Kingsley.

Bolton, G., Field, V., & Thompson, K. (2011). *Writing routes: A resource handbook of therapeutic writing*. London: Jessica Kingsley.

Cixous, H., & Calle-Gruber, M. (1994/1997). *Rootprints: Memory and life writing*. London: Routledge.

Douglas, K., & Carless, D. (Writers). (2016). *Qualitative conversations: Tony E. Adams*. Retrieved from www.Youtube.com

Etherington, K. (2003). *Trauma, the body and transformation*. London: Jessica Kingsley.

Field, V., Bolton, G., & Thompson, K. (2006). *Writing works: A resource handbook for therapeutic writing workshops and activities*. London: Jessica Kingsley.

Haig, M. (2015). *Reasons to stay alive*. Edinburgh: Canongate Books.

Holman Jones, S., Adams, T. E., & Ellis, C. (Eds.). (2013). *Handbook of autoethnography*. Walnut Creek, CA: Left Coast Press.

Josselson, R. (2007). The ethical attitude in narrative research. *Handbook of Narrative Inquiry: Mapping a Methodology*, 537–566. doi:10.4135/9781452226552.n21

Lengelle, R., & Meijers, F. (2014). Narrative identity: Writing the self in career learning. *British Journal of Guidance and Counselling*, *42*(1), 52–72.

O'Faolain, N. (2003). *Almost there: The onward journey of a Dublin woman, a memoir*. New York: Riverhead Books.

Pelias, R. J. (2015). The end of an academic career the desperate attempt to hang on and let go. *Qualitative Inquiry*. 10.1177/1077800415603398 (https://doi.org/10.1177/1077800415603398)

Richardson, L., & St Pierre, E. A. (2005). Writing: A method of inquiry. In N. K. Denzin & Y. S. Lincoln (Eds.), *Handbook of qualitative research* (pp. 959–978). Thousand Oaks, CA: Sage.

Rogers, N. (1993/2000). *The creative connection - expressive arts as healing*. Palo Alto: Science and Behaviour Books/PCCS Books.

Speedy, J. (2015). *Staring at the park: A poetic autoethnographic inquiry*. Walnut Creek, CA: Left Coast Press.

Thompson, K., & Adams, K. (Eds.). (2015). *Expressive writing: Counseling and healthcare*. London: Rowman & Littlefield.

Tullis, J. A. (2013). Self and others: Ethics in autoethnographic research. In S. Holman Jones, T. E. Adams, & C. Ellis (Eds.), *Handbook of autoethnography* (pp. 244–261). Walnut Creek, CA: Left Coast Press.

Williamson, C. (2015). Writing as a way of becoming. *Writing in Education*, *65*(Spring). Retrieved from https://www.google.co.in/url?url=https://www.theatlantic.com/education/archive/2015/12/fear-islam-tennessee-public-schools/420441/&rct=j&frm=1&q=&esrc=s&sa=U&ved=0ahUKEwjEnsuFrevYAhUbSY8KHY0pAa8QFggTMAA&usg=AOvVaw1vnhA8THmic6xH_cwtxk_4

Williamson, C., & Wright, J. K. (In press). How creative does writing have to be in order to be therapeutic? A dialogue on the practice and research of writing to recover and survive. *Journal of Poetry Therapy*.

Wright, J. K. (2003). Writing for protection: Reflective practice as a counsellor. *Journal of Poetry Therapy*, *16*(4), 191–198.

Wright, J. K. (2009). Autoethnography and therapy writing on the move. *Qualitative Inquiry*, *15*(4), 623–640.

Wright, J. K. (2012). Write, read, share, reflect. *Therapy Today*, *23*(9), 22–25.

Wright, J. K., & Bolton, G. (2012). *Reflective writing in counselling and psychotherapy*. London: Sage.

Wyatt, J., & Adams, T. E. (Eds.). (2014). *On (writing) families: Autoethnographies of presence and absence, love and loss*. Rotterdam: Sense.

Enter centre stage, the case study …

Deborah A. Lee

ABSTRACT
This existentially informed person-centred paper argues that current conceptualisations of 'case studies' (beloved of psychotherapy training and beyond) can reduce complex/beautiful human beings to flat/objectified characters defined by 'presenting problems' – 'presenting problems' which clever therapists 'fix'. In response, the paper develops an arts-based approach: a collaborative, respectful/ethical, narrative 'case study', written as a play – a piece of public psychotherapy available for the audience's responses. The play seeks particularly to convey the warmth of encounters between two rounded/unique characters, Deborah and Kate, offering a challenge to the 'us' and 'them' approach of many 'case studies'; it contends that if this is achieved, it is this – rather than narrow/sterile advice about 'assessment', 'formulation' and 'interventions' – which establishes the usefulness of the work.

Prologue

Narrator:
'Prepare to welcome the "case study"!
A fictional/academic/ethnotheatre hybrid!
A narrative approach – person-centred and existentially-informed!
Magical encounters in relational ethics and shared humanity!
A public psychotherapy for the stage!'

*

Playwright's notes: A name in bold means that person is on-stage; more than one audience member is being signified by **AM**; artistic licence has been taken with the cast!

*

Act 1
(The curtain rises.)
McLeod (2010), standing in a spotlight, muses: 'There has been relatively little methodological innovation within the narrative approach … ' (p. 27).
Zeldin (2015) enters, observing: 'Each meeting between two people that is not merely superficial is an opportunity to enlarge [life] beyond the banal, through discovery and invention' (p. 395).
Bourriaud (1998) (introduced with a flourish by **Jones**, 2006, p. 72) takes both their hands and declares: 'Relational art … [is] a set of artistic practices which take as their theoretical and practical point of departure the whole of human relations and their social context' (p. 133).
('Clinical' bright light blinds the audience; it's freezing cold …)
Voice off: 'It's the CASES!'
The 'cases' enter; signs covering their faces.

'I'm borderline'
'I'm depressed'
'I'm anxious'
... 'I'm a healthy control's' sign doesn't obscure his smile.
(The lights soften. The cast list appears on-screen.)
'The "case" – forty-six+ audio-recorded fifty-minute encounters, between Kate Smith (a self-chosen pseudonym) (38, female, heterosexual and in a relationship) (the "client") and Deborah Lee (44, female, heterosexual and in a relationship) ("the psychotherapist-in-training"). In the wings, an experienced/enigmatic female supervisor (her choice of words). All encounters are UK-based'.
'And here, a supporting cast of many (Ayckbourn's, 2002 rule that "economy often equals better art" [p. 13] is cast aside!)'
(The screen displays the following.)
'Assessment of the "presenting problem"? People are "a dynamic flow, continually changing over time" (Cooper, 2015, p.55). Worsley (2006) says of Levinas: "we cannot know others or ourselves for we are creatures of inexhaustible possibility" (p. 213)'.
Ayckbourn (2002) interjects: 'A good DSM is like gold' (p. 157). The only DSM here is the Deputy Stage Manager!
'The intervention? "Dialogical exchange" (Cooper, 2015, p.73).
How was the case study done? It was a collaboration.
The outcome? The relationship is ongoing; Kate's judgement is paramount.'
AM: 'She's ... HUMANISED the case! She doesn't know how to do assessment and formulation! Where's she studying?'
Two cognitive-behavioural therapy (CBT) therapists, **Shorey and Stuart** (2012) read from their assessment/formulation: "Henry" was a 26-year old, single, non-Hispanic Caucasian male who was self-referred ... for possible treatment for symptoms related with anxiety. Henry lived alone, was employed part-time as a cashier at a local retail company and was also a full-time student .... Henry's presenting diagnosis was SAD ["social anxiety disorder"]. The therapist was a 2nd year male undergraduate student in clinical psychology supervised by a licensed clinical psychologist' (p. 36).
Shorey and Stuart (2012) add: 'He reported living alone ... ' (p. 37).
AM: 'We heard you the first time'.
Shorey and Stuart (2012) continue, after treatment: 'he was currently engaged to be married' (p. 44).
AMs: 'Didn't you do well!'
The therapists smile.
Cooper (2003) shakes his head: 'It-ification' (p. 134).
Friedberg, Tabbarah, and Poggesi (2013) object, declaring 'presence' ('a way of being' which 'enables authentic connection' [Tannen and Daniels, 2010, p. 1]) important in CBT: when 'therapists add presence, immediacy and transparency ... increased patient involvement and therapeutic momentum is likely to be realised' (p. 2).
AM: 'Feels like a technique'.
Person-centred therapists, **Stephen, Elliott, and MacLeod** (2011) share 'their' social anxiety case. 'Lucy ... was 40 years old. ... A Scottish female, living alone, Lucy was employed in a professional role ... The therapist assigned to work with Lucy was trained as a psychologist and a PCT psychotherapist, with 12 years' post-training experience' (pp. 57–58). After therapy, 'she had developed a lasting relationship'! (Stephen et al., 2011, p. 60).
(Confetti rains down.)
AM: 'Was Lucy white? How old was the psychologist?'
A voice off muses: '"presence" was probably there in the *encounter* with *"Lucy"*, but it feels like the "clinical case study's" structure jars with person-centredness?'
'Yes!' says **Madison** (2010): 'The pathology-centred form of encounter gives rise within psychotherapeutic literature to medical attitudes expressed in adjectives such as "clinical". [Then] the therapist

takes an objective quasi-physician role in order to deliver the experimentally derived intervention' (p. 194).

Deurzen (2010) tweets: 'existential therapy does not consider anxiety to be evidence of pathology, but rather an essential reminder of our vibrant and dangerous aliveness' (p. 238).

AM: 'McLeod (2010) says "it is the most troubling, embarrassing or shameful aspects of [a client's] life that are being most closely scrutinised [in a case study]" (p. 54), so maybe there's better to come ... '

MacLeod and Elliott (2014) muse that the 'skeptic' stance of their hermeneutic single-case efficacy design (HSCED) studies ... may be problematic '[because] the client may access and read public accounts of their experience' (p. 308).

McLeod (2010) concurs, clients 'may discover what their therapist really thought about them' (p. 55).

(Offstage, women laugh.)

A psychodynamic therapist, **Jacobson** (2000) introduces the 'case' of 'Pierre': '[My supervisor said] "I should let him leave if he needed to, since two years is about as long as these kinds of borderlines remain in treatment"' (p. 4).

Geller and Greenberg (2012) assert that psychodynamic therapy 'emphasise[s] the importance of creating a lively, genuine relationship with the patient' (p. 20) to effect change.

AM: 'The "genuine relationship" sounds good ... But "these" borderlines? Are we seeing how the "clinical case study" can objectify? Is this ethical? Does it prize diversity? Is this what psychotherapists-in-training need to hear?'

Leavy (2015) says that arts-based research (ABR) work (like this) can 'jar people into seeing and thinking differently' (p. 25).

(It starts warming up.)

Narrator:

'We've started to see "case studies" questioned, with regard to diversity (or "intersectionality" [Collins and Bilge (2016)] explain that "power relations are to be analysed both via their intersections ... as well as across domains of power, namely structural, disciplinary, cultural and interpersonal" (p.27) and "relational ethics" ("a co-constructed ethical and moral encounter, with associated relationship experiences and processes, that both influences and in turn is influenced by the complex multidimensional context in which the relationship occurs" [Gabriel & Casemore, 2009, p. 1]), so let's take a closer look at "case studies".

McLeod (2010) identifies five 'genres' (p. 17): (i) 'single subject studies ... an observable and measurable target behaviour would be identified, and the frequency of this behaviour would be monitored' (McLeod, 2010, p. 19); (ii) 'theory building case studies' (McLeod, 2010, p. 21); (iii) 'pragmatic case studies [in which] the practitioner is required to collect as much information as he or she can on a case' (McLeod, 2010, p. 24); (iv) 'HSCED studies ... [which ask] is this a good outcome case? Can the outcome be attributable to therapy?' (McLeod, 2010, p. 26); and (v) 'narrative case studies ... [which look at] what the therapy was like' (McLeod, 2010, p. 27). In addition, there have been 'autobiographical and fictional narrative case studies' (McLeod, 2010, p. 203), which haven't been received with great interest (McLeod, 2010, p. 204).

'Single subject studies' raise questions in viewing a case 'as if it were an experiment' (McLeod, 2010, p. 20); 'theory building case studies' challenge therapists who fear questioning 'conceptual edifices' (McLeod, 2010, p. 23); 'pragmatic case studies' imply that there are 'different types of client' (McLeod, 2010, p. 25) when Worsley (2006) draws on Levinas to talk of people as 'infinite' (p. 218); and the 'judicial framework' (McLeod, 2010, p. 26) of HSCED studies makes the client 'a key witness' (MacLeod & Elliott, 2014, p. 296) rather than the judge. Of the 'narrative approach', McLeod (2010) says 'much more needs to be done, in terms of method development ... ' (p. 206) or work may be unpublishable. As we saw just now, 'case studies' can reduce clients to first names, their identities encapsulated selectively – and meaninglessly. That 'Lucy' is '40' (Stephen et al., 2011, p. 60) signifies nothing in the text. People become 'presenting problem(s)' which clever therapists (identified by their experience) 'fix' – preparing them for (more) social control. For is a 'lasting relationship' (Stephen et al., 2011, p. 60) really the pinnacle of therapeutic success? Are we hearing a distasteful suggestion that 'Lucy' was gathering dust? Samuels (2015) talks of psychotherapy's 'fairly bad record' (p. 9) in relation to 'diversity'.

McLeod (2010) explains that: 'there has been little work on case study ethics' (p. 58). Therapists' decisions must not just be about 'ethical procedures' advises McLeod (2010, p. 71) but about 'moment-by-moment ethical decision making'. Carroll & Shaw's (2013) conceptualisation of 'ethical maturity' (p. 137) – to be able to make/implement 'good or better' decisions, to take responsibility for them, and to learn/grow from them – involves 'relational ethics': 'with such importance on human relationships for life, development, growth and happiness, is it any wonder that a relational ethics should find its way into the heart of ethical maturity?' (Carroll and Shaw, 2013, p. 103).

The narrative/ABR approach offers a relationally-ethical approach which respects complexity. Leavy (2015) defines ABR as 'an engaged, moral, and at times political activity' (p. 29). Leavy (2015) contends that public ABR can generate 'empathy' and 'self-reflection' (p. 2). Willis, Bondi, Burgess, Miller, and Fergusson (2014) says that this sort of approach is now 'attracting increasing attention in the field of counselling and psychotherapy' (p. 526), citing Meekums' (2011) special issue of the *British Journal of Guidance and Counselling* as one example. Speaking of ethnotheatre, Saldana (1999) explains that only editing which 'will not affect the integrity of the voice or quality of the data' (p. 63) is permitted. This is what Deborah has done here. Such work calls for 'new and more ambiguous [evaluation] criteria' (Gergen and Gergen, 2011, p. 8). Leavy (2015) declares that 'usefulness' (p. 27) is highly important.

Deborah is committed to the British Association of Counselling and Psychotherapy's (BACP's) (2016) ethical principles: being 'trustworthy', '[respecting] the client's right to be self-governing', 'promoting the client's wellbeing', 'avoiding harm to the client', being 'fair' and self-caring (p. 2). There was 'no inducement or pressure' (McLeod, 2010, p. 64) for Kate to participate (informed consent for the work went through two negotiated iterative informed consent forms). The 'ongoing' (Abrahams, 2007, p. 241) nature of Kate's consent was recognised.

Bond (2013) refers to an 'ethically mature' research as involving 'discussion with clients' (p. 339), but he doesn't suggest collaborating. MacLeod and Elliott (2014) refer to a client undergoing a 'battery of quantitative measures' (p. 296), which sounds like an imposition. Here, Deborah and Kate spent time dialoguing about their relationship (prior to, or after therapy sessions). For one dialogue, 'helpful/unhelpful' events (Elliott 1986, p. 307) was used. All dialogues were audio-recorded (McLeod, 2010, p. 69), with consent; material selectively quoted was transcribed, and approved by Kate. Kate approved the final version of the work.

As the focus is upon process, personal material was kept minimal. While 'intersectionality' demonstrates 'complexity', revealing all of anyone's identity jars with ethics: instead, Kate chose how she wished to be described, and Deborah mirrored her choices. There are some personal identity similarities evident in these descriptions (above) but clearly Deborah and Kate are different (Lago & Christodoulidi, 2013, p. 116), and the social structures in which they are located matter even if they are not explored here in order to be respectful of ethics.

Deborah feels this approach is consistent with her therapy room encounters. Adame and Leitner (2011) point out that Buber's meaning of 'dialogue' is 'literal spoken conversation but also how our choices and actions in life are a way of dialoguing or being-in-the-world' (p. 44). She follows Yalom (2002), seeing client/therapist as 'fellow travellers' (p. 8).

Kate is a current, not ex-client (in comparison with Etherington, 2000). This means that issues arising may be processed in the relationship'.

Voice off: 'We know that clients can defer to therapists, how do we know that Kate didn't defer to Deborah in this study?'

(The screen displays messages from the enigmatic supervisor.)

(Before the research) 'Kate is a unique client. I believe she will benefit a lot from a deep reflective process and she will equally be able to decline things she does not want to do'.

(During the research): 'I listened to the research dialogue and noticed that while Deborah was in the role of researcher as well as being Kate's therapist, Kate remains Kate as she is in a therapy session; and Deborah had no difficulty in resuming only the therapist role afterwards'.
(After the research): 'While doing research will take a client in a direction that they aren't going in spontaneously, you'll see something therapeutically interesting come out of this collaboration!'
Deborah: 'There's, of course, a power dynamic here, in that I need to quote my supervisor's support of my decisions ... But I also trusted my internal supervisor!'

*

Act 2
Noises off: POLICE SIRENS, CAR DOORS SLAMMING, PEOPLE SHOUTING (but no-one blinks an eyelid). A clock appears on the screen, and time passes very quickly.
(Two women appear in a soothing cream light.)
Deborah: (a professional statement, addressed to **Kate**).
'Until recently, I saw myself as a 'classical-client centred' (CCT) psychotherapist-in-training.
I like CCT's political nature: Rogers (1978) talks of challenging inequalities (p. 273). I've also always liked 'the model's elegant economy' (Barrett-Lennard, 1998, p. 104). It emphasises, as I do, the relationship (Merry, 2012, p. 21). I concur with Geller and Greenberg (2002) that 'presence' (being 'fully there' [Schmid & Mearns, 2006, p. 176]) is 'the foundation of ... empathy, congruence and unconditional positive regard' (p. 83).
I believe that being 'genuine', 'the more helpful [the relationship] will be' (Rogers, 1961, p. 33), and 'the more acceptance and liking I feel towards [an] individual, the more I will be creating a relationship which [she] can use' (Rogers, 1961, p. 34); and I feel 'a sensitive empathy with each of the client's feelings and communications' (Rogers, 1961, p. 34). Like Rogers (1961, p. 35), I believe in people's tendency to actualise. Like Franke, Rachlin, and Yip-Bannicq (2012), I notice that 'nondirective therapy' 'directs' (p. 205).
I agree with the CCT 'rejection of diagnostic assessment and labelling' (Merry, 2012, p. 21); and I am increasingly confused by a perceived mismatch between this and Rogers' (1961) ideas of 'psychological maladjustment' (p. 37).
This has led me towards existentially-informed person-centred therapy. Above, Deurzen (2010) (a prolific tweeter) said: 'existential therapy does not consider anxiety to be evidence of pathology, but rather an essential reminder of our vibrant and dangerous aliveness' (p. 238). I agree.
I'm increasingly questioning 'certainties', so with any approach to therapy I'm aware how: 'the theory's "gaze" ... both opens up and reflects realities and closes down and deflects realities' (Goodman, 2016, p. 81). The most exciting work I read recently is Madison (2010), explaining an experiential-existential model. Madison (2010) says: 'the body, rather than an inert object, is an experiential process interacting with and responding to its environment' (p. 192). As such, 'therapists offer invitations to the client to stay with what is felt but not being paid attention to' (Madison, 2010, p. 196). This speaks to me'.
Kate (who is the only one qualified to assess the impact of Deborah's therapeutic responses): 'I've felt quite open to the way that you work, and kind of trust the way that you have worked with me, for it to work ... '
(Then ... we go back in time ...)
'Phase A: the beginning phase' (Barrett-Lennard, 1998, p. 106)
Deborah (wrote notes after listening again to session 2, and Kate read them): 'I heard a lot of the processes [or interventions] that are still present. (They came naturally "embedded within a fluid, dialogical exchange" [Cooper, 2015, p. 73] rather than being "intents"): "active listening", (Cooper, 2015, p. 76) "if a therapist comes in too quickly ... it may interrupt clients from connecting at [a deep] level"; "minimal encouragers" (Cooper, 2015, p. 76), "brief interjections that let clients know that they are being listening to, received and understood"; "reflecting, paraphrasing and summarising" (Cooper, 2015, p. 76) which show clients that "their experiences are intelligible" (Cooper, 2015, p. 77); and "asking open-ended questions" (Cooper, 2015, p. 78)'.

Deborah: ' … you were sharing a lot with me (some types of therapists might have "asked for" what you said, to do an "assessment" … my intention was not to "ask for" anything, only to receive whatever you wanted to say – your "assessment", in fact, of whether you wished to share with me) … '
Kate: 'I've always felt very comfortable with you'.
Sexton, Littauer, Sexton, and Tommeras (2005) comment: 'the early client-therapist connection was largely established in the first session. The level of the client-therapist connection was quite stable from the first to the second session' (p. 112).
Deborah: 'At 8.16 minutes into the session, you say (rather profoundly) that: "now is all we have" and observe that might sound "a bit poncey". You then tell me, laughingly, that "you're shaking your head", I say: "it's not poncey!", and you agree. It felt like there was already a connection developing between us'.
Barrett-Lennard (1998) observes that at the end of the 'beginning phase', there's a move from 'monologue to duologue … communicating with a person now felt and coming into view as a distinctive other person' (p. 107).

The middle

Deborah: 'Something that stood out for you [in our relationship] later? I know what mine is [laughing]'.
Kate: 'You tell me what yours was [laughs]'. (**Deborah**: 'ok')
Deborah: 'There's a bit of self-disclosure in it, I hope that's going to be ok, and we can talk about it afterwards. I nearly didn't train for psychotherapy in case people brought a certain thing and there was a day when you did bring that thing and the relational depth [explored below] took over and I facilitated you saying more about the thing I probably didn't want to hear about and I think you cured me'.
Kate: [pause] 'Oh gosh. (**Deborah:** 'yes') I don't know what to say. (**Deborah:** 'mmm') Oh, I might cry. I feel quite emotional hearing that'.
Barrett-Lennard (1998) says: 'personal realness and transparency works to disarm and evoke trust in the other' (p. 113).
Deborah: 'Rapport/alliance building, assessment, interventions – they're ongoing processes. New patterns emerge from relating'.
'Phase D … clients now experience new levels of personal change' (Barrett-Lennard, 1998, p. 117).
Kate: 'There's been a lot of reflection on how some of the processes in me are changing, particularly this [deleted] element. And I remember when I first started coming to see you, that I couldn't put my finger on what I was missing (**Deborah:** 'mm'), it was almost like grasping at candy floss, or ether, and it's become clearer, it's become clearer what it was that was missing, and then what's happened is that I feel the [deleted] now, I'm more connected with it'.
Barrett-Lennard (1998) observes, 'a helping relationship does not literally produce change but works by releasing or nourishing inbuilt recuperative and actualising tendencies' (p. 89).
Edgar (2009) observes that 'clocks' are a regular theatrical 'device', (p. 156) but here, time seems to be passing at the speed of light!

*

Act 3

Noises off: POLICE SIRENS, CAR DOORS SLAMMING, PEOPLE SHOUTING (but no-one blinks an eyelid). A clock appears on the screen, and time passes very quickly.

Narrator:

'Let's now fully unpack the meaning of the clocks and the noises off.
Geller and Greenberg (2002) define 'presence', as: 'the ultimate state of moment-by-moment receptivity and deep relational contact' (p. 85).
In Geller and Greenberg's (2002) work, 'therapists [from a variety of modalities] described actively clearing a space [for presence]' (p. 77). In 'presence', therapists felt 'flow, energy and calm' (Geller and Greenberg, 2002, p. 80); 'time and spatial boundaries seem[ed] to drop away' (Geller and Greenberg, 2002, p. 81).

'[Presence] involves being with the client rather than doing to the client' (Geller and Greenberg, 2002, p. 85); this raises questions about whether 'presence' is really present in some of the modalities now explored.

Geller and Greenberg (2012) say that: Freud referred to 'receptivity, and described it as emerging from an impartial, non-judgemental, evenly applied attention' (p. 18); it was not communicated to the analysand. As we saw earlier, current psychodynamic work uses the relationship instrumentally. Gauna, Roibal, Ruiz, Fernandez, and Bleichmar (2015) talk of 'moments of high receptiveness' in clients, when therapists can 'produce change' (p. 65).

CBT now also values how relationship affects outcomes (Geller & Greenberg, 2012, p. 34) (see Friedberg et al. [2013, p. 2] above). But Geller, Greenberg, and Watson (2010) compared 'presence' in CBT, process-experiential and process-experiential/client-centred therapists; CBT therapists scored lowest (p. 607).

'Presence', in existential theory, 'helps people confront, accept and tolerate ... the inevitability of the conditions of living' (Tannen & Daniels, 2010, p. 2). For Yalom and Bugental, 'the cultivation of presence' (Krug, 2009, p. 330) 'goes beyond, experiences or moments of deep connection with self and other' encompassing also 'that each person's past is present in the here-and-now' (Krug, 2009, p. 331). Therapy then involves 'connection' and recognition of 'how specific behaviours and attitudes block [a client] from these deeper connections' (Krug, 2009, p. 331).

In person-centred therapy, Schmid and Mearns (2006) say that: 'we are looking for a deeper sense of meeting than simply a working alliance' (p. 178). For Focusing-oriented therapists, 'presence of the therapist is central to clients who are learning to listen to their own emotional experience' (Geller & Greenberg, 2012, pp. 29–30). Geller and Greenberg (2012) note that: 'even though humanistic therapists espouse the value of presence, they have not clarified how to be fully present' (p. 34).

Geller (2013) feels that therapist 'presence'/inviting client 'presence' 'can allow for moments of relational depth' (p. 175). Variations of 'relational depth' occur across modalities (Wiggins, Elliott, & Cooper, 2012, p. 140). Mearns and Cooper (2005), person-centred therapists, define 'relational depth' as 'a feeling of profound contact and engagement with a client' (p. 1); it is 'fundamentally dyadic' (Mearns & Cooper, 2005, p. 113); it can be 'moments' or 'enduring experiences' (Mearns & Cooper, 2005, p. 1)'.

Kate: (to whom Deborah had previously said she didn't notice time passing in their meetings, and who had just read some notes about 'relational depth' written by Deborah) 'So, it's a "thing"!' [**Deborah:** 'mmm!'] [both laugh].

Narrator:

'Wiggins et al. (2012) contend that there being a "timeless atmosphere" seemed to be about "moments" only (p. 150)'.

Deborah: 'The reason I put bold around "enduring" (in the notes), is because that's the one they don't write about as much, but that is what I feel here, it's not every now and again, to me, it feels enduring. I don't know how it is for you?'

Kate: 'I'm not aware of what's happening outside, not aware of anything else'.

Narrator:

'Knox and Cooper (2011) say that their interviewees compared experiencing relational depth with not experiencing it with previous therapists (p. 68)'.

Kate: 'Whereas all the other times [of having person-centred therapy], yes I've connected with people on a level, and, you know, I've got a lot from it, it's not been the same connection, I don't think, as it has been with us'.

Narrator:

'When relational depth didn't happen for clients: "a recurring theme was the unwillingness of the client to 'let go'" (McMillan & McLeod, 2006, p. 288)'.

Deborah: 'I wrote that (on the materials Kate read) because there were a few sessions where you said you were censoring ... I was thinking [pauses] perhaps this [what has been written before] isn't quite

right, that you *can* still be censoring and still have relational depth, there can still be some things that you're thinking how you can say it for your own ... '
Kate: ' ... safety, yes'.
Deborah: 'Yes, and it doesn't mean you can't have connection. They might have missed something'.
Kate: ' ... when I've been holding things back, it's not been because I don't t-rust you, it's maybe because I don't trust myself with it, what those feelings mean and then get carried away with it, and open Pandora's box. ... But, that doesn't mean to say that I'm not engaged'.
Bazzano (2014) observes of ideas of clients not 'letting go' that: 'the therapist's frustration can be a great teacher' (p. 210).
Narrator:
(She throws her script aside): 'Deborah and Kate, I find your interpretation more interesting!'
Kate: ' ... that's a whole other paper!'
Deborah: 'It is!' [both laughing].
Narrator:
'Bazzano (2014) introduces the term "togetherness", referring to "aloneness, autonomy and conflict alongside relatedness and interdependence"' (p. 205).
(Off-script again; she's building up her part.) 'That doesn't jettison relational depth, and it offers the existentially-informed approach that you're developing, Deborah'.
AM: 'Doesn't time fly?'

*

Epilogue
Narrator:
'When Deborah and Kate reflected upon their research dialogues, something interesting happened ... '
Deborah: 'We've been doing what we do, but before [this process], we hadn't sort of done a review of how we are doing it, to me it feels a very helpful thing to know more about how you feel about it'.
Kate: 'Yes, definitely. I've had quite a lot of counselling and stuff and I've not had that kind of dialogue'.
Deborah: 'Would you like for us to reflect on being together more often?'
Kate: 'Yes, maybe, yes, I think that would be good'.
Deborah: 'How would you like that to be initiated?'
Kate: 'Shall we do it every month. Does that sound ok?'
Narrator:
'Bond (2013) distinguishes between therapy/research, contending that research "is primarily for the benefit of people other than the patient" (p. 338). As has just been shown, that need not necessarily be so.
This outcome suggests a pluralistic framework. Cooper and McLeod (2007) explain that it: 'maintains that the client's view on what is helpful and not helpful in therapy is as valid as the therapist's' (p. 139). This development is available to Deborah and Kate because of Deborah's personal work on 'certainties' – previously she would have been too 'classical client-centred' for 'reviews'!'
Deborah:
'I've written this case study in a way that might not have been expected, as a piece of ABR in which Kate and I collaborated.
Leavy (2015) explains that evaluation of ABR provokes 'much debate' (p. 266), with people considering if it should be assessed like qualitative work, or if something different is needed.
Leavy (2015, p. 267) is opposed to a 'gold standard' of evaluation for ABR, for she judges assessment of ABR to be 'a messy terrain' (Leavy, 2015, p. 268).
Nevertheless, Leavy (2015, p. 266) says that 'there is no question that we need ways to evaluate this work'. Evaluation methods may reflect researchers' locations in the sciences/arts (Leavy, 2015, p. 267–8) and are outlined in Leavy (2015, pp. 266–289).

Earlier, McLeod's (2010, p. 203) misgivings about 'autobiographical and fictional narrative case studies' were cited. Those preferring more usual 'case studies' may be challenged by the collaborative approach and the ABR here. But, as Leavy (2015, p. 285) observes: 'no research product can be all things to all people'.

Taking Leavy's (2015, p. 267) advice that any 'individual criteria' for evaluation need to be applied 'as appropriate to a specific project', I follow Leavy (2015, p. 273) in being particularly drawn to the concept of 'usefulness' as a means of evaluating this present work.

I perceive (as explained above) that psychotherapy 'case studies' usually tend to define people attending by their 'problems' and psychotherapists by their training/experience, and that this creates flat/objectified characters, an 'us' and 'them' situation of deep inequality – in which some people are deficient and others 'fix' them - rather than revealing complex human beings who have more in common than might be supposed. Such writings create a sterility to psychotherapy which does not resonate with me, and a situation in which I feel 'ethical practice' (Leavy, 2015, p. 280) is compromised.

In contrast, in collaborating with Kate to explore our sessions together and drawing on that material here, I hope the warmth of the encounter between us two 'multi-dimensional' (Leavy, 2015, p. 281) human beings has been shown. In editing this work for publication, I have repeatedly agreed with Meekums (2011) that ABR provokes 'emotional/embodied reactions' (p. 382): I have felt/feel deep honour and pleasure that I meet with Kate. And if I have been able to convey at least some of the warmth of the relationship and its relating then this is primarily, for me, how this work should be evaluated – a 'usefulness' (Leavy, 2015, p. 272) which I would also hope might influence ethical principles in psychotherapy 'case study' research (see Leavy's [2015, p. 274] comments on influencing policy) – for I feel that psychotherapists need to take all opportunities available to stop seeing 'clients' as 'other', including in writing; I believe that ABR has enabled me to start to develop this 'research goal' (Leavy, 2015, p. 273).

Bourriaud (1998) says art has a 'co-existence criterion … does this work permit me to enter into dialogue?' (p. 1089). Bringing many voices on-stage, I sought/seek to encourage the voices of you, the audience, maybe particularly those of you who are in psychotherapy training or delivering it. Might you conceive of 'case studies' differently through this arts-based research?'

(The curtain falls.)

Acknowledgements

The author would like to thank Glenda Melville, Deanne Gardner, Ambika Erin Connelly, Michelle J. Cooke, Michelle Oldale, Suzanne Keys, Jason Wood, and, of course, Kate Smith. The author would also like to thank the Editors – Frans Meijers, Reinekke Lengelle, Deirdre Hughes, Liane Hambly, and the two anonymous reviewers.

Disclosure statement

No potential conflict of interest was reported by the author.

Funding

This work was approved by the Sherwood Psychotherapy Training Institute (SPTI).

ORCID

Deborah A. Lee http://orcid.org/0000-0001-9971-3542

References

Abrahams, H. (2007). Ethics in counselling research fieldwork. *Counselling and Psychotherapy Research, 7*(4), 240–244. doi:10.1080/14733140701707068

Adame, A., & Leitner, M. (2011). Dialogical constructivism: Martin Buber's enduring relevance to psychotherapy. *Journal of Humanistic Psychology, 51*(1), 41–60. doi:10.1177/0022167810379959

Ayckbourn, A. (2002). *The crafty art of playmaking*. London: Faber & Faber.

Barrett-Lennard, G. (1998). *Carl Rogers' helping system. Journey and substance*. London: Sage.

Bazzano, M. (2014). Togetherness: Intersubjectivity revisited. *Person-Centred & Experiential Psychotherapies, 13*(3), 203–216. doi:10.1080/14779757.2013.852613

Bond, T. (2013). The ethics of research. In M. Carroll, & E. Shaw (Eds.), *Ethical maturity in the helping professions* (pp. 329–349). London: Jessica Kingsley.

Bourriaud, N. (1998). *Relational aesthetics*. Dijon: Les presses du reel.

British Association for Counselling and Psychotherapy (BACP). (2016). *Ethical framework for the counselling professions*. [Online]. Retrieved from http://www.bacp.co.uk/ethics/EFfCP.php.

Carroll, M., & Shaw, E. (2013). *Ethical maturity in the helping professions*. London: Jessica Kingsley.

Collins, P. H., & Bilge, S. (2016). *Intersectionality*. Cambridge: Polity.

Cooper, M. (2003). "I-I" and "I-Me": Transposing Buber's interpersonal attitudes to the intrapersonal plane. *Journal of Constructivist Psychology, 16*, 132–153. doi:10.1080/10720530390117911

Cooper, M. (2015). *Existential psychotherapy and counselling: Contributions to a pluralistic practice*. London: Sage.

Cooper, M., & McLeod, J. (2007). A pluralistic framework for counselling and psychotherapy. *Counselling and Psychotherapy Research, 7*(3), 135–143. doi:10.1080/14733140701566282

Deurzen, E. V. (2010). *Everyday mysteries*. London: Routledge.

Edgar, D. (2009). *How plays work*. London: Nick Hern Books.

Elliott, R. (1986). Helpful and non-helpful events in brief counselling interviews: An empirical taxonomy. *Journal of Counselling Psychology, 32*(3), 307–322.

Etherington, K. (2000). *Narrative approaches to working with adult male survivors of child sexual abuse*. London: Jessica Kingsley.

Franke, M., Rachlin, H., & Yip-Bannicq, M. (2012). How nondirective therapy directs: The power of empathy in the context of unconditional positive regard. *Person-Centred & Experiential Psychotherapies, 11*(3), 205–214. doi:10.1080/14779757.2012.695292

Friedberg, R., Tabbarah, S., & Poggesi, R. (2013). Therapeutic presence, immediacy and transparency in CBT and youth: Carpe the moment! *The Cognitive Behaviour Therapist*, 6(12), 1–10. doi:10.1017/S1754470X13000159

Gabriel, L., & Casemore, R. (2009). Introduction. In L. Gabriel, & R. Casemore (Eds.), *Relational ethics in practice* (pp. 1–8). London: Routledge.

Gauna, M., Roibal, M., Ruiz, J., Fernandez, J., & Bleichmar, H. (2015). Active change in psychodynamic therapy: Moments of high receptiveness. *American Journal of Psychotherapy, 69*(1), 65–86.

Geller, S. (2013). Therapeutic presence as a foundation for relational depth. In R. Knox, D. Murphy, S. Wiggins, & M. Cooper (Eds.), *Relational depth* (pp. 175–184). Basingstoke: Macmillan.

Geller, S., & Greenberg, L. (2002). Therapeutic presence: Therapists' experience of presence in the psychotherapy encounter. *Person-Centred & Experiential Psychotherapies, 1*(1-2), 71–86. doi:10.1080/14779757.2002.9688279

Geller, S., & Greenberg, L. (2012). *Therapeutic presence*. Washington, DC: American Psychological Association.

Geller, S., Greenberg, L., & Watson, J. (2010). Therapist and client perceptions of therapeutic presence: The development of a measure. *Psychotherapy Research, 20*(5), 599–610. doi:10.1080/10503307.2010.495957

Gergen, M., & Gergen, K. (2011). Performative social science and psychology. *Forum: Qualitative Social Research, 12*(1), 1–11.

Goodman, D. (2016). The McDonaldization of psychotherapy: Processed foods, processed therapies and economic class. *Theory and Psychology, 26*(1), 77–95. doi:10.1177/0959354315619708

Jacobson, G. (2000). Case presentation – A perfect transference. *Psychoanalytic Social Work, 7*(3), 3–18. doi:10.1300/J032v07n03_02

Jones, K. (2006). A biographic researcher in pursuit of an aesthetic: The use of arts-based representations in "performative" dissemination of life stories. *Qualitative Sociology Review, 11*(1), 66–85.

Knox, R., & Cooper, M. (2011). A state of readiness: An exploration of the client's role in meeting at relational depth. *Journal of Humanistic Psychology, 51*(1), 61–81. doi:10.1177/0022167810361687

Krug, O. (2009). James Bugental and Irvin Yalom: Two masters of existential therapy cultivate presence in the therapeutic encounter. *Journal of Humanistic Psychology, 49*(3), 329–354. doi:10.1177/0022167809334001

Lago, C., & Christodoulidi, F. (2013). Client-therapist diversity: Aspiring towards relational depth. In R. Knox, D. Murphy, S. Wiggins, & M. Cooper (Eds.), *Relational depth* (pp. 114–124). Basingstoke: Macmillan.

Leavy, P. (2015). *Method meets art: Arts-based research practice.* New York, NY: Guildford Press.

Macleod, R., & Elliott, R. (2014). Non-directive person-centred therapy for social anxiety: A hermeneutic single-case efficacy design study of a good outcome case. *Person-Centred & Experiential Psychotherapies, 13*(4), 294–311. doi:10.1080/14733145.2011.546203

Madison, G. (2010). Focusing on existence: Five facets of an experiential-existential model. *Person-Centred & Experiential Psychotherapies, 9*(3), 189–204.

McLeod, J. (2010). *Case study research.* London: Sage.

McMillan, M., & McLeod, J. (2006). Letting go: The client's experience of relational depth. *Person-Centred & Experiential Psychotherapies, 5*(4), 277–292. doi:10.1080/14779757.2006.9688419

Mearns, D., & Cooper, M. (2005). *Working at relational depth in counselling and psychotherapy.* London: Sage.

Meekums, B. (2011). Editorial. *British Journal of Guidance and Counselling, 39*(5), 379–384. doi:10.1080/03069885.2011.617146

Merry, T. (2012). Classical client-centred therapy. In P. Sanders (Eds.), *The tribes of the person-centred nation* (pp. 21–46). Ross-on-Wye: PCCS Books.

Rogers, C. (1961). *On becoming a person.* London: Constable.

Rogers, C. (1978). *Personal power.* London: Constable.

Saldana, J. (1999). Playwriting with data: Ethnographic performance texts. *Youth Theatre Journal, 13*(1), 60–71. doi:10.1080/08929092.1999.10012508

Samuels, A. (2015). *A New therapy for politics?* London: Karnac.

Schmid, P., & Mearns, D. (2006). Being-with and being-counter: Person-centred psychotherapy as an in-depth co-creative process of personalisation. *Person-Centred & Experiential Psychotherapies, 5*(3), 174–190.

Sexton, H., Littauer, H., Sexton, A., & Tommeras, E. (2005). Building an alliance: Early therapy processes and the client-therapist connection. *Psychotherapy Research, 15*(1-2), 103–116.

Shorey, R., & Stuart, G. (2012). Manualised cognitive-behavioural treatment of social anxiety disorder: A case study. *Clinical Case Studies, 11*(1), 35–47. doi:10.1177/1534650112438462

Stephen, S., Elliott, R., & Macleod, R. (2011). Person-centred therapy with a client experiencing social anxiety difficulties: A hermeneutic single case efficacy design. *Counselling and Psychotherapy Research, 11*(1), 55–66. doi:10.1080/14733145.2011.546203

Tannen, T., & Daniels, M. H. (2010). Counsellor presence: Bridging the gap between wisdom and new knowledge. *British Journal of Guidance and Counselling, 38*(1), 1–15. doi:10.1080/03069880903408661

Wiggins, S., Elliott, R., & Cooper, M. (2012). The prevalence and characteristics of relational depth events in psychotherapy. *Psychotherapy Research, 22*(2), 139–158. doi:10.1080/10503307.2011.629635

Willis, A., Bondi, L., Burgess, M. C., Miller, G., & Fergusson, D. (2014). Engaging with a history of counselling, spirituality and faith in Scotland: A readers' theatre script. *British Journal of Guidance and Counselling, 42*(5), 525–543. doi:10.1080/03069885.2014.928667

Worsley, R. (2006). Emmanuel Levinas: Resource and challenge for therapy. *Person-Centred & Experiential Psychotherapies, 5*(3), 208–220. doi:10.1080/14779757.2006.9688410

Yalom, I. (2002). *The gift of therapy.* London: Piatkus.

Zeldin, T. (2015). *The hidden pleasures of life.* London: Quercus.

Walking in a fairy tale forest in search of a second primitivity with the help of Little Red Riding Hood

Michiel de Ronde

ABSTRACT
In our modern society, self-reflection is valued as an important tool to work on a positive and lasting self-identity and to find and define our own path in life. Self-reflection can be seen as the fruit of the scientific approach, which has taught us to divide reality into subject and object. The reflecting person looks at him- or herself as an object that can be observed and analysed in order to reach a conclusion. However, this division between human and nature, and between the person and him- or herself, can also be a source of alienation and depression, because it fractures a more primitive connection between the self and nature. The article documents a coaching workshop that seeks to restore, to an extent, the undivided self in unity with nature. To do so, it uses the fairy tale of Little Red Riding Hood, a story that stems from a time long before the rise of objective thinking and cognitive reasoning. It presents a method that combines the telling of the fairy tale, walking in a forest with old oaks, and talking about life events. Twelve participants, all career counsellors, take part. Their reflections demonstrate that through connecting the walk in nature with our absorption into the fairy tale, we are able to accomplish a state of *second primitivity* where cognitive control and reflective observation temporarily give way to sensitivity, vulnerability, and susceptibility to the symbolism that is linked to pre-reflexive experience. The interplay between the symbolism of the fairy tale, the lived story of the walking experience in the woods, and the mutual storytelling between the participants enhances the emergence of new insights and new (self-)acceptance.

Introduction

To us, modern people inhabiting a world shaped by scientific thinking and technologically-informed action, it has become second nature to differentiate between subject and object, between the perceiver and the thing perceived, between the thinking individual and formulated thought. We have been taught to objectivise the world, to reason over its laws and regularities, and to use it in our pursuit of certain objectives (Dijksterhuis, 1961).

The natural sciences have provided a role model in this respect. This branch of science has, very successfully, implemented the scientific method of objectification by eliminating our influence, as perceiving subjects, as much as possible. This scientific mastery of reality has led to technology's comprehensive and ubiquitous impact on human life (DeWitt, 2010). The social sciences are treading the same path: the aspiration there is to master the knowledge of human behaviour in order to discover predictable dependencies and manipulatable, objective laws in order to regulate our own thoughts, feelings, and actions. This way of thinking is not without consequences for the practice of professional coaching.

Alienation

This objectifying view of the world is ingrained in our minds to such an extent that, even when communicating with ourselves we are unable to observe ourselves unless from a distance. We have termed this *reflexivity*. The idea is widespread – and it's partly due to the coaching guild – that such positioning of the observer with regard to one's own self is essential for accomplishing self-regulation and self-navigation in dealing with emotional events and making correct choices in life (Goz & Barnes, 2013). We have learned to divide the self into an observing part and an observed part.

By objectifying our world, we divide reality into two halves: the one that knows, and the one that is known. Western thought has separated humans from nature, and by internalising these objectifying attitudes in dealing with our own selves, the very nature of the human mind itself has also been split. Using a paradox, we could say that, thanks to reflexive thinking, humans have become alienated from themselves, as Horkheimer and Adorno (2002) argue in their *Dialectic of Enlightenment*. The direct and natural connection with our inner feelings has become mediated by self-observation and self-reflection, which Hoffman (2016) states "has led to a consciousness that is fundamentally alienated through the genesis of consciousness itself."

These philosophical deliberations are not only of theoretical importance. Korthagen and Vasalos (2010), for example, analyze 30 years' worth of developments concerning the concept of reflection in teacher education. They conclude that the dominant view of self-reflection in education posits a cognitive and rational approach to self-related questions. Students are taught to observe, to analyze, and to deduce in regard to their personal questions: that is, to handle them in an objectifying manner. The consequences of this way of thinking in the practice of coaching and education have become clear in evaluation studies. Boud and Walker (1998) showed that reflection in education often has the character of an obligation, performed by the students according to a given procedure that the students follow in an instrumental (i.e. not fully engaged) and rational way. Mittendorff (2010) underscores this conclusion with her finding that students often dislike reflection tasks and reflexive career conversations. Only more recently has the concept of self-reflection in education been broadened and has also become oriented on presence, feeling, and awareness, according to Korthagen and Vasalos (2010). However, other studies indicate that there still is a gap between this way of conceptualising reflection and the practice of teachers who have to coach their students (Kuijpers & Meijers, 2017).

More in general Lengelle, Luken, and Meijers (2016) maintain that self-reflection is not without danger. When reflection is unilaterally cognitive it can result in worrying and depressive thoughts. Kross (2009) also warns about alienating forms of self-reflection, reporting the results of a research programme on adaptive and maladaptive ways of reflection. All these authors state that self-reflection, in order to be adaptive and to enhance well-being, should not primarily be a kind of rational and instrumental thinking to control thoughts and feelings, but rather be a receptive and creative activity that requires a state of surrender to the stream of consciousness.

Primitive embeddedness

We learn from the cultural anthropology of non-western peoples that an objectifying and distancing attitude towards nature and towards ourselves is far from universal. In their depictions of the so-called primitive societies, anthropologists from the beginning of the twentieth century talk about *participation mystique,* as a mystical, pre-reflexive connectedness with nature and community (Levy-Bruhl, 1922/2015). They use this concept to describe a way of perceiving reality in which humans are an immediate and inseparable part of nature and, in their senses, real phenomena are completely merged with the experience of the symbolic and magic emanation of these phenomena. Thus, for instance, in the noise of the wind we hear the voices of ghosts, and ploughing up the field and performing a fertility ritual are one and the same. By wearing a mask, a person evokes and embodies the spirit of that mask. Within *participation mystique*, providing a chain-of-causation explanation of things is unnecessary because their meaning is corporeal and their connection to all other things is mystical. Both humans and nature are part of both a supreme force and a sacred order; together they are subjected to them and united with them. Earth is our mother, for we originate from it, are part of it, and share its fate.

By contrast, in our modern, scientific world, we have won a technological mastering of our lives to a high degree, but at the same time in this struggle we have lost a deep sense of meaningful embeddedness within life itself (Wulff, 1996). In our search for meaning in life, the pre-reflexive connectedness with the whole is broken. Life itself has become a project in which we have to make personal sense where before that sense was "given" through culture stories and archetypal meaning-making. Nevertheless, in our modern world, nature is still important to help us to construct a positive and lasting self-identity and a sense of well-being (Olivos & Clayton, 2016). Windhorst (2016) describes the discovery of this relationship as a process of remembering the ecological self. In this article we will work on a guiding method we can use to restore, to some extent, our primitive connection with nature, and which can help us to experience the connection between self and nature as filled with pre-reflexive meanings on the one hand without loss of our self-conscious thinking on the other.

Symbolic narratives

In the world of fairy tales and ancient myths, we sense the echo of that life in an undivided reality where inner feeling and external world were one, and where the actual manifestations of things was not yet separated from their symbolic meanings (Du Toit, 2016; Welman, 2001). In fairy tales and myths, animals can speak because, emotionally, they possess the power to be messages, and objects and characters may transform themselves because they change in our conception of the world. When reality and perception are the same, the sensation of things shifts the moment that they take a different shape – and vice versa – reality changes depending on the alteration of our own moods.

Erich Fromm (1951) examines dreams, fairy tales and myths as a universal language in which, in accordance with the laws of intensity of perception and of association (and contrary to the laws of logic and causality), things transfer their meaning to the surrounding world – through sensory perception that causes bodily association. If we should once again begin to understand the language of symbolism in fairy tales and myths, this, according to Fromm, would bring us to "the deepest sources of worldly wisdom", and in learning from them, we would touch "the depths of our personality" (p. 17).

Extending the idea of *participation mystique*, telling and listening to fairy tales grants us access to the sensation that we are one with ourselves and with the surrounding world. Allowing ourselves to be guided by the associative power of symbolism – where shapes transform, meanings merge, and the personality of the listener is identified with the characters of the narrative – it is possible to explore our moral space and to regain knowledge of the world and of ourselves from the depths of our spiritual mind (Bolton, 2016).

We can establish a deeper connection between ourselves and life if we abandon the position of observers, rid ourselves of reflexivity and the empiricism of the autonomous, thinking subject, and surrender ourselves to the momentary sensation, unite with the world we inhabit, and absorb all impressions it imprints in our senses and all associations and meanings it awakens (Bolton, 2016). The path of rationality and of reflexivity may take us to logical conclusions and explanations, but that does not yet equal comprehension from within or the experience of meaningful insight. These are not the fruit of logical thought and cognitive reflexivity, they are gifts of mind; they yield themselves not to analysis and arguing – we can only surrender ourselves to them (De Ronde, 2015).

Second primitivity

To us, people of the modern world, it is impossible to begin living as ancient peoples did. Thinking in terms of cause and effect, reflexivity and deduction, analysis and expedience, has conquered us irrevocably. We can no longer rid ourselves of these. This article is, by itself, an example of the empirical approach to the question of empathetic knowing and connectedness between our spirituality and the surrounding world. All of this, however, does not necessarily mean that we are completely unsusceptible to the influence of things as defined by *participation mystique*.

Studying the nature of the creative artist, Erik Erikson (1977) speaks about "regression in service of the ego": supervised by the stern look of the reality principle, this same reality principle is abandoned for a moment. Han Fortmann (1974) introduces the concept of "second primitivity" to designate that also modern humans are capable of opening up their consciousness to the meaning of the world in the present moment here and now – in the form of a lived experience that precedes the intrinsic act of reflexivity. "Critical distance ought to give way to a restored proximity from time to time", he writes. "Criticism corrects empathy (participation), and empathy corrects criticism" (p. 557).

In *Phenomenology of Practice*, Max van Manen (2014) calls for a study of lived experiences. The aspiration to such a study is paradoxical because a lived experience is something that we can experience but cannot completely grasp if we should try to study it. Having hardly begun to talk about it, it has already slipped away, transforming itself from an experienced tale to a told experience, from a lived story to a told story (Stern, 2004). Like Fortmann, Van Manen makes an essential connection to modern natural sciences, where it is now accepted to regard reality to possess two (or more) manifestations that are mutually exclusive: like particle and wave, matter and energy. Both manifestations are real but cannot be harmoniously nested together within the same framework at the same time. In a similar way, lived experience and conscious reflection are incompatible in the same moment, but both are nevertheless real, existing positions of the human mind.

The narrative approach of the dialogical self theory (Hermans & Hermans-Konopka, 2010; Vassilieva, 2016) provides a conceptual framework that helps us understand these different positions as the alternating perspectives of the teller and/or listener on the one hand, and of the inhabiting character of the tale on the other. In one moment, we are part of the story and in the other, we are its teller or listener. The theory of the dialogical self, in which the self is conceptualised as a multivocal whole of I-positions, can help us to permit and to understand the pre-modern experience of the participation mystique as a certain I-position within the dialogical space of the self. This way, again paradoxically, the experience of *wholeness* can become *part* of our life.

Walking in a fairy tale as a work approach

In coaching practice, much attention is paid to the mutual influence of the two manifestations of reality in the human mind. As coaches, we try to invoke lived experiences within the people turning to us, and we try to let them into themselves, accept themselves, as well as grasp their own message while looking at themselves from a distance and thinking about themselves. In this article, I develop and present an approach that explores the combination of the sensation of participation mystique with the ability to reflexively find one's own path of life. In this exercise, a narrative space is created (Breuer, 2008). During an actual walk in the wood, the participants listen to the Little Red Riding Hood fairy tale and, from time to time, together with a partner and led by the plot of the fairy tale, they exchange thoughts and memories of experiences from their personal past or current emotions. In the pages that follow, I will describe how this workshop progresses and will briefly present the reactions of the participants. I shall conclude with a concise review of the psychological meaning of fairy tales and the idea of participation mystique within it.

Participants

The starting point of the development of this workshop was an encounter with a colleague. I told her about my ideas of combining storytelling and taking a walk in the woods. Spontaneously, she proposed to bring together a group of interested career counsellors working in educational settings by sending out a call to their professional network. Thirteen women responded and twelve of them actually participated. We agreed that they would take part in my workshop and, afterwards, they would provide me with their experience-based feedback.

Within the fairy tale forest of little red riding hood

The workshop begins in a restaurant near the woods where the participants and the workshop leader have agreed to meet. Here, I tell them about the plan for the forthcoming walk in the Little Red Riding Hood fairy tale. It includes several stages: going to the wood; four stages inside the wood; returning to the place of our first meeting. We shall walk in a group and within this group each member will have one permanent partner; at each stage I shall tell a part of the fairy tale that will invariably end in a question that is relevant to participants, and which will form the topic of their conversation.

I continue explaining while walking out of the restaurant. I invite the participants to choose a buddy and, on their way to the wood, tell each other how they have grown up with fairy tales and stories, in order to become acquainted with each other. "Little Red Riding Hood is a fairy tale for mothers, daughters, and grandmothers", I explain. "Perhaps you can share with each other how you've grown up with fairy tales and stories, and also how you've raised your children with fairy tales, how you told and read stories to them, and to what talks these stories led" (cf. Lykke, 1993). I look at the group: a brief moment of silence and concentration ensues. Then I say: "Well, off we go!" And the group is on the move.

The forms of work in which a narrative space is applied require a correct introduction. The participants need to be gradually introduced to the fairy tale atmosphere (De Ronde, 2015). The pairs are given the chance to become acquainted with each other and create a feeling of mutuality. By referring to the intergenerational perspective, I introduce the idea of the path of life, of origin, and of continuity. The initial stage of getting to the wood is intended to create an atmosphere of trust. We are still not inside the fairy tale but we are getting closer to it.

Stage one: the mother's errand

After some fifteen minutes we have reached an old oak wood. I summon the group, raise my index finger knowingly, lower my voice, and start speaking:

> Here, at the fringe of the wood, our fairy tale begins ... Once upon a time, long ago, at the end of a great forest with tall trees, a girl lived in a tiny house. Everybody loved her very much, for she was lively and jolly. Her grandmother, who lived further in the wood, had knit a red hood for her and that is why everyone called the girl Little Red Riding Hood. One day, early in the morning, her mother called her. "Come, Little Red Riding Hood. I learnt that your grandmother is sick. Go to her and bring her this basket with cake and wine. But do not leave the path or you might lose your way, and you might meet the Wolf!" Little Red Riding Hood took a firm hold of the basket and went on her way.

After this first excerpt, I invite the participants to share with each other how they have entered the the world beyond their parents' homes, and to tell each other what was, symbolically, in the basket they received from their parents, and what errands and what warnings accompanied them from their homes along the paths of their lives. From a methodical point of view, I consciously touch upon several motives. I emphasise the contrast between the big woods and the little girl. I interpret the fringe of the woods as a metaphor of the transition between childhood and adulthood.

Using my voice, gestures, and facial expressions, I do two things. First, I tell the fairy tale evocatively. I conjure up the fairy tale world and the feeling of mysticism, lowering my voice to a whisper, playing with the effect of silence and quietness: in this way, I create expectation in the participants. Second, my voice is restored to a normal timbre and I then invite the group to pair up and continue their conversations, answering my questions about the basket and the errands.

Stage two: flowers in the wood

We walk among the tall trees. I overhear snatches of conversation, but I try not to watch them; I can feel that they are quite lively, though. After twenty minutes, we stop again. In one larger clearing, the group gathers around me: the pairs now turn into the circle for a while. The fairy tale continues.

> Little Red Riding Hood is walking through the woods happily and joyfully. The sun's rays are shining through the branches, the sky is blue, and birds are singing. How pretty is the forest! What lovely flowers grow beside the path! Oh, what a beautiful flower! I shall pick it for Granny! Oh, there's one more over there ... and another! Without knowing, Little Red Riding Hood is carried away, picking the most alluring flowers. And over there, ah, farther down, are even more beautiful flowers! And how sweet they smell! Attracted by these pretty flowers, she picks a large bouquet.

Here I interrupt the fairy tale and, returning to my normal tone, I turn to the participants, enjoining them to

> Continue the story from where you stopped before, and gradually progress to the question of the flowers you have encountered in your life. What beautiful things have happened on the path of your life? Which of these flowers did you pick and which did you perhaps overlook?

I am silent for a few seconds, then urge them: "And on we go!"

Stage three: the wolf

The pairs start deep conversations and spread out even more, separating from the other pairs. The occasional phrases I hear suggest that cherished memories are being shared. After some twenty minutes, we stop again. We wait until everyone is gathered around me. I take a look at the group, let the silence create expectation, and continue telling the story.

> Suddenly, Little Red Riding Hood raised her eyes. It looks like it's getting dark. Clouds have covered the sun. Little Red Riding Hood is startled when she remembers she was actually headed for her Granny's and that it's high time she continued down her path. She looks around and is seised with fear. Where did the path go? And in that very moment, behind a tree, the Wolf appears. "Are you looking for something, little girl? Are you lost perhaps?" Little Red Riding Hood is frightened, but responds bravely, saying, Yes, I am going to my Granny's, but I've lost the path. She lives yonder, in a small house, and she is sick. When I arrive, she always says, "Just press the latch and the door will open." "Right, so ... ", says the Wolf. "Yeah, I can help you, little girl, because I see you've really strayed from the path ... "

Here I interrupt my story again and look at the participants. "Sometimes", I explain, "We have the feeling we are wandering in life and we doubt we're on the right path. Sometimes we connect with people without being sure it's wise. Continue your story from where you stopped earlier, and tell your partner about what you've searched for along the path of your life, and perhaps also about the wanderings in some of your undertakings."

Stage four: at granny's

The third stage of the workshop I make shorter than the previous ones, because the fourth stage is a direct extension of the third. After ten minutes I once again summon the group around me.

> You know how the fairy tale goes: the Wolf pointed Little Red Riding Hood to a roundabout path to her Granny's house and she, cheerful and happy, hurried along. The Wolf, however, took the shorter path through the woods and it was not long before he got to the door of the house. He knocked and heard Granny's voice from within. "Just press the latch and the door will open." The Wolf did not hesitate, rushed into the room and devoured the Grandmother. He then put on her nightcap and slid under the duvet. Not long after, Little Red Riding Hood

knocked on the door. "Just press the latch and the door will open," a hoary voice was heard from the inside. Gasping for her breath because she had been running, Little Red Riding Hood was astonished when she saw her Grandmother in bed. "Oh, Grandmother, what big eyes you have!" Said she. "All the better to see you with." The strange voice replied. "Oh, Grandmother, what big ears you have!" The little girl exclaimed. "All the better to hear you with." "Oh, Grandmother, what a big teeth you have!" "All the better to eat you with!" – the wolf jumped from the bed, dove onto Little Red Riding Hood, and swallowed her.

Again I switch from the tale to the reasoning.

Sometimes in life situations arise that overwhelm us, that, as it were, swallow us up, and sweep us over like a giant wave. "You", I pause then continue, "Talk with each other about your experiences along your path of life. Continue your conversation and consider if you might also dwell on any such moments".

As the leader of this workshop, I am aware that my question will touch upon some raw spots. It is important that the participants feel invited to such intimacy, yet at the same time, are free to decide how much of their souls to lay bare. "What do I share and what do I keep silent about?" It is in this respect that reciprocity plays a vital part: the confidence one partner inspires in the other generates the propensity in that other to also be discreet. Each pair has built their own type and extent of familiarity.

Stage five: freed by the hunter

Meanwhile, an hour and a half has passed since we began our walk. Innermost secrets and existential questions have been shared. I take a look around so I can pick a suitable spot for the finale of the fairy tale. The wood co-operates, and we find ourselves very close to a hut with an imposing old tree next to it. The pairs, who have long been moving at a great distance from one another, gather in a circle once again, and I start speaking in a loud voice.

The fairy tale continues. You all know how it ends. The Wolf climbed back into bed with a heavy belly, fell asleep, and began to snore very loudly. He was snoring so loudly that the Huntsman, who was passing by, heard him and immediately realised that something was not right in Granny's house. "I should check out this strange thing", he said, and walked in. Seeing the fat wolf sleeping in the bed, he wasted not a moment, but cut open the Wolf's belly. Little Red Riding Hood and her Grandmother jumped out, sound and well, and gave the Huntsman a happy hug for saving them. The Huntsman filled the Wolf's belly with stones and sewed it up. When he awoke, the Wolf was so thirsty that he jogged on to the well. He leaned down to drink but the heavy stones inside his belly dragged him down, he fell into the water, and forever disappeared on the bottom of the well. The Huntsman saw Little Red Riding Hood off to her home, and she would remember her adventure long afterward.

I step aside to emphasise the transition from narrator to instructor.

In the fairy tale, Little Red Riding Hood and her Grandmother are released by the Huntsman, and the Wolf disappears at the bottom of the well. Tell each other how the things you have just shared between yourselves have fallen into their places in your life, how you've "ordered" them in it. Just like the basket at the start of the path, so are the flowers and the Wolf metaphors of the things you have been given, or that you have encountered along your path, and similarly perhaps the Huntsman-liberator and the well also have their symbolic places in your life. Share what you feel like sharing with your partner.

Finally, I tell them this is the last stage of the walk with the pairs grouped as they are. "Shortly, we will reach the fringe of the wood again, and then I will ask you to thank your partner for whatever they have shared, and then walk the rest of the path to the restaurant together with another participant. Agreed?" I ask rhetorically. "Let's go!"

The way back: the end of the fairy tale

Eventually we reach the spot where the fairy tale began. The circle of the story is now closing. The meeting of the partners who have shared intimate experiences from their childhood and adolescent years is now over, and the transition to the ordinary world must be made. To finalise with a ritual, I recite a poem by the Dutch poet Neeltje Maria Min to the group, which, in only a few words, explores the relationship between daughter, mother, and grandmother. In a short ceremony, I then invite the participants to thank each other for their candour and trust. This moment of closing the personal encounter is important. The workshop is not yet over, but the intimate sharing has ended now. Therefore I ask them to look for a different partner to share, in a more methodological way, their impressions from the workshop: its emotional value for them and its impact on them. This last part of the wandering has two functions. On the one hand, it helps to release and leave the intense emotional atmosphere and on the other it contributes to comprehension of how the method works. The task thus assigned, we all advance towards the restaurant where we began our trip.

Impressions

A few weeks after the workshop, the participants send me their reflections, I asked for by an e-mail message. The feeling of integrity and unity discussed earlier is felt in these responses. The participants describe the act of abandonment of objective thinking and indulging in the momentary lived experience as follows:

- It was as if something dragged me with enormous power back to my childhood. I could hear my mother's voice.
- Walking there was like getting closer to one's own self. I've now grasped the meaning of the messages my parents had been sending me off with back then.
- The fairy tale stirred my imagination. Letting my thoughts take their own course, literally walking inside the fairy tale, the wood as a metaphor of life, the flowers along the path – all of this has moved me deeply.
- The symbolism of the wood, the fairy tale in general, elevates you to a higher level of sensitivity.
- You follow the fairy tale and, without having to think, you stumble upon all sorts of curious things. And everything around us – the wood, the air, and weather – played in tune with the context.
- In some miraculous way, it turns out that you are comfortable talking about things that difficult and delicate …
- It was a demonstration of strength for me to go deeper and deeper into my own life. The Little Red Riding Hood tale is a popular one and this is why I could feel, my curiosity and eagerness growing, the arrival of each new motif. This could be the reason why the questions seemed natural to me, rather than embarrassing.

The participants' impressions of the workshop show that the components of the workshop: walking in the woods, listening to the fairy tale, and sharing with each other, all intensified the effect of their impact. It seems that something like participation mystique has transpired: the personal past, the fairy tale symbolism, and the natural surroundings of the wood have united in a harmonious whole, formed a stable combination, created a pattern (Gestalt), and this wholeness is something more than the sum of its parts.

What the participants share about their conversations also substantiates the emotional value of the workshop. They touched upon personal and intimate moments, which is evident from the following responses:

- "To me the flower picking motif stood as a symbol of my resistance – to stray from the right path so I can have a taste of freedom."
- "The fairy tale is a metaphor of the great big world, of my own entry in life when I was 18. The woods are not simply enticing, they are big and often impenetrable, you could get lost in no time. The flowers reminded me of the temptations of excessive freedom – it was hard to deal with them and that is why I wandered in my relationships with people, with men in particular."
- "The fairy tale made me recall many sad moments of my life. Without going into detail, this was a period of my life when I was really at a loss, when I had actually lost myself. A time when I did not know who I was, what I wanted, and which way I wanted to go."

- "The fairy tale made me realise that there are quite a few wolves in my life, and it looks like it is I who's been attracting them. Perhaps (to use another metaphor) I promise some of them an abundance of food … "
- "To me the most important insight was found at the end of the fairy tale. I realised that everything that had happened to me I could just throw away like stones in the well. Old heartaches, but at least my soul will be tidy."

Finally, many participants point out that reciprocity in the confidential conversations was an extremely important aspect of the workshop:

- "What I enjoyed was that we were talking in pairs – and this helped me get 'deep' into it.
- Thanks to others also sharing intimate things, I was able to bear my own pain more easily. It is a sort of consolation to feel that both of you are equally vulnerable."

Playing in the narrative space

"Man (…) is only completely a man when he plays," writes Friedrich Schiller (1795/2016), pondering over the tension between prudence and spontaneity in man. It is only in the area of play that these two unite and humans are capable of harmoniously combining the moral (guided by rules and norms) with the spontaneous, the free, the sensual within themselves. In a similar manner objective, reflexive thinking is, on the face of it, opposed to lived experience. Owing to this unconventional approach of walking in the fairy tale forest, we seem to have found a way to get the momentary lived experience and the reflexive insight of reasoning into proximity. The lived story, the wandering with each other in the wood, and the stories they share are both constantly enriched and deepened.

The aforementioned excerpts of participant reactions illustrate the interplay of the fairy tale narrative and the participants' narratives. Characters and metaphors have their own significance in the fairy tale, they also have their equivalents in the participants' lives. What's more, the fairy tale characters and metaphors assume a "flesh" as they are "filled" by the personal story of each participant. The personal story adds depth to the fairy tale story; the story of the fairy tale, on the other hand, helps reconsider and give new meaning to the personal story (Echols, Gravenstine, & Mobley, 2010; Parkin, 2010).

The conversations between partners are characterised by mutuality, not only with respect to the sharing of intimate things but also with respect to listening and hearing what the other person has to share (Cf. Coplan, 2004). A constant process of shifting from the present to the past and back is observed. The fairy tale recalls childhood and adolescent memories that we are talking about in the present moment. This is due to the evocative nature of the fairy tale: it is both past, as an old, well-known story, and present, as a story told at this very moment. The setting – the woods as the venue of both the fairy tale and the workshop – contributes greatly to achieving this effect. Although the fairy tale begins with the invariable "Once upon a time", its plot unfolds in the here and now.

What is interesting is the play between light and darkness in the fairy tale and in the feelings it stirs, between the effort to face painful memories from the past and the courage to accept our own life lessons learned from past suffering. For example, a number of the participants told about the tension between the feelings of closeness and intimacy of their parental homes and at the same time the necessity and inevitability of relieving themselves of those feelings. Another instance of the interplay between light and darkness, or good and evil, is the enjoyment of the beauty and pleasure the flowers offer, which gradually transforms into threat and confusion, and thus becomes the image of the Wolf. Conversely, the heaviness and darkness that the Wolf embodies also turn out to be the things we cannot do without along the path of our lives: the things that help us mature and grow, gain our own freedom and build our own independence (Cf. Kast, 1987).

The venue of the walk as a kind of playing, the meeting of the participants and the fairy tale itself, turn out to be a transitional space (Winnicott, 1971), that area of transition that phenomenologists see as the birth of a new sense of meaning and a renewed relationship of belonging to the lives we live. It is in this transitional space that our moods are filled with experiences from outside and at the same time that the outside world is meaningfully loaded with our thoughts and feelings. The fairy tale, as it is told, is interpreted in the context of our life experiences. Conversely the story of our life is re-told in a new way by that comprehension. It is the transitional space of the walked narrative in which new insights are born and a new sense of meaning is embraced.

Conclusion

In our modern society, the construction of a positive and lasting self-identity is one of the most important personal challenges (Taylor, 1989). Self-reflection is widely regarded as an important tool to find our way and to define ourselves in an uncertain and precarious world and to give meaning to our lives. At the same time, this self-reflection can also be a source of alienation when it is comprehended and practised in an overly cognitive way.

Being the children of the Enlightenment, we have learned to objectify the world and to think about ourselves. As a consequence, we are incapable of being one with nature in the way our ancestors once were. Those very same ancestors have, however, bequeathed to us, in their fairy tales and myths, an immense treasure trove of symbolism that speaks to us in the language of sensory images, of metaphors borrowed from nature, of fantasies filled with sensitivity. These can help us to reach beyond an unduly rational approach to life's questions.

Searching for the path in the fairy tale forest as a working method demonstrates that, in connecting the walk in nature and becoming absorbed into the fairy tale, we still manage to enter a state of *second primitivity,* where cognitive control and reflexive observation temporarily give way to sensitivity, vulnerability, and the susceptibility to symbolism that is linked to pre-reflexive experience. In the interplay between symbolism and the personal story, between identifying with the fairy tale and formulating one's own experiences, between the search for the path in the woods and the search for the correct destination in our own lives, the *narrative space* emerges in which new insights appear, we experience a new acceptance, and we find a new inner balance.

Of course, many questions can be asked. How sustainable is the self-acceptance that emerges? What is the depth of our new insights? Can we generalise from this example, in which we walked with counsellor colleagues, to our work with other clients? Are these career counsellors able to transfer these experiences to their own practices in educational settings? Much research is needed if we want to design an evidence-based method. In this article, my sole intention was to present an exploration of a creative and inviting method to stimulate the interplay between lived stories and the told stories of people with whom we work. The method described can be seen as an endeavour to use reflexive thinking while at the same time overcoming objectifying reflexivity in our search for meaning in life.

Acknowledgement

My thanks goes to Stefan D. Stefanov, Veliko Turnovo, Bulgaria, and to Andrea Hankinson, Edmonton, Canada, for their assistance with translation of this article.

Disclosure statement

No potential conflict of interest was reported by the author.

References

Bolton, E. M. A. (2016). *Exploring the moral space in literacy practices: A fluid model for the actions of the emotive self in adults' responses to fairy tales*. Toronto: ProQuest Dissertations Publishing.

Boud, D., & Walker, D. (1998). Promoting reflection in professional courses: The challenge of context. *Studies in Higher Education, 23*(2), 191–206.

Breuer, F. (2008). Playing in the narrative space. In L. de Caluwé, G. J. Hofstede, & V. Peters (Eds.), *Why do games work? In search of the active substance* (pp. 117–129). Deventer: Kluwer.

Coplan, A. (2004). Empathetic engagements with narrative fictions. *Journal of Aesthetics and Art Criticism, 62*(2), 141–152.

De Ronde, M. A. (2015). *Speelruimte voor ervaring en reflectie. Een praktijkgericht onderzoek naar het gebruik van spel in begeleidingssituaties*. Delft: Eburon.

DeWitt, R. (2010). *Worldviews. An introduction to the philosophy and history of science*. Oxford: Wiley Blackwell.

Dijksterhuis, E. J. (1961). *The mechanization of the world picture*. Oxford: Clarendon Press.

Du Toit, D. H. (2016). Utilizing symbolic expressions, art, myths, dreams and fantasies in coaching. In L. van Zyl, M. Stander, & A. Odendaal (Eds.), *Coaching psychology: Meta-theoretical perspectives and applications in multicultural contexts* (pp. 299–314). Cham: Springer Verlag.

Echols, M., Gravenstine, K., & Mobley, S. (2010). Using story in coaching. In C. Wahl, C. Scriber, & B. Bloomfield (Eds.), *On becoming a leadership coach. A holistic approach to coaching excellence* (pp. 53–59). London: Palgrave McMillan.

Erikson, E. H. (1977). *Toys and reasons. Stages in the ritualization of experience*. New York: Norton.

Fortmann, H. (1974). *Als ziende de onzienlijke. Een cultuurpsychologische studie over de religieuze waarneming en de zogenaamde religieuze projectie*. Hilversum: Gooi en Sticht.

Fromm, E. (1951). *The forgotten language. An introduction in the understanding of dreams, fairy tales and myths*. New York: Rinehart.

Goz, A., & Barnes, B. K. (2013). *Self-Navigation: A compass for guiding your life and career*. CA: Johari Press Publication.

Hermans, H. J. M., & Hermans-Konopka, A. (2010). *Dialogical self theory. Positioning and counter-positioning in a globalizing society*. Cambridge: Cambridge University Press.

Hoffman, L. (2016). *Adorno and Augustine; parallel conceptions of alienation and the self*. Colorada: University of Colorado.

Horkheimer, M., & Adorno, T. W. (2002). *Dialectic of enlightenment*. Stanford: University Press.

Kast, V. (1987). *Sprookjes als therapie*. Rotterdam: Lemniscaat.

Korthagen, F. J., & Vasalos, A. (2010). From reflection to presence and mindfulness: 30 years of developments concerning the concepts of reflection in teacher education. In N. Lyons (Ed.), *Handbook of reflection and reflective inquiry* (pp. 529–552). New York: Springer.

Kross, E. (2009). When the self becomes other: Toward an integrative understanding of the processes distinguishing adaptive self-reflection from rumination. *Annals of the New York Academy of Sciences, 1167*, 35–40.

Kuijpers, M., & Meijers, F. (2017). Professionalising teachers in career dialogue: An effect study. *British Journal of Guidance and Counselling, 45*(1), 83–96.

Lengelle, R., Luken, T., & Meijers, F. (2016). Is self-reflection dangerous? Preventing rumination in career learning. *Australian Journal of Career Development, 25*(3), 99–109.

Levy-Bruhl, L. (1922/2015). *How natives think*. New York: Martino Fine Books.

Lykke, N. (1993). Questing daughters: Little Red Riding Hood, antigone and oedipus complex. In J. van Mens-Verhulst, K. Schreurs, & L. Woertman, (Eds.), *Mothering and daughtering. Female subjectivity reanalysed* (pp. 15–25). New York: Routledge.

Mittendorff, K. M. (2010). *Career conversations in senior secondary vocational education* (PhD-thesis). Eindhoven University of Technology, Eindhoven.

Olivos, P., & Clayton, S. (2016). Self, nature and well-being: Sense of connectedness and environmental identity for quality of life. In G. Fleuri-Bahi, E. Pol, & O. Navaro (Eds.), *Handbook of environmental psychology and quality of life research* (pp. 107–126). New York: Springer.

Parkin, M. (2010). *Tales for coaching. Using stories and metaphors with individuals and small groups*. London: Kogan Page.

Schiller, F. (1795/2016). *Briefe über die ästhetische Erziehung des Menschen*. Berlin: Verlag Contumax.

Stern, D. (2004). *The present moment in psychotherapy and everydag life*. New York: Norton.

Taylor, C. (1989). *Sources of the self. The making of the modern identity*. Cambridge: University Press.

van Manen, M. (2014). *Phenomenology of practice. Meaning-giving methods in phenomenological research and writing*. Walnut Creek, CA: Left Coast Press.

Vassilieva, J. (2016). *Narrative psychology. Identity, transformation and ethics*. London: Palgrave McMillan.

Welman, A. J. (2001). *De menselijke levensloop. Een psychologische benadering met behulp van sprookjesbeelden*. Zeist: Christofoor.

Windhorst, E. (2016). Re-membering ecological self: A personal narrative autoethnography. *Ecopsychology, 8*(4), 264–270.

Winnicott, D. (1971). *Playing and reality*. London: Routledge.

Wulff, D. (1996). *Psychology of religion. Classic and contemporary views*. New York: John Wiley.

Cures for the heart: a poetic approach to healing after loss

Patricia A. McClocklin and Reinekke Lengelle

ABSTRACT

Writing creatively, expressively, and reflectively to aid the grieving process is founded on the idea that in order to survive and thrive after loss, personal meaning must be made of what has been suffered. The individualisation and secularisation of society has put the onus of meaning making on the individual while an abiding reservation about speaking openly about death in Western culture complicates this task. In this article we examine how metaphors are used to make sense of loss and its ensuing emotions and how they help the writer move from a 'first' (i.e. anguish, pain) to a 'second' story (i.e. healing). We argue also that evoking the beloved through writing is part of healthy grieving. We conclude that *nudging, thread* and *crystalising* metaphors as well as 'poetic conversations' – that help locate and position oneself in relation to the loss – together make constructing new life-giving (i.e. second) stories possible. The safety and privacy of writing is also key in making space for the voice of the bereaved. We note that grieving individuals 'write about' and 'write to' and thus evoke the person who has died. In this paradoxical way the bereaved face the reality of death by *retaining* the loved one.

Introduction

Grief theorists emphasise the importance of finding personal meaning after the death of a loved one and research indicates that people adapt more positively if they are able to make sense of their loss. Indeed, more complicated grief may ensue from lengthy, frustrated struggles to find meaning (Currier, Holland, & Neimeyer, 2006; Hall, 2014; Smit, 2015). Pain from witnessing a fading life, the shock of unexpected death, comprehending finality, musing over life's meanings and contributions can linger for months, for years, occasionally forever. However, such distress may remain troublesome until it is truly felt, reflected upon and made sense of, and writing can offer a way to do so (Anderson & MacCurdy, 2000; Furnes & Dysvik, 2011).

Writing in the face of loss is not a new phenomenon: the field of poetry therapy thrives and offers solace (Mazza, 2003) and there is extensive research now showing that writing is a powerful means of healing and personal transformation (Bolton, 1999; Hunt, 2000; Pennebaker, 2011). Studies show that the healing combination of writing entails the expression of both facts and emotions. A beneficial narrative is one that is 'under construction' and is characterised by a narrative thread (DeSalvo, 1999; Pennebaker, 2011, 2012). Based on recent research on the change processes within narrative guidance, we propose that metaphors play an important role in meaning making (Lengelle, Meijers, & Hughes, 2016). We also see confirmed that 'talking' – in person or on paper – about and to the deceased and in this sense *retaining* them is a beneficial part of healing (Parkes, Laungani, & Young, 2015; Walter, 1996).

Before we describe the healing process through writing and illustrate with a personal case study and analysis, we will present several key problems that make the act of grieving more difficult in contemporary society.

Grief: the individualised journey of healing and death as 'unsayable'

Traditional rituals and customs that surrounded death and which offered solace to the bereaved and helped channel the difficult emotions surrounding loss have largely disappeared in our individualised and secularised society (Parkes et al., 2015). In the past, mourning entailed a religious or culturally prescribed ceremony and was a communal undertaking, whereas in contemporary Western society, grief and bereavement are increasingly viewed as an individual and psychological experience. In the literature on bereavement, grief is frequently described as an individualised undertaking (Arnold & Gemma, 2008) where the experience of grief is felt and interpreted in a uniquely personal way (Furnes & Dysvik, 2011, p. 16) and emphasis is put on the personal needs of those left behind (Hardy-Bougere, 2008). Though contemporary scholars do not ignore the sociological dimensions of grieving, they point out that the individual is in the process of 'meaning making' and constructing a new 'self narrative' which is later 'negotiated in the intimate interpersonal domain of family and close associates' (Neimeyer, Klass, & Dennis, 2014, p. 485). This shift in part has it origins in Freudian thinking and became particularly visible in the second half of the twentieth century and continues today (Smit, 2015). The purpose of grieving, it seems, is the 'reconstitution of an autonomous individual' and is achieved through the 'construction of a durable biography that enables the living to integrate the memory of the dead into their on-going lives' (Walter, 1996, p. 7). This individualised view is also evident in the way that ceremonies are tailor-made or 'personalised' (Schafer, 2012) and in the language that is used in examinations of death and dying. In sum: the onus to make sense and engage in meaning making after loss is increasingly the task of a person as opposed to a process based on the grand theories that dominated before post-modernism (Walter, 1996).

A complicating factor is that while in many cultures expressive mourning is still built into communal rituals, Western cultures 'tend to discourage the overt expression of emotion at funerals' (Parkes et al., 2015, p. 5). Although a wider understanding of psychology affirms the positive aspects of feeling, cultural programmes that emphasise control and composure are deep-seated. Many people simply don't know what to do with the painful emotions that erupt after a loved one has died and the conversation about death is therefore not an easy one. Social scientists have proposed that Western society may in fact be 'death denying' or alternatively that society is simply creating a calming practice to confine the fear and turmoil of death and dying (Zimmermann & Rodin, 2004).

Fear of the unknown, linked to medicalised approaches that relegate illness and death behind closed doors have also lead to the difficulty many have in dealing with loss. Science is focused on preventing death and having the 'death talk' is a challenge for patients and clinicians alike (Zimmermann & Rodin, 2004). Medical staff may experience anxiety for various social, cultural, or religious reasons or because of other gaps in their preparedness to engage in such dialogue (Charon, 2006; Nia, Lehto, Ebadi, & Peyrovi, 2016). Dying is frequently prolonged with drugs and state-of-the-art interventions that can conflict with other more internal concerns of those caring for the terminally ill (Charon, 2006; Zweig & Oliver, 2009).

Reasons for discomfort in discussing death can be traced to social taboos that may have initially sought to shield the terminally ill but eventually served to protect relatives and then society from the messiness of death. 'Death in the abstract … remains easier to discuss than one's own death or the death of a close friend, a relative or a patient one has cared for' (Zimmermann & Rodin, 2004, p. 123). Dying is often an isolated event in hospital rather than at home amongst one's family (Teno et al., 2004; Zimmermann and Rodin, 2004 cited in Zweig & Oliver, 2009). Rational, technical or medical approaches to illness and death are often disconnected from more sagacious, instinctive, or symbolic responses (Charon, 2006). Paired with an oft unwitnessed death or unobserved final moments, the embodiment of spiritual, philosophical or scientific sense-making may often be denied to the bereaved (Valentine, 2007). 'Narrative methods can help to bridge … these divides' (Charon, 2006, p. 35).

Although a variety of (model-based) theories about grieving have appeared in the last fifty years, their assumptions and limitations are being called into question. Freud, for instance, defined grief as a natural response in the face of loss. However, he theorised that normal grieving involves breaking emotional ties with the deceased '… so that their emotional energy can be re-invested elsewhere' (Smit, 2015, p. 34). This is now a contested notion (Walter, 1996; Buglass, 2010; Goss & Klass, 2005; Hall, 2014; Smit, 2015).

Other theorists hypothesised that grief follows a path of stages or phases (Hall, 2014; Smit, 2015). Kübler-Ross proposed a model based on the 'anticipatory grief' of palliative patients (Kübler-Ross, 2009) that transformed into five stages of grief: shock and denial; anger, resentment and guilt; bargaining; depression; and acceptance. These indicators soon became associated with bereavement and were considered relevant to other forms of change. However, later it was found not everyone went through each stage and the order of the stages was also called into question (Goldsworthy, 2005; Hall, 2014; Smit, 2015).

Worden (2002) proposed a four-phase model: acceptance, working through pain, adapting to new situations and, finally, establishing a new connection to the deceased. Others concurred by suggesting grieving, instead of a quest for closure, leads towards new ways of relating to the deceased: 'They did not see bereavement or grieving as ever being fully resolved, culminating in closure or recovery' (Smit, 2015 p. 35).

The dual-process model of grieving suggested that most people move back and forth between two domains. During 'loss-orientation', grief and emotional issues are addressed; during 'restoration-orientation', the focus is toward specific problems and the practical issue of new routines (Buglass, 2010). Individuals may have found comfort in 'stage models' of grief. Anxiety is perhaps alleviated by the belief that bereavement was a common journey toward a 'final' phase and resolution. However, in reality grief does not follow a predictable or rigid path. Suggesting patterns of 'normal' behaviour does not account for the complicated process of each individual's bereavement (Buglass, 2010) that is impacted by unique physical, psychological, social and spiritual needs (Hall, 2014).

In sum: the cultural realities described above and the critiques on model-based grieving theories mean that the processing of loss requires an individual search for meaning – which requires an internal and external dialogue (Hermans & Hermans-Konopka, 2010, Meijers & Lengelle, 2012) – yet must be undertaken in a society that stigmatises death and is ill at ease with such a conversation. Writing provides a safe and private way to begin the work that intends to: 'reconstruct a world of that has been challenged by loss, at every level from the simple habit structures of our daily lives, through our identities in a social world, to our personal and collective cosmologies, whether secular or spiritual' (Neimeyer et al., 2014, p. 486).

In this article we propose that writing is a way in which a 'first story' surrounding loss – characterised by difficulty in dealing with the loss – can be transformed into a 'second story' where meaning is made of what has happened (Lengelle & Meijers, 2009).This process is aided by the help of metaphors. Three types of writing are involved: *expressive writing*, as defined by Pennebaker (2011) refers to the writing done about one's deepest thoughts and feelings surrounding a loss or trauma. *Creative writing* refers to the use of the imagination in describing the loss (in this case through poetry) and *reflective writing* in our context refers to the ability to view the lived experience from some distance and comment on its meanings and process (Lengelle & Meijers, 2009). Ultimately, the writing done by someone who is grieving can be shared with important others when it feels right to do so and invites them into a conversation.

The illustrative case and points of analysis

The first author of this article shares the story of the death of her husband. She did the writing here as part of a graduate course, entitled *'Narrative Possibilities: The Transformative Power of Writing, Story, and Poetry in Personal and Professional Development'* (Lengelle, 2008), during which time she continued the poetry writing she began during her spouse's illness and death. We note that the second author was the professor of the course and recognised the story as a source of further research on the process of grieving through writing.

The coursework included theories of reflective and transformative writing, narrative and poetry therapy, and investigations of literary forms that revealed additional perspectives. Armed with fresh viewpoints, the first author began to create a 'second story' – one filled with a richer appreciation and nuanced meanings about life and death, love and loss, and what it means to grieve. Although not all the poems, or accompanying reflections, from the original project are included here an attempt was made to retain the essence and order of the grief narrative that demonstrates the writer's progression from despair to healing.

The analysis of the case study will see whether the three key metaphors associated with using writing for narrative self development, as identified by Lengelle et al. (2016), can be found. These are: *nudging, thread,* and *crystallizing* metaphors. In the process of examining this particular case we will also see if we can identify the presence of 'poetic conversations' as attempts to sort out 'where I am now'. Such poetic conversations while being part of the internal dialogue, also represent an imagined external dialogue that is continued with the beloved and is a precursor to new dialogues about the deceased and about one's own life. Indeed, both forms of dialogue, which segue into one another, are the motor in the creation of new narratives (Meijers & Lengelle, 2012). *Nudging* metaphors are 'small' metaphors that stand on their own but are useful in exploring the territory in order to move forward incrementally. *A thread* metaphor often appears early on and is expanded and revisited throughout the storying process and serves to connect the fragments of insight into a new narrative. It bridges the gap between the past, the present and the future. *A crystallizing* metaphor articulates an insight, solution, (temporary) image or idea that represents a kind 'product' of the process. The *crystallizing* metaphor can serve as a source of comfort in contemplating the future. 'Poetic conversations' which represent external and internal dialogues shape the narrative through exploring 'placement and positioning' enabling a grieving writer to relocate from immobilising loss into the current struggle, in part, by speaking 'about' and 'to' the beloved, to oneself, and eventually to living others.

Patricia's story

The following poems and reflections were written following my husband's death until the present. Never having written poetry before, I was astonished how deeply compelled I was to write the words that bombarded me from the inside. Having since completed two courses on transformative writing, I now understand it was my intuitive attempt to make sense of a meaningful life event.

My poems are presented, loosely, in the form of an elegy that flows with the passing of time. Elegiac poetry is a reflective poetry of mourning; sorrow and love are the primary themes. The traditional elegy is one poem comprised of three stages: lament, praise and admiration, and finally consolation and meaning. This elegy, however, consists of several poems laid out in a timeline that begins after *Dusk*, the 'end' of a day. Dusk becomes 'midnight', the darkest hour; midnight drifts into a seemingly endless 'middle of night'. But inevitably, as in life, 'dawn' emerges and brings with it light, renewed hope, and unanticipated wonder.

The passing of a day is a significant *thread metaphor* that sutures the broken 'self' into a new 'second story'. Moreover, it.connects my memories – characterised by the poetry in my time of Dusk and Midnight – with current emotions (Middle of the Night) and contemplations about the future (Dawn). The timeline is also a *crystalising metaphor* that links my personal loss to the grander narrative of life itself: birth, life, death and rebirth. Additionally, each separate part of the day (E.g. 'Dusk' below) acts as a *nudging metaphor* that prods towards 'dawn' and back 'into' life.

Cole (2005) postulated that the bereaved might find relief by writing elegies. He argues that through the poetic task of wrestling with the effort of finding suitable words to paint the painful picture of misery and mourning, one may reconcile loss and move towards less 'complicated' grief. Initially I thought my poetry might fit neatly into the elegiacal stages and into a linear representation of time. I also imagined I might observe a decisive shift in the style and content of my writing as my emotions softened or perhaps waned. But, although differences were noted, as is explained by grief theorists, emotionally reconciling oneself with loss is not a simple, straightforward process. It is, in fact, a course of ups and downs; it may move towards a resolution about life and an acknowledgment of death. That said, grief is never 'gotten over' or 'done with'. The reader will understand then, why a sorrowful lament may appear a year and a half later just when 'dawn' might be expected to break.

The reflection that occurs above, before the presentation of poems, already contains metaphors worth exploring. The *thread* metaphor in Patricia's references to dusk, night and dawn appear throughout her story. She also *crystallises* for herself how the grieving process works saying 'Ups and downs' as if to prepare herself. Her reference to a 'shift' or the 'softening' or 'waning' of emotions point to an exploration of how she might move forward; these *nudging* metaphors imply movement and change.

Dusk: As a metaphoric symbol, dusk implies a fading life. In 2014, I drove 50 kilometres, each way from hospital to our home every day from February until April. Over that time, I watched my husband enduring his first round of chemotherapy treatment for leukaemia, initially strong and hopeful but then, after the unexpected discovery of colon cancer and resulting surgery, growing ever more weary, frail and filled with despair. As mentioned previously, 'Dusk' serves as a *thread* metaphor related to the passage of time and weaves the moments experienced into a cohesive second story. On its own, it is also a *crystalising* metaphor reflecting back to personal memories combined with current insights of how the end was in sight even then.

Although I didn't write the following poem until nine months after Don died, the words 'don't look at me' had circled incessantly around in my head on the evenings I walked from his room to the parking lot. I didn't realise at the time that I had started thinking in poetic terms and that writing poetry is a common response to grief.

The anguish of the downed

Don't look at me!
This skinned-boney, slackly muscled body in the bed is not me!
This skeletal creature with mock veins projecting from his arm and plastic conduits
    worming their way to his heart –
This frail, feeble, fellow – is not me.
That man shocking me from the mirror – watching me with black-ringed eyes agog,
With oversized elfish ears jutting from his unfamiliar head,
With sparse feather-down wisps poking from his sickly velvet dome,
With down-turned gaze, and mouth, and gait –
That pallid person is not me.

Don't look at me!
This man who trembles to stretch a band between his puny arms,
who pants after a rising and sitting down again,
who gags when meals arrive,

who struggles to greet each dawn and each visitor alike,
who dreams chimera and suspects chemo conspiracy –
This distorted, delusional, doppelganger is not me.
That man reflected in your distressed, pitying gaze –
That man whose hand you hold,
Whose despair you wrap with fragile hope,
Whose body has been sliced, re-sectioned and rearranged from inside out –
That miserable man is not me.

Look at me!
I am concealed underneath this chemical camouflage.
I am strong!
        I am scared.
I am determined!
        I am uncertain.
I am a thinker but I don't want to think.
I want to sleep.
I want to weep.
I want this life to end.

The words of this first poem convey uncertainty, vulnerability, and sense of looming tragedy. I had watched my husband live this poem and seen his eyes express these thoughts. Looking back, I understand that these words, appearing of their own accord, were an attempt to articulate what I was witnessing. Writing allowed me to finally cry out loud and was an intellectual endeavour to make sense of the silence, pain, and distress I had observed. Writing poetry requires emotion, intellect and action. It gives understanding and some measure of control over troubling circumstances. (Mazza, 2001, p. 35).

Don't Look at Me is a 'poetic conversation'. Don is talking to me and to the world – but through my voice. Much of my earliest poetry is a conversation with Don. Later my poetry is often to an unseen audience. I believe 'poetic conversations' with the deceased come up early as we think through ideas and 'sort' our thoughts. We do it 'with' them – not by ourselves – because we are only beginning the lone journey – and we are checking in with them – testing our feelings about them first before we share with others and, as the theorists posit, creating new relationships with them (Smit, 2015). The 'skeletal creature' and 'camouflaged' man are metaphors for a ravaged body. They are *crystalising* metaphors in that they connect what I witnessed in the past to what I have now come to understand (an internalised belief) about my husband's journey.

Midnight: At 'the darkest hour', my poems expressed grief and sorrow most profoundly: numbing confusion, painful loss, and a raging resistance against my husband's death. This earliest writing exposes pain – and a lament that parallels the first stage of an elegy. The idea of midnight maintains the *thread* metaphor, linking this next part of the story with previous perceptions; it grounds my experience and my sense of self within the narrative.

Why, Dylan Thomas?

Why did he move so 'gentle into that good night'?
Why did he not rant against the injustice of it all?
        Or roar: 'Why me'? Where was his fight?
It's hard to understand how he slipped out of focus
        and into my dreams – so gently, – so swiftly.
I expected him to cry out for me to tie him to the life raft.

But as waves crashed higher 'cross the bow, he didn't hold his breath
        or quake with fright.
He did not 'rage against the dying of the light'.
After his vessel was altered – became something new – something he never knew,
        after dream-like reflections curdled into a thick, foggy gloom
                and the recognisable shore no longer appeared on his horizon,

he contemplated the after-life.
After life became a turbulent, unfamiliar, moiling, boiling, seemingly endless sea,
        from inside a craft with endless seams –
                threatening imminent collapse,
he slipped into the briny and floated soundlessly away.

I wrote this poem using published verse as a starting point for reflection. Therapists and facilitators often begin therapeutic writing using published text (Field, 2006). Ideal poems, are those with the potential to elicit strong emotional responses that vary among participants who rewrite lines to fit their own stories – revealing multiple perspectives that have similar beginnings: tone, setting, environment, or plot. Each rewrite, however, is unique and personalises the emotional theme in the writer's own voice.

The poem I rewrote, by Dylan Thomas, is well known and often chosen for memorials to reflect life well lived and not easily 'given up'. My words flip the poem toward my own despair. I question whether missing rage would have prolonged my husband's life. I express my own incredulity at the dignified strength with which Don faced inevitable death. I am trying to comprehend his quiet acceptance of the 'end' when I could not and did not consent.

Illness pathographies contain common myths. The 'battle' myth attributes a military metaphor to fighting an illness. Research shows that patients who internalise a battle myth seem inspired by an increased sense of dignified self towards more active participation in their treatment, resulting in more positive outcomes. Contrary to the fight narrative, however, are stories of other patients who are unconcerned with winning or losing (Hunsaker-Hawkins, 2000).

> "Hon", he says weakly. Each word is an effort but I sense what he wants to say is most important. I lean in close to hear the gasping whispers.
>
> "Whatever you say, don't say I fought a brave battle. Or anything like that."
>
> "I wouldn't say that," I reassure him. And in the saying - I know it's true. What I will say must feel like him. And so the obituary in the paper reads: *He faced death as he faced life, with thoughtful determination and quiet strength.*

After writing the poem and reflecting upon the 'battle myth' I have come to understand how truly remarkable Don's determination to live his final days without showing weakness was. He remained, until the end, true to the man he was: one who spent his life accepting challenges and, rather than setting sights on wealth or power, took pride in serving people (family, friends, clients) in the best possible way. That kind of man does not fight a battle but faces illness and then, unbearably, faces impending death with strength characterised by restrained emotion.

In *Why Dylan Thomas?* The boat ('vessel', 'craft') is a metaphor for Don and for his failing body. The disappearing 'shoreline' metaphor acknowledges his recognition of approaching death. That he 'floated soundlessly away' affirms my belief that Don died in the way that he lived – meeting challenges without fanfare – clearly recognising the inevitable with internal courage. These metaphors are all *crystallizing;* they bridge the gap between what I witnessed as an outside observer (failing health and then death) to what I internalise as 'truth' about how it might have been for him and how he approached both life and death.

Solitary Hiking

I stumble over rocks and twisted branches on an unfamiliar path.
Another voice, now silent, once linked our separate journeys –
        called out to keep me from wandering too far off the trail.

But now in this shrill silence it's too easy to veer off course,
        to find myself, suddenly, amidst a tangled scrub
                that chokes me, trips me, catches me unprepared.

I've worn good boots, warm socks and gloves.
I've wrapped myself in fleece and down
        but I am chilled and flustered off the track.

Occasionally, echoes resonate from hidden spaces.
I get my bearings and stagger, weakly, back onto the route.
to find my stride again
        before exhaustion halts my shaky step.

The setting and plot of *Solitary Hiking* are told in the first person voice in real time. They describe event specific details: 'rocks', 'branches', 'boots', 'socks' and 'fleece' that refer to the familiar trappings of past experience. I describe myself as 'stumbling', 'unprepared', 'chilled' and 'flustered' and acknowledge the missing companion of those hikes. Here I examine a past partnership that no longer exists and admit the difficulty of being on my own although I begin to comprehend that 'echoes' (from the past) help to steady me. Cole (2005) explains that through the process of mourning one re-examines self-identity and the relationships and shared events that contributed to that identity.

Solitary Hiking nudges me metaphorically forward to hesitantly contemplate a future alone. But it is also a *crystalising* metaphor in that it allows me to recognise the present reality as disparate to a past memory. I express my fear and my new shaky existence but also sense a tentative ability to find my way back on to the path. The metaphor bridges the gap between my 'hiking' past and future. 'Hiking' (also 'trail' and 'path') are metaphors for my life journey (my personal narrative)].

It's Hard, Grief

Inner clock-workingly,
        Cog-wheeling jerkily.
Spinning incessantly nervily jangles.
Heartedly trying to
        Thought locker-downwardly.
Failingly stopping un-merry go-rounds.
Driving one witlessly
        Forward all murkily.
Grippingly, hopingly, sorting un-tangles.
        Clinging beliefessly
Life forcing faithfully.
Out-focused gazing insidedly pounds.

This poem connects to the time *thread* metaphor, however, the nonsense word 'inner clock-workingly' indicates that time is not proceeding smoothly forward but, rather, is 'spinning', 'wheeling jerkily' and caught in incessant 'un-merry go-rounds'. At the time of our loss, my son and I noticed that others, not so deeply tied to 'our beloved', although saddened by his death, seemed to be able to laugh and continue with their daily lives easily. However, we thought the world should stop and 'take note!' because we did – we stopped – we could hardly breathe – we could hardly take a step. Grief stuck us to the present and we couldn't comprehend how everything and everybody else seemed to keep moving. Grief makes it hard to move forward. It is painful to look back on what was and is now gone; it is impossible to think about anything beyond the small space you curl up in. Mourning, through the creative process of poetry writing, *nudges* one forward from that painful event back into life that moves through 'time'. The *thread* metaphor here is described as tangled mess; in other words, for me time had stopped. I had paused and stepped out of my story. By describing it, I took the first tentative step back into my narrative – my 'second story'.

In the original project, the poetry that followed linked into the *thread* metaphor under the heading: 'Middle of the Night', a metaphor for deepest sense making where, often, my verses expressed fear of the unknowable future. During this second stage of the elegy, the writing also began to acknowledge Don with appreciation and respect. I no longer seemed to be 'on pause' but found myself having many 'poetic conversations' through which I re-established my relationship, revisited memories, and tested my impressions of what was to come. I was cautiously moving back into the story of now. Part of one such 'poetic conversation' is included below.

In early December I found myself immobilised, unable to muster up excitement for the upcoming Christmas season, the second one since Don's passing. When overwhelming emotion struck, I wrote a poem called *'Well It's Been a Year'* (below is the first stanza) that, on this occasion, I also hummed to music. Unusually, I sent the poem to each of my four sons inviting them to understand. I felt, somehow, that I was letting them down.

Well it's been a year

and I still ache with sorrow
and I fall asleep each night not thinking of tomorrow
so I stay close beside you feel you linger in our spaces
knowing you have disappeared from all of my dreamed faces
and I understand
that this won't end
that it's the end

Soon after, at a holiday gathering, eight of my oldest and dearest women friends offered to help me decorate the bare tree that was standing 'undressed' in my living room. With that loving, caring gesture, by a community inviting me to re-join life in the fullest sense, Christmas was back on track. *Well it's been a Year* is a 'poetic conversation' Significant people, places, things and dates (included in the original longer version) can trigger distressful emotional reactions after loss even after a period of calm acceptance. Talking to the deceased helps to 'sort out' those feelings. It is noteworthy that this poem was written after the delight of a sunny, garden-filled summer and fall. Metaphors and 'poetic conversations' are companionable navigators and mapmakers on the switchback trail of mourning. The poetry links the painful bodily-felt emotion to intellectual understanding. This conversation *nudges* me to acknowledge 'the end'.

The next poem was a way of recreating a narrative from a muddle of emotional memories (Cole, 2005) as I began to reconstruct my sense of self and my past relationship in a new way. This poem takes an unusual and more creative form. It is not a personal lament but a biography of sorts. I no longer discuss just my own thoughts, in the first person, but reveal the ways we said: 'I love you' over a lifetime.

Saying I Love You With …

… *Gazes*
Gazes tell stories
Stares filled with words
Flashing, Laughing, Flatly Observing
Misread in low winter's light; read between lines in the glaring sun
1968
Wanted: A Creative Interpreter and Language Lessons.
… *Words*
Words disguise messages
Indicating impenetrable secrets
Unintentional hints given and guessed during life's game of Charades
Building courage to take turns.
1996
Wanted: A Game Coach and Analyst
… *Eyes*
Your blue eyes
Spilling out involuntary messages
Breaking free of your vulnerability
A love song bound within a toneless glance
2014

Wanted: A Healer and Wizard
… *Songs*
Love Songs
Hummed without melody
A lyrical lament, uplifting requiem, painful and joyous
Sung so clearly; Heard so unmistakably
2014
Wanted: A Time Traveller and Biographer

The years signify a lifetime in the poem above. The 'want ads' are *crystallizing* metaphors for all the complications we bump up against in our relationships. Despite the difficulties, death brings with it the realisation that only unconditional love and acceptance matter. The poem expresses a personal view but may reveal meaning for others in that it connects comprehension about 'was', 'is' and 'will be'.

In the poem *Life and … Death*, below, I try to construct more universal meanings by linking both those concepts to the wind and the action of scooping a hole in the sand or the scree.

Life and …

on a sandy beach we dig a hole
the sea breeze tossing words
across the sparkling water
incoherent sentences
become chuckles, indistinguishable from gulls cries
choppy waves fill the hole
as fast as we scoop, impossible to empty

… *Death*

on a rocky cliff I scrape a nook
a wailing wind whips anguish
into the moaning canyon
drowning out whispers and the cries of the jays
incessant gusts sweep beloved fragments from the hollow
leaving it forever empty

Over a lifetime our conversations may be heard clearly or, alternatively, drowned out by distraction, avoidance or interference; our actions ('scraping a nook' or 'digging a hole') fluctuate between being productive and having to begin all over again. Using metaphors and visualising familiar settings helped me construct this core meaning following bereavement (Neimeyer, 2010). Because 'human beings live in a richly symbolic world as well as a literal one [they] register loss at the level of meaning as well as in terms of physical separation' (Neimeyer, Torres, & Smith, 2011, p. 647).

We identify the 'nook' and 'hollow' as *crystallizing* metaphors that represent life and death respectively. Symbolic actions are described: digging a hole at the beach with someone special; or scrapping a hollow on a mountaintop for beloved ashes. The poem grounds a personal understanding about the cycle of life. It spans the sorrowful disconnect between activities done together in past life and acts we must perform alone after a death.

In the original project, the final poetry came under the heading of 'Dawn'. And, just as in stage three of the traditional Elegy, the last few poems (one of which is included below) convey comfort and new insight. The *thread* metaphor comes full circle here. 'Dawn' as it connects to time is the start of a new day and, as such, signifies the on-going self-narrative: different but, as yet, incomplete.

Kintsugi

I am flawed –
Cracked
Shattered
Missing pieces – crucial pieces;
Bits that held me together;

Lost parts that have altered me – inside and outside.
Ancient scars:
        Life, loss, transition.
Recent wounds:
        Life, loss, transition.

But I am intact
        Mended
                Restored
Golden stiches frame my fractured lines,
        Binding with delicate glimmering lacquer;
Altering me within and without.
Love reconstructs the splintered faults.
        Compassion caresses the golden joinery.
                Caring eyes reflect a wondrous, imperfect soul.

The art of Kintsugi refers to the Japanese art of fixing broken pottery with gold or silver dust and lacquer to give it new life. Damage, however, is illuminated rather than hidden. My poem is meant to parallel that Japanese philosophy that embraces imperfection and values the scars of life. (Keulemans, 2016). Though I have been broken by loss, I can be restored and made whole again. The missing pieces will be filled with the love and compassion of those closest to me.

Kintsugi is a *crystalising* metaphor. It represents the experience of being formerly, an intact piece of pottery, and now broken. But it will be pieced together again albeit with beautiful imperfection. The flaws are significant because they define the 'me' in my 'second story'. The piecing together is also important because it can only be done with the help of other gentle and compassionate hands – family, friends and those who read this work, discuss and view the journey from their unique and considerate perspectives.

My intuitive responses to grief, and the resulting poetry, support the notion that creative, expressive, and reflective writing can lead to sense-making and transformation. My own path of mourning attests to the complexity of loss, and fits with current grief theories that confirm the unique and circuitous journey of individual experience. Grief has led me to search for meaning, to articulate my emotions and perceptions metaphorically, and to revisit my relationship in 'poetic conversations' and from a distanced perspective in order to reimagine how it must now be. Writing has allowed me to cry and to contemplate.

My poems expose my internal dialogue: both feelings and understandings. I invite the reader into my emotional external expressions to witness 'a powerful transformative connection' of intersubjectivity (Charon, 2006, p. 52) and to consider grief: a universal human response we will all, someday, experience.

Discussion

If healthy grieving can be described as a meaning-making's process that uses metaphorical language to articulate pain and construct a new narrative (i.e. a 'second story'), one in which the deceased in dead but not lost, writing is shown here to be a promising creative method. Of course, one might argue that the case we presented to illustrate the process is only one and one written by an articulate person who demonstrates a strong reflective ability. Is writing about loss something anyone can just sit down and do?

The authors propose, based on their joint experience in social professions and in transformative writing, that this creative method can be used by anyone who can write – and that, in the face of loss, words often erupt spontaneously and compel someone to articulate them in spoken or written voice. Skilled facilitation for the individual or group may aid the process for those inexperienced in reflective analysis and for those seeking more professional guidance after loss. One of the most essential roles of the facilitator, however, is not to 'teach' but to be a benevolent witness, one the writer knows will offer a close and expert reading of the grief and trust the writer's process. The theoretical perspectives Patricia gained from the course readings, along with the knowledge that her story would be read and received by a compassionate witness/reader were essential for a deeper understanding. It should be clear that 'writing for healing' is not achieved simply by a cathartic 'dump' on the page; the course, in which Patricia participated, was structured, offered a variety of particular writing exercises, and was founded on the theoretical writing and healing model developed by Lengelle and Meijers (2009).

If poetry is a vessel for safely containing the emotions of grief, then metaphors allow for the unique expression of and give personal meaning to those emotions. *Nudging* metaphors prod one forward, bit by bit, from a 'first' story of loss into a 'second' story of life. *Thread* metaphors serve as the link whereby events and memories from the past are integrated into the present life and an imagined future after loss. Memories, rewritten as poems, serve to revive and revisit the beloved. *Crystallizing* metaphors transform bodily felt pain into thoughtful reflections and attempts to create meaning. Metaphors and poetic conversations help one move into the new reality where 'gone forever' can be recognised and acknowledged.

As the authors worked on this joint article, an additional level of reflection (and healing) was noted – Patricia spoke about gaining an even deeper appreciation of her process and was able to accept editing of the original poems and reflections without it feeling like a painful exercise. We remained mutually aware and spoke of the need to have thoughts and feelings continue to align as we wrote. We met at Patricia's home where we sat outside overlooking the beautiful space she and Don had created. We also had several phone conversations to ensure that our intellectual efforts stayed in tune with the pace and proprioceptive sense of Patricia's experience. Our academic activity became the compassionate inter-subjective reflection of a common journey that embraced the 'instinctive, sagacious and symbolic responses' we observed earlier are often missing in contexts dominated by rationality (i.e. medical world, academia). The academic discourse, which can be dividing, as noted in Bochner's (1997) work on grieving, can also be made to be enriching.

Several additional advantages of writing (over talking) also make this creative method promising in grief recovery. First, writing can be done privately; when the conversations one yearns for cannot (yet) be had with others, writing allows for the dialogical process to begin anyway. What is written, moreover, can be shared when the 'timing is right' as in this case: Patricia shared her course paper with her four sons, who in turn chose to read it in private moments when their own time was 'right' for doing so. Later each shared back with her how he had received it; the text becoming an object of reflection. The internal dialogue fostered through the writing, in other words, can ease the transition into the external dialogue. The comfort one cultivates in talking about death and accompanying feelings lowers the threshold in sharing with others; it normalises grief (e.g. 'If I can admit to myself how I felt, it's easier to share it with my sons').

Conclusion

Writing expressively, creatively and reflectively can aid grieving because the process is inherently dialogical and narrative in structure and healing metaphors appear which serve to guide the bereaved towards new (i.e. second) stories. The act of writing about the facts and emotions of what has and who has been lost, allow the bereaved to evoke the beloved in a way that reintegrates them into the life story. Indeed, the beautiful paradox is that by writing, death is acknowledged, but the beloved is 'retained' and becomes part of a new, life-giving story that moves us forward.

To encourage those facing loss to begin to put words or poems on a page is not as scary as it sounds. Poetry therapists are adept at using existing poems of love and loss to get the process going and our personal courage to 'voice' loss – first on paper and then out loud as Patricia has done here – gives others courage too. Whether we are encouraging our students, our clients, our friends and kin, or ourselves to heal with the pen, we know that we need not explore alone, unsupported, or feel unheard as we delve into poetic encounters with 'that good night'.

Disclosure statement

No potential conflict of interest was reported by the authors.

References

Anderson, C., & MacCurdy, M. (2000). *Writing and healing: Toward an informed practice*. Urbana, IL: National Council of Teachers of English.

Arnold, J., & Gemma, P. B. (2008). The continuing process of parental grief. *Death Studies, 32*(7), 658–673. doi:10.1080/07481180802215718

Bochner, A. P. (1997). It's about time: Narrative and the divided self. *Qualitative Inquiry, 3*(4), 418–438. doi:10.1177/107780049700300404

Bolton, G. (1999). *The therapeutic potential of creative writing: Writing myself*. London: Jessica Kingsley Publishers.

Buglass, E. (2010). Grief and bereavement theories. *Nursing Standard, 24*, 44–47. doi:10.7748/ns.24.41.44.s46

Charon, R. (2006). *Narrative medicine: Honoring the stories of illness*. Oxford: Oxford University Press.

Cole, A. H. J. (2005). Elegiac poetry: A pastoral resource with complicated grief. *Pastoral Psychology, 53*(3), 189–206. doi:10.1007/s11089-004-0553-6

Currier, J. M., Holland, J. M., & Neimeyer, R. A. (2006). Sense making, grief and the experience of violent loss: Toward a mediational model. *Death Studies, 30*, 403–428. doi:10.1080/07481180600614351

DeSalvo, L. A. (1999). *Writing as a way of healing: How telling our stories transforms our lives*. Boston, MA: Beacon Press.

Field, V. (2006). Writing from published poems. In G. Bolton, V. Field, & K. Thompson (Eds.), *Writing work: A resource handbook for therapeutic writing workshops and activities* (pp. 97–118). London: Jessica Kingsley Publishers.

Furnes, B., & Dysvik, E. (2011). Results from a systematic writing program in grief process: Part 2. *Patient Preference and Adherence, 5*, 15–21. doi:10.2147/PPA.S15155

Goldsworthy, K. K. (2005). Grief and loss theory in social work practice: All changes involve loss, just as all losses require change. *Australian Social Work, 58*(2), 167–178. doi:10.1111/j.1447-0748.2005.00201.x

Goss, R., & Klass, D. (2005). *Dead but not lost: Grief narratives in religious traditions*. Lanham, MD: Rowman Altamira.

Hall, C. (2014). Bereavement theory: Recent developments in our understanding of grief and bereavement. *Bereavement Care, 33*(2014), 7–12. Web. doi:10.1080/02682621.2014.902610

Hardy-Bougere, M. (2008). Cultural manifestations of grief and bereavement: A clinical perspective. *Journal of Cultural Diversity, 15*(2), 66–69.

Hermans, H. J. M., & Hermans-Konopka, A. (2010). *Dialogical self theory: Positioning and counter-positioning in a globalizing society*. Cambridge: Cambridge University Press.

Hunsaker-Hawkins, A. (2000). Pathography and enabling myths. In C.M. Anderson, & M. McCurdy (Eds.), *Writing and healing: Towards and informed practice* (pp. 222–245). Urbana, IL: National Council of Teachers of English.

Hunt, C. (2000). *Therapeutic dimensions of autobiography in creative writing*. London: Jessica Kingsley Publishers.

Keulemans, G. (2016). The geo-cultural conditions of kintsugi. *The Journal of Modern Craft, 9*(1), 15–34. doi:10.1080/17496772.2016.1183946

Kübler-Ross, E. (2009). *On death and dying: What the dying have to teach doctors, nurses, clergy and their own families*. Oxon: Taylor & Francis.

Lengelle, R., Meijers, F., & Hughes, D. (2016). Creative writing for life design: Reflexivity, metaphors and change processes through narrative. *Journal of Vocational Behavior* (in press).

Lengelle, R., & Meijers, F. (2009). Mystery to mastery: An exploration of what happens in the black box of writing and healing. *Journal of Poetry Therapy, 22*, 57–75. doi:10.1080/08893670903072935

Lengelle, R. (2008). *Narrative possibilities: The transformative power of writing, story, and poetry in personal and professional development (MAIS 621 course)*. Athabasca, AB: Athabasca University.

Mazza, N. (2001). The place of the poetic in dealing with death and loss. *Journal of Poetry Therapy, 15*(1), 29–35. doi:10.1023/A:1012962923701

Mazza, N. (2003). *Poetry therapy: Theory and practice.* New York: Psychology Press.

Meijers, F., & Lengelle, R. (2012). Narratives at work: The development of a career identity. *British Journal of Guidance and Counselling, 40*, 157–177.

Neimeyer, R. A., Klass, D., & Dennis, M. R. (2014). A social constructionist account of grief: Loss and the narration of meaning. *Death Studies, 38*(8), 485–498. doi:10.1080/07481187.2014.913454

Neimeyer, R. A. (2010). Reconstructing the continuing bond: A constructivist approach to grief therapy. *Studies in Meaning, 4*, 65–91.

Neimeyer, R. A., Torres, C., & Smith, D. C. (2011). The virtual dream: Rewriting stories of loss and grief. *Death Studies, 35*(7), 646–672. doi:10.1080/07481187.2011.570596

Nia, H. S., Lehto, R. H., Ebadi, A., & Peyrovi, H. (2016). Death anxiety among nurses and health care professionals: A review article. *International Journal of Community Based Nursing and Midwifery, 4*(1), 2–10.

Parkes, C. M., Laungani, P., & Young, W. (Eds.). (2015). *Death and bereavement across cultures.* New York, NY: Routledge.

Pennebaker, J. W. (2011). The secret life of pronouns. *New Scientist, 211*(2828), 42–45. doi:10.1016/S0262-4079(11)62167-2

Pennebaker, J. W. (2012). *Opening up: The healing power of expressing emotions.* New York, NY: Guilford Press.

Schafer, C. (2012). Corpses, conflict and insignificance? A critical analysis of post- mortem practices. *Mortality, 17*(4), 305–321. doi:10.1080/13576275.2012.731724

Smit, C. (2015). Theories and models of grief: Applications to professional practice. *Whitireia Nursing & Health Journal, 22*, 33–37. 5p.

Teno, J. M., Clarridge, B. R., Casey, V., Welch, L. C., Wetle, T., Shield, R., & Mor, V. (2004). Family perspectives on end-of-life care at the last place of care. *JAMA, 291*(1), 88–93.

Valentine, C. (2007). The "moment of death". *OMEGA - Journal of Death and Dying, 55*(3), 219–236. doi:10.2190/OM.55.3.d

Walter, T. (1996). A new model of grief: Bereavement and biography. *Mortality, 1*, 7–25. doi:10.1080/713685822

Worden, J. W. (2002). *Grief counseling and grief therapy: A handbook for the mental health practitioner* (3rd ed.). New York: Springer.

Zimmermann, C., & Rodin, G. (2004). The denial of death thesis: Sociological critique and implications for palliative care. *Palliative Medicine, 18*(2), 121–128. doi:10.1191/0269216304pm858oa

Zweig, S. C., & Oliver, D. P. (2009). Returning from the total institution to a home environment: A journey for birthing and dying. *Journal of Housing for the Elderly, 23*(1), 116–129. doi:10.1080/02763890802665064

Construction of narrative identity based on paintings

Katarzyna Garwolińska, Piotr K. Oleś and Anna Gricman

ABSTRACT
This article presents a new method for encouraging clients to articulate and explore their narrative identities. The method combines the advantages of perception of art and of construction of narrative identity. It is inspired by McAdams 'Life Story Interview' and Hermans and Hermans-Jansen's Self-Confrontation Method. The material is a set of 100 colour copies of paintings that introduce a spectrum of life experiences and symbolic scenes. The person is asked to choose as many pictures as he/she needs to present his/her life story and to tell this story looking at the pictures. The clients construct their stories and they assume units of meanings in valuations (sentences). Afterwards they create life themes referring to sets of pictures or valuations.

Introduction

Narrative therapy engages both a client and a therapist in a narrative mode of thinking specific to telling and retelling stories (Bruner, 1990). Numerous functions of self-narratives make this approach not only attractive for the therapist but also very friendly for clients. Telling and listening are natural elements of interpersonal contact, interesting the participants in interaction and fulfilling basic needs of affiliation and self-esteem. Being listened to means being important for another person. Self-narratives make expression of apparent and hidden emotions possible in order to share a unique experience with another person, to gain a sense of being understood and to understand oneself better (Carr, 1998; Freedman & Combs, 1996). Moreover, it enables the person to construct his/her story about the self, other people and the external world and to determine how it fits with reality. A life story that connects a person's past, present and future and gives a sense of meaning and continuity in life constitutes narrative identity (McAdams, 1993). Telling and retelling one's own story, stimulated by good questions, can increase personal ability to get proper distance on personal experience or events and their interpretations. Moreover, narrative identity is always a kind of personal myth, so retelling it or trying other versions or interpretations of the events and experiences broadens the personal perspective of self-understanding and may influence particular decisions, goals or forms of activity in the future. According to psychological research, forming a story or self-narrative guided by self-reflection and inspiring even deeper self-reflection can contribute to personal maturity or wisdom, coping with difficult life events and post-traumatic personal growth (Hermans & Hermans-Jansen, 1995; McAdams, 1993; McAdams & Olson, 2010; Neimeyer, 2006; Ramirez-Esparza & Pennebaker, 2006).

We propose a new method for inspiring a client to construct a personal life story based on pictures. The method combines advantages of perception of art and construction of narrative identity. The method is inspired by studies on aesthetic perception of beauty in art, by McAdams (1993) theory of narrative identity and his Life Story Interview, and by Hermans (2003) valuation theory and the Self-Confrontation Method (Hermans & Hermans-Jansen, 1995).

The method refers to intuitive assessment of the aesthetic value of the picture and to analytical reflection on life experiences, important life events, turning points and in general, one's life story. Looking at the pictures implies affective engagement that stimulates biographical memory and activates the system of personal meanings. In fact, paintings, sculptures and other pieces of art used in work with clients help them understand their difficult experiences such as illness (White, Perlman, Fantona, & Kumagai, 2010).

Why do we propose pictures? How do they influence the quality of self-narratives? As Clovis (2012) and Strydom (2007) argue, our perception of beauty is connected to our identity, which means art can inspire self-reflection on identity but also opens us up to intrinsic values when our own desire for pure value meets external expressions of associated value in paintings, sculptures or any other piece of art. Pictures release the imaginative and iconic representations of common myths and thus enrich the self-understanding of the person.

Looking at small reproductions of paintings diverts one's attention from personal problems and inhibitions during a therapeutic session and encourages paying attention to universal icons of human experiences in which one can identify one's own experiences. It allows perceiving personal problems as inevitable and sometimes even important parts of life. In this way, the person gains additional motivation to tell his/her life story and reduce internal obstacles to doing so.

Paintings like in a lens, introduce universal human experiences and in this way may evoke imagination and episodic memory to (re)produce important personal meanings. Thus, we consider if using pictures instead of questions can inspire people to tell their stories. Questions are abstract and not emotional in their nature, and the pictures are concrete or abstract, but nevertheless full of connotative (affective) meanings.

Description of the method

Materials

We propose a set of small reproductions of 100 paintings showing different scenes and human experiences. The pictures are more or less balanced in content according to sex and age of figures in them and interactions between people of the same and different age groups. Some pictures present nature or the countryside, places, trees, forests, fields, houses or streets. The paintings are printed in colour and printed as about 8 cm × 5 cm reproductions with the original proportions (see: Appendix).

In addition, we use some parts of the Self-Confrontation Method, the interview schemata and original list of 24 affect terms with a six-point rating scale (from 0 – not at all; 5 – very much). The entire Self-Confrontation Method includes three sets of questions related to personal past, present and future. A common task for a client is to formulate valuations as sentences that represent important parts of their personal story. The valuation is a unit of meaning: important, personal (e.g. expressed in a unique way by the person) and specific, that is, related (directly or indirectly) to defined time and space. The Self-Confrontation Method is used in counselling and research as a method of assessment and stimulation of change. It allows to explore a system of personal valuations as well as their affective meanings (Lyddon, Yowell, & Hermans, 2006).

In this application of the method, we propose using a few open-ended questions encouraging the person to tell a personal story associated with a given picture. Each picture is chosen for story construction and each valuation is rated across a standard list of 24 affect terms (Hermans & Hermans-Jansen, 1995, p. 277). Relationships among affective profiles, computed as Euclidian distances or Pearson's correlations, allow understanding their mutual – and for the person, not so obvious – similarities and differences among personal experiences and perceptions of the pictures.

Procedure

The procedure consists of six stages. First, a helper introduces the method by showing a set of 100 pictures and inviting the person to choose several pictures associated with their important experiences or life events. At this stage, participants usually select a few, a dozen or so (the most common) or even over 25 pictures. They often spontaneously put the pictures in an order.

In the second stage, the person is asked to tell his/her personal stories connected to the pictures. The most common approaches use a one by one picture technique, sometimes combining a group of pictures for a more complex story. In this stage, the participant creates a narrative about his/her life with the paintings. While telling about their own experiences, the participants are formulating valuations.

The helper asks about adequate valuations (sentences) representing significant part(s) of each story. Most often, one picture evokes one valuation, but sometimes, one picture can stimulate more valuations (e.g. the person looking at a couple in the picture tells about falling in love, sharing time and souls, conflicts and jealousy, and leave-taking and thus needs four valuations to express all necessary personal meanings). The person may also need more than one picture for one valuation (e.g. looking at a nice house in one picture and at ruins in another, he/she tells about a shift from happy family life to the divorce of parents). Thus, the goal of this stage is twofold: to tell personal stories and to reflect them at an angle that provides the most important personal meaning of them – construction of valuations.

A goal of the third stage is to explore affective meaning of paintings as well as valuations by rating them (pictures and valuations) with affect terms and a six-point rating scale. In this stage, the helper or psychotherapist computes affective indices of each valuation and each picture. The affective profile consists of 24 ratings because of the number of affect terms. The profiles are then compared by mean correlations that result in clusters of valuations or pictures having similar affective profiles.

There are also four indices characterising each valuation or picture: P – the sum of the ratings of eight positive affects (e.g. joy or satisfaction); N – the sum of the ratings of eight negative affects (e.g. anxiety, anger); S – the sum of the ratings of four affect terms related to the self-enhancement motive (S motive, e.g. self-esteem, strength); and O – the sum of the ratings of four affect terms related to longing and union with the other (O motive, e.g. love or care). A combination of high P and high motive means gratification of that motive, while a combination of high N and high motive means frustration and activation of the motive.

During the fourth stage, the person knows affective climates (meanings) of the valuations and pictures. The helper or therapist introduces correlations among valuations (pictures) and explains the meanings of affective indices (S, O, P, N). Then, valuations or pictures are introduced to the client as groups according to their affective similarities respectively. The therapist or helper asks the client about his/her interpretation of such similarities. These questions are posed in a specific way for the valuations (pictures) that have common affective meaning and may represent significant life themes (or plots). The questions are: What is a common meaning of these valuations (pictures) for you? Do they represent any theme currently important in your life? What do they, as a group, mean for you?

Two short examples can clarify this stage. First, providing that affective profiles of valuations concerning unhappy love, longing for parents in childhood and a stressful relationship with a friend correlates with each other to a high degree, their common meaning may represent growing autonomy emerging from difficult life conditions. Second, if the pictures no. 7, 9, 31, 44, 57 and 86 (see Appendix) have common affective meaning (high correlations among their affective profiles), their common meaning may be expressed as: 'A close relationship helps to overcome loneliness.'

The participant can try to construct or discover his/her life motto based on the pictures and/or the valuations. Theme extraction via the received correlations of the affective climates of the valuations or paintings help people express, discover or understand what is crucial for their life stories. Moreover, the person has a chance to compose various experiences into a complex but integrated whole, which helps him/her gain a bird's-eye view of his/her life stories. The person can also compare life themes generated on the basis of valuations as well as on pictures. When there is more than one cluster of mutually related valuations (pictures), the person can generate more than one life theme.

Short case studies

Case 1. Adam: To be one's own man is to decide, but also to feel closeness.

Adam is a 24-year old man, graduated in physics, just finished his studies. He seems to be active, engaged in life desires and interested in gaining a deeper insight. His main motivation was not to resolve any special problem or to overcome a difficult situation, he just intended to know more about himself and to combine different personal experiences and meanings. A characteristic feature of his life-narrative was an almost perfect chronology from the past through present to future. Altogether he chose 17 pictures, 14 beautiful (82%) and 3 not beautiful.

Using 17 pictures, Adam constructed 17 valuations introducing his life story (Table 1). In general, he formulated one valuation in reference to one picture, as most people do. However, in two cases, he formulated two valuations in association to one picture (valuations 2 and 3; 7 and 8) and in one case, he used three pictures for one valuation (10). Adam's story seems full of meaningful experiences. He reflected on his childhood, finding positive and negative experiences, and the same is true for his adolescence and emerging adulthood. Interestingly enough, even if a valuation is positive (P > N), negative affects still exist to some degree and the same is true for negative experiences, as even if a valuation is negative (N > P), positive affects still exist to some degree. Some valuations are ambivalent (11 and 2). Adam is able to confront himself with various aspects of his past and current life, reflecting positive sides of negative experiences as well as negative aspects of positive experiences. Moreover, he is aware of different kinds of experiences like being a winner (10, 12) or loser, love (3) and *fugit amor* (1), power and unity (e.g. 6, 15), or powerlessness and isolation (14) (see Hermans & Hermans-Jansen, 1995). One can say that his story is rooted in reality, which does not preclude that it may represent personal myth (see McAdams, 1993). When rating ideal experiences, Adam used

Table 1. Adam's valuations and their affective indices.

No.	Valuations	S	O	P	N
1.	When I was in the nursing home, I realised the importance of my parents' taking care of me at home. (picture 53)	4	9	6	21
2.	The sense of carelessness connected with my childhood and exploring the world. (83)	8	13	30	40
3.	When I was a child, I was bored for most of the time. I was asking adults a lot of questions. (83)	7	11	25	11
4.	I was really happy with the fact that I had a sister and I enjoyed playing with her. (41)	9	12	24	5
5.	I was jealous because I was not the apple of my parents' eye any more – Ann took my place. (65)	3	8	10	24
6.	Family trips to the mountains made me happy. (71)	12	14	32	3
7.	During one of the holidays, I was playing a chess with Tom, which I recollect with a smile. (93)	14	3	20	7
8.	Tom is mentally ill. I am not able to keep in touch with him. I feel very sad when I think of him. (93)	8	7	5	18
9.	Pride and self-confidence arising from successes achieved in high school and participation in physics Olympiad. (39)	19	2	20	14
10.	The feeling of alienation in high school and loneliness that transformed into sense of dominance. (14, 51, 6)	11	1	12	27
11.	While I was lonely and walking by the sea during holidays, I realised that people spend their time playing and dancing, but I prefer to walk and think about different things. (24)	14	5	18	16
12.	Problems during my third year at university, being satisfied with learning more and more complicated things, feeling integrated with colleges from the university. (47)	15	4	27	3
13.	At the beginning of the relationship with Barbara, something new appeared. I fell in love. (96)	11	13	26	6
14.	A crisis during learning in the fourth year of studies, hard and difficult work, feeling that physics might not be good for me. (20)	2	0	4	25
15.	Realizing the importance of my decision about the wedding, the vision of a shared life with B. (37)	13	14	25	4
16.	The sensed aspect of a life with Barbara, admiring her feminine beauty. (54)	12	18	23	8
17.	The aspiration of self-realisation, the pursuit of passion. (21)	16	4	27	11
18.	How are you feeling recently?	12	10	21	7
19.	How would you like to feel?	17	14	30	0

positive affect terms, omitting all negative ones and emphasising both basic motives and a motive for self-enhancement a little bit more.

A general impression emerging from these valuations is that Adam could manage or cope with difficult experiences and transform them into autonomy and self-directed behaviour: ability to love and work. In fact, when he referred to a set of valuations which had high correlations among their affective profiles (6, 15, 2, 13 and 4), he formulated their common topic as follows: 'I perceive my life as the realisation of new goals, often with the help of hard work and determined input – until recently alone, now and in the future with Barbara.' When he referred to pictures similar in their affective climates (39, 24, 71, 21 and 96), he said something different but complementary: 'The thing that is always important is the presence of my loved ones because of their understanding and happiness.' This necessary condition of happiness originates from childhood experiences of carelessness and adolescent experiences of loneliness, as well as current experiences of love and sharing a common world with a close person. Telling his life story and looking at the pictures, and reflecting on personal valuations made Adam clearly aware of his history, conditions of optimal functioning and ability to share life with another person.

Case 2: Aga: A life story should be positive.

Aga is a 24-year old woman, who following college where she studied economy got a job in a company. She is single and not ready to have a close relationship with another person. Her childhood was difficult and stressful due to permanent conflicts between parents. Her parents lived separately, however, at the same house and both had tried to play their daughter – Aga – one against another. So, Aga felt split between mother and father. Aga used 25 pictures, but she constructed only 10 valuations to describe her life story (Table 2), using 23 beautiful pictures and only 2 not beautiful. She told her story in a specific way: first, she divided the pictures into 10 groups and then she formulated one valuation for each group; second, she avoided the present, telling only about her past or future; third, she expressed emotions in a direct way, crying when she told about the past and laughing when telling about the future.

Almost all valuations (except 10, which is a little bit ambivalent) are strictly positive (P > N). The story resembles wishful thinking in a way and it certainly functions in the service of well-being, optimism and faith in a good future. One can also find signs of continuity from childhood ('When I was miserable, my mum hugged me'), through positive expectations and desires concerning the future, to symbolic extension of one's life ('My grave should be kept in order. I would like people to respect me after my death'). This last valuation seems unexpected in this story which clarifies life priorities. A theme of a life story based on paintings – 'We live in order to match ourselves with someone, to give birth, to take care of this new-born' – illustrates such a function very well. However, a theme created on valuations seems as unexpected as the last valuation concerning the grave: 'Sex is necessary in life, because it gives us babies who make our life meaningful.' Probably both are symptoms of a

Table 2. Aga's valuations and their affective indices.

No.	Valuations	S	O	P	N
1.	When I was miserable, my mum hugged me. (pictures 69, 70)	11	16	30	2
2.	In the future, I would like to have a lot of babies who will play together and will be happy. (9, 65, 67, 31)	12	13	34	0
3.	A marriage with a man with whom I share a life, problems, and time. I feel calm and carefree. There are no arguments or serious troubles. (15, 63, 37, 17)	15	19	34	1
4.	I would like to have a house by the sea, where I would be able to observe the sunrise and sunset among many animals. (95, 48, 3, 5)	12	15	37	0
5.	Financial stability that lets me feel safe. (74)	7	0	26	0
6.	There are important friends around me with whom I can have fun, talk and share time. (57, 94, 81)	12	9	36	0
7.	Passion, sex, desire and romance with my husband. (54, 42, 27)	12	18	34	0
8.	When I was young, I was always waiting for my parents to take care of me. (62, 83)	7	11	23	9
9.	Motherhood, taking care of my baby. (53)	11	18	34	0
10.	My grave should be kept in order. I would like people to respect me after my death. (33)	3	11	21	15
11.	How are you feeling recently?	10	16	29	7
12.	How would you like to feel?	15	20	40	0

hidden narrative structure related to real life dilemmas. Note that no one valuation expresses engagement in everyday activity, current concerns or personal problems. Instead, the person justifies intimate or sexual relationships and wonders about the condition of her grave. Both probably are important personal signs of deep existential dilemmas that need further discussion with a helper. One more observation: both general and ideal affective states are positive and emphasise fulfillment of both motives; a little bit more longing for contact and union with the other, and a little bit less for self-enhancement. Readiness and the need for a close emotional relationship plays a role in the most important life plot in an actual life situation, which is another starting point for counselling.

Modifications and extensions

The method is flexible. Some changes and/or extensions are possible. One is to include one blank white 5 × 8 cm card at the end of the therapeutic session with a question: Is there any experience, life event, person or reflection that is significant for your story but has been omitted up until now? Is something necessary to complete your story or to understand it properly that you would like to add? If yes, please tell me about it as it would be symbolised in that picture.[1]

One can also use figurative and abstract paintings, both black and white and coloured. According to our experiences, people deal with abstract pictures in a very similar way as they do with figurative pictures, but abstract pictures are especially inspiring for stories about the future. Most participants are able to tell personal stories while looking at abstract paintings almost as well as when they are referring to figurative paintings. Moreover, when we ask specifically about personal futures, abstract pictures seem very friendly objects for such self-narratives. We believe this is due to their form, which is open to flexible interpretations, just like perspectives on open futures. This fits very well to an important function of narrative therapy, namely construction of alternative stories that are sometimes more adaptive than current and strictly personal stories (Angus & McLeod, 2004; Dimaggio, Salvatore, Azzara, & Catania, 2003; Freedman & Combs, 1996; Morgan, 2000). We find indirect confirmation that stories constructed in reference to abstract pictures are more varied than stories constructed in reference to figurative paintings. However, figurative paintings can also inspire various and flexible interpretations like in Adam's case where picture 93 led to two quite different valuations: positive (7) and negative (8), due to power of imagination as well as uniqueness of personal experience and associations.

Last but not least, one can work with valuations as in a regular Self-Confrontation Method, remembering, however, that they originated from pictures combined with life memories but not from regular sets of questions about personal past, present and future. Self-narratives based on pictures are especially suitable to exploring given aspects of a personal life story which are particularly intriguing for the person and not necessarily the life story as a whole (as in Aga's case). However, using valuations for modal analysis raises a question about similarities and differences regarding possible results of such analyses based on pictures or valuations. It could also lead to comparisons of affective profiles of the pictures and the valuations. According to our results, the emotional climate of the pictures and of personal valuations constructed in association with the pictures corresponded quite well, but the affective structure of the valuations did not replicate the affective structure of the pictures.

The method is also open to other modifications, for example pictures selected for gender research, identity or midlife crisis, or career development.

What are the advantages of pictures in contrast to telling the story? First, the person looking at the pictures and associating them with his/her own memories has a special kind of experience. On the one hand, he/she confronts his/her own affects and thoughts evoked by an external visualisation of human experience of the same or very similar kind as his/her own. It means that he/she finds himself in a larger context of universal human experience. Something which has been regarded as unique as well as strange or threatening in a personal story has become familiar. It encourages the person to explore his/her cognitive-affective experience. Second, in finding himself/herself in a piece of art, one can distance himself/herself and simultaneously feel indirectly socially supported because somebody has experienced something similar. Third, many people have inhibitions or obstacles when they are asked about their life stories, even if they want to share that story. A picture works as a distraction because the person is interested in its content and meaning and can have an impression that refers to the picture telling a personal story. He/she can also go beyond personal problems in creating a story that relies on a continuation of current life events and personal situations (Batory, 2014; Kunnen, 2006). Abstract paintings especially stimulate such phenomena. This seems quite parallel to stories created in a thematic apperception test (Murray, 1943/1971), in which people are asked what would happen next.

In contrast to McAdams (1993) approach in which the questions indirectly emphasise continuity of the life story, in our approach, each picture is different to encourage telling different parts of the life story from different perspectives or so-called I-positions like for example in Aga's case (Hermans, 2003; see also Angus & McLeod, 2004; Holstein & Gubrium, 2003). Such changes allow reflection on one's life from various points of view to broaden insight and construct a multidimensional model of life experience that is one of the functions of metacognition (Dimaggio & Lysaker, 2010). Moreover, it increases chances to overcome shortcomings caused by not adopting a fixed I-position (or perspective), if it exists. Through facing universal human experiences in the pictures, one can change his/her mind about how to evaluate a given event, personal relationship or experience from quite new perspectives. We argue that while McAdams' questions evoke convergent rather than divergent thinking, the pictures as a basis for personal stories evoke divergent rather than convergent thinking. Thus, the proposed approach is open for creation of a saturated as well as integrated self (Gergen, 1991). This does not mean that it could lead to disintegration of various parts or plots of a personal story, as all those parts or plots constitute a complex story of a unique person. It means that the person confronts himself/herself with a real challenge about how to integrate various plots and experiences in his/her life. By having a bird's-eye view of one's personal history, one is able to retell one's personal story or reflect on it.

Our clients reported significant personal experiences, insight and self-understanding as well as showing authentic emotions. When we reflect on their personal expression during life story construction, from a point of view of our clinical and research experience, we would like to suggest higher engagement in story telling based on pictures than in McAdams' life story interview. This aspect should be explored more systematically. The paintings (probably) engage both intuition and analytical thinking and episodic memory, while questions from the life story evoke mainly the analytical system and semantic biographical memory. The paintings invite participants into a universal world of happiness and suffering, longing, fighting and love, thus helping them anchor their individual meanings in a broad scope of human experiences.

It can be concluded that the participants were very involved when they created life stories with the use of paintings. They looked for values they believe in, ideological thoughts, secret dreams or important personal experiences. The stories were very different and interesting. The respondents were willing to talk about their childhood memories, important people in their lives or dreams connected with having a family, experiencing happiness, professional careers, self-development or a calm and cheerful old age. Sometimes, they were even quite enigmatic for the researcher, who was not able to understand a particular valuation. Some participants cried or recognised meanings of the facts about their life or their decisions. The paintings stimulate memories and help one to express one's experiences, thoughts, emotions and dreams. They also stimulate a person in an affective, cognitive and behavioural way. Constructing a narrative identity is more than a set of facts or life situations. During sessions, participants looked for answers related to their identities. They tried to find meaning or unity in their lives. What is also interesting is that people were able to extract a main theme of a life story based on paintings. Moreover, their themes were complementary.

Possible applications

The main function of this approach to open the person to a new and inspiring interpretation of a personal life story. It does not imply changing narrative identity but rather an extension of personal understanding of it and modification of future aspects of it. Thus, the method can be applied for all who need to understand themselves better or those who want to change themselves. It seems particularly useful for adolescents looking for identity formation and for young or middle-aged adults looking for inspiration for personal development (Arnett, 2000; McLean, 2008; Pals, 2001; Waterman, 1999). The method can also be applied in clients experiencing emotional crises, facing difficult life decisions, coping with personal events influencing their lives, experiencing difficulties typical for identity crisis, or interested in personal development or insight.

A similar method has been used in Uganda to make people more aware of common stories shared in their culture, but telling stories inspired by illustrations, paintings or sculpture which not only inspired common identity but also personal identity (Palmo, 2010). This seems to be an important function of art; opening people to self-transcendence by overcoming one's point of view and participating in the universe of human meanings.

The method is proposed for psychological counselling and stimulation of self-reflection as well as personal development towards optimal functioning (Sheldon, 2004) or psychological well-being (Ryff, 1995). It can be included in narrative therapy or combined with other approaches.

Note

1. This proposal originates from Murray's (1943/1971) thematic apperception test and from McAdam's fresh version of the 'Life Story Interview'.

Disclosure statement

No potential conflict of interest was reported by the authors.

Funding

This study was inspired and supported by [grant number UMO-2013/11/B/HS6/01816], 'Psychological and neurophysiological determinants of aesthetic judgments' founded by National Science Center, Poland.

References

Angus, L., & McLeod, J. (2004). Self-multiplicity and narrative expression in psychotherapy. In H. J. M. Hermans, & G. Dimaggio (Eds.), *The dialogical self in psychotherapy* (pp. 77–90). Hove and New York: Brunner–Routledge.

Arnett, J. J. (2000). Emerging adulthood: A theory of development from the late teens through the twenties. *American Psychologist, 55*(5), 469–480.

Batory, A. (2014). Reorganization of personal identity in the context of motivational dynamics and internal dialogical activity. *Scandinavian Journal of Psychology, 55*, 362–370.

Bruner, J. S. (1990). *Acts of meaning*. Cambridge: Harvard University Press.

Carr, A. (1998). Michael White's narrative therapy. *Contemporary Family Therapy, 20*(4), 485–503.

Clovis, D. (2012). Issues of beauty through identity: The works of three artists in studio practice and their interpretations into art and language. *Dissertation Abstracts International Section A: Humanities and Social Sciences, 73(2-A)*, 448.

Dimaggio, G., & Lysaker, P.H. (Eds.). (2010). *Metacognition and severe adult mental disorders: From research to treatment.* New York: Routledge/Taylor & Francis Group.

Dimaggio, G., Salvatore, G., Azzara, C., & Catania, D. (2003). Rewriting self-narratives: The therapeutic process. *Journal of Constructivist Psychology, 16,* 155–181.

Freedman, J., & Combs, G. (1996). *Narrative therapy. The social construction of preferred realities.* New York: Norton.

Gergen, K. J. (1991). *The saturated self: Dilemmas of identity in contemporary life.* New York: Basic Books.

Hermans, H. J. M. (2003). The construction and reconstruction of a dialogical self. *Journal of Constructivist Psychology, 16,* 89–130.

Hermans, H. J. M., & Hermans-Jansen, E. (1995). *Self-narratives: The construction of meaning in psychotherapy.* New York: The Guilford Press.

Holstein, J. A., & Gubrium, J. F. (Eds.). (2003). *Inside interviewing. New lenses, new concerns.* London: Sage.

Kunnen, E. S. (2006). Are conflicts the motor in identity change? *Identity: An International Journal of Theory and Research, 6* (2), 169–186.

Lyddon, W. J., Yowell, D. R., & Hermans, H. J. M. (2006). The self-confrontation method: Theory, research, and practical utility. *Counselling Psychology Quarterly, 19*(1), 27–43.

McAdams, D. P. (1993). *The stories we live by: Personal myths and the making of the self.* New York: William Morrow.

McAdams, D. P., & Olson, B. D. (2010). Personality development: Continuity and change over the life course. *Annual Review of Psychology, 61,* 517–542.

McLean, K. (2008). Stories of the young and the old: Personal continuity and narrative identity. *Developmental Psychology, 44,* 254–264.

Morgan, A. (2000). *What is narrative therapy. An easy-to read introduction.* Gecko: Dulwich Centre Publication.

Murray, H. A. (1943/1971). *The Thematic apperception test: Manual.* Cambridge, MA: Cambridge University Press.

Neimeyer, R. A. (2006). Narrating the dialogical self: Toward an expanded toolbox for the counselling psychologist. *Counselling Psychology Quarterly, 19,* 105–120.

Palmo, M. (2010). The artistic process in community development: Disclosing cultural narrative and identity through art practices in Uganda. *Dissertation Abstracts International Section A: Humanities and Social Sciences, 71(6-A),* 2118.

Pals, J. L. (2001). Identity: A contextualized mechanism of personality continuity and change. *Psychological Inquiry, 12,* 88–91.

Ramirez-Esparza, N., & Pennebaker, J. W. (2006). Do good stories produce good health? Exploring words, language and culture. *Narrative Inquiry, 16,* 211–219.

Ryff, C. D. (1995). Psychological well-being in adult life. *Current Directions in Psychological Science, 4,* 99–104.

Sheldon, K. M. (2004). *Optimal human being. An integrated multi-level perspective.* Mahwah, NJ: Lawrence Erlbaum Associates, Publishers.

Strydom, M. (2007). Five daughters of eve are painting an angel: The use of therapeutic art in the realisation of spiritual identity in the young adult woman. *Dissertation Abstracts International Section A: Humanities and Social Sciences, 67(8-A),* 3032.

Waterman, A. S. (1999). Identity, the identity statuses, and identity status development: A contemporary statement. *Developmental Review, 19,* 591–621.

White, C. B., Perlman, R. L., Fantona, J. C., & Kumagai, A. K. (2010). The interpretive project: A creative educational approach to fostering medical students' reflections and advancing humanistic medicine. *Reflective Practice, 11,* 517–527.

Appendix

	PICTURES	Artist	Link
1	The Proud Ship	Montague Dawson	https://www.allpainter.com/montague-dawson/the-proud-ship-handmade-oil-painting-reproduction-280670.html
2	Tree in Autumn	Jenish Pansuriya	https://stock.adobe.com/pl/images/tree-in-autumn/324465282?as_campaign=tineye&as_content=tineye_match&clickref=1100lxNxPCso&mv=affiliate&mv2=pz&as_camptype=backlink&as_channel=affiliate&as_source=partnerize&fbclid=IwAR3zFzTDZvh9dFlbgHlYcl3uA7MBlxF1X96hASkVaMOUgtaZLVetWgWQDmc
3	The Road	Grazyna Jezak	Droga, Malarstwo autorstwa Grazyna Jezak | Artmajeur
4	The Apple Spas	Wacław Sporski	Spas jabłkowy - Wacław Sporski - Galeria sztuki Advena-art
5	The End of a Perfect Day	Thomas Kinkade	The End Of A Perfect Day | Thomas Kinkade Carmel, Monterey & Placerville
6	Still Life	Sporski Wacław	http://www.interarte.pl/artist_edit22.html
7	Zwei Kätzchen Im Korb Mit Blauem Tuch	Julius Adam	Julius Adam Zwei Kätzchen Im Korb Mit Blauem Tuch Stockfotografie - Alamy
8	The Lovers	René Magritte	René Magritte. The Lovers. Paris 1928 | MoMA
9	Repairing The Little Cart	Edmund Adler	Edmund Adler (1876–1965, Austrian) | I AM A CHILD (wordpress.com)
10	Palm Sunday	Zdzisław Jasiński	Plik:Zdzisław Jasiński Palm Sunday 1891.jpg – Wikipedia, wolna encyklopedia
11	River Gum	Graham Gercken	River Gum Painting by Graham Gercken - Fine Art America
12	Voyeur	Oleg Shuplyak	Amazing Illusions by Oleg Shuplyak | Digital PhotoPix
13	Natalie	Mario Teodosio	https://www.deviantart.com/marioteodosio/art/Natalie-266590067
14	A frame from the movie "Shame"	Steve McQueen's	https://www.hollywoodreporter.com/movies/movie-reviews/shame-film-review-231114/
15	The Happy Family	Eugenio Zampighi	https://www.mutualart.com/Artwork/THE-HAPPY-FAMILY/752473121B21FE99
16	The Happy Violinist with a Glass of Wine	Gerard van Honthorst	File:Gerard van Honthorst - The Happy Violinist with a Glass of Wine - WGA11668.jpg - Wikipedia
17	The Waltz by Anders Zorn	Biltmore House	https://pl.pinterest.com/pin/the-waltz-by-anders-zorn-hangs-in-the-second-floor-living-hall-at-biltmore-estate--137008013640620724/
18	Fishing the Nile	Feliks Michał Wygrzywalski	„Nad ciepłym morzem" - wystawa F.M. Wygrzywalskiego - Essey (galeria-essey.pl)
19	A Young Maiden filling an Oil Lamp	Jan Baptist Lodewyck Maes	File:Jan Baptist Lodewyck Maes – A young maiden filling an oil lamp.jpg - Wikimedia Commons
20	Vanitas still life	Pieter Claesz	https://kjgcop.wordpress.com/2014/01/14/the-essay/pieter-claesz-vanitas-still-life-with-oil-lamp-and-writing-utensils-1628-levin-rodriguez/
21	Horse Riding	Vishal Lakhani	https://fineartamerica.com/featured/1-horse-riding-vishal-lakhani.html
22	Frame from the movie "Modigliani", the Passion to Create	Mick Davis	https://media2.woopic.com/api/v1/images/1825%2Faudiovisual%2Fmovie%2F1b7%2Ffe5%2F99a4e4e01ca65c673978821c7d%2Fmovies-54208-18385830.jpg?facedetect=1&quality=85
23	True Emotions	Anna Orbaczewska	https://www.laznia.pl/wystawy/anna-orbaczewska-niedzielska-emocje-prawdziwe-62/
24	Autumn Park	Graham Gercken	https://pixels.com/featured/autumn-park-graham-gercken.html?fbclid=IwAR3Y4IVbkykMDDcegjy6zt1WdSi6zqFGv8X_Nr_0qU7KART-e5QoiDZd5sk
25	Dred2010	Wooden boat ashore	Zdjęcie Stock: Wooden boat ashore | Adobe Stock
26	Young girl making chapati (Indian Bread)	Chitrakala Academy Exhibition	http://sankriti.blogspot.com/2013/03/chitrakala-academy-exhibition.html
27	Bea	Marek Szczęsny	Marek Szczęsny, Bea, 2005 - Aukcja internetowa / Licytacja online - Cena - OneBid

(Continued)

	PICTURES	Artist	Link
28	Poppies	Małgorzata Rawicka	Malarstwo, Maki, Małgorzata Rawicka, Łąka Na Pulpit (na-pulpit.com)
29	Fire and water, inspired by the photography of Rafal Makiela	Wiola Gaszka	Ogień I Woda, Z Inspiracji Fotografią Ra, Painting by Wiola Gaszka | Artmajeur
30	The Still Point	Ladislav Záborský	https://www.tumblr.com/dramoor/190406121817/i-worship-in-silence-your-holy-will-i-offer
31	Glückliche Kinder	Paul Barthel	File:Paul Barthel - Glückliche Kinder.jpg - Wikimedia Commons
32	Temples	Yvette Lentz	https://pl.pinterest.com/pin/308496643195504095/?fbclid=IwAR00K2qi2gwbBTdnj5n9MKiAHr3gkHXw3d4DCcazZvxAEixRDjGEFHvEOEE
33	The Cross	Józef Chełmoński	Krzyż (artyzm.com)
34	Dinner with crickets	Izabela Morlak-Pyżyńska	artpub galeria: Izabela Morlak-Pyżyńska - Malarstwo
35	Friends II	Marta Lipowska	https://twitter.com/EyauukArt/status/836215482818560002/photo/1
36	Study for a Portrait (Portrait Oil Painting of a Young Man in Silver Leaf Frame)	Mark Beard	https://www.1stdibs.com/art/paintings/portrait-paintings/mark-beard-study-portrait-portrait-oil-painting-young-man-silver-leaf-frame/id-a_1892033/
37	Flamenco Dancers	Mark Spain	https://www.tuttartpitturasculturapoesiamusica.com/2018/01/Mark-Spain.html
38	Voices of the prisoners victims of torture	Despina Papadopoulou	https://fineartamerica.com/featured/voices-of-the-prisoners-victims-of-torture-acryl-auf-tuch-150-x-150-cm-despina-papadopoulou.html
39	The Night Train Wall Art	Lionel Walden	https://www.etsy.com/pl/listing/1225935775/lionel-walden-the-night-train-wall-art
40	Tango	Fabian Perez	Tango painting | Fabian Perez Art
41	Interior of a Cottage in Polesie	Józef Chełmoński	https://slideplayer.pl/slide/431162/1/images/10/%E2%80%9EWn%C4%99trze+chaty+na+Polesiu+%281909%29.jpg
42	The Lovers	Domenic Cretara	erotyzm w sztuce | Szkiełka w kalejdoskopie (wordpress.com)
43	Stay	Kristina Toxicpanda	https://abstract.desktopnexus.com/wallpaper/1613062/
44	The Cossacks near a mountain river	Franz Alekseevich Roubaud	Franz Alekseevich Roubaud The Cossacks near a mountain river: Description of the artwork | Arthive
45	Lanscape	Author unknown	http://tse3.mm.bing.net/th?id=OIP.mR7-3jRz9Fj-nH5AS1qCQQEsEs
46	Alexa's Portrait	Ruslana Levandovska	https://pixels.com/featured/alexas-portrait-ruslana-levandovska.html
47	Defend Sevastopol	Vasily Igorevich Nesterenko	https://www.reddit.com/r/BattlePaintings/comments/hjjc8j/vasily_igorevich_nesterenko_1967_russia_pavlograd/
48	My Village	Elena Michajłowna Samarskaja	https://stihi.ru/2013/11/18/905
49	Tangerine sea	otoart.pl	https://www.otoart.pl/produkt/bez-tytulu-332/
50	Transition to a better life	Jem Bendell	https://aktv.st/%D0%BB%D1%83%D1%87%D1%88%D0%B0%D1%8F-%D0%B6%D0%B8%D0%B7%D0%BD%D1%8C/reform-devolution-bendell-deep-adaptation/
51	Damian Marley Smoking	Luka Vadachkoria	https://www.deviantart.com/lukach/art/damian-marley-smoking-357575169
52	Flamenco Dancers	Renata Brzozowska	Renata Brzozowska, 1977 | Flamenco dancers | Tutt'Art@ | Pittura * Scultura * Poesia * Musica (tuttartpitturasculturapoesiamusica.com)
53	Hand in Hand	Miki De Goodaboom	https://www.peakpx.com/en/hd-wallpaper-desktop-nuicj

(Continued)

	PICTURES	Artist	Link
54	Vera	Jowita Kotów	https://art-fund.pl/product/vera/
55	Melody Of The Night	Leonid Afremov	Plakat, Obraz Leonid Afremov - Melody Of The Night | Kup na Posters.pl
56	Trainwreck	Simon Birch	https://www.hongkonghustle.com/art-design/388/simon-birch-art-exhibit-chai-wan/
57	Landscape	Author unknown	Rzecz o naprawie małżeństwa - Adonai.pl
58	Cossack on a horse (Commuter)	J Chełmoński	Plik:J Chełmoński - Kozak na koniu (Dojeżdżacz) (1907).jpg – Wikipedia, wolna encyklopedia
59	At the threshold of oblivion	dark_spider	https://www.fanpop.com/clubs/fantasy/images/17376812/title/threshold-oblivion-photo
60	A Travel	Alina Picazio	https://goldenmark.com/pl/podroz/
61	It's Grandma And Grandpa	Author unknown	pain-1.jpg (1024×826) (diaforetiko.gr)
62	It's Grandma And Grandpa	Donald Zolan	Donald Zolan (1937 – 2009) « AMERICAN GALLERY (wordpress.com)
63	In Love	Marcus Stone	https://www.meisterdrucke.uk/artist/Marcus-Stone.html
64	At Rest	Pino Daeni	PINO ARTIST | Bedroom Scenes by Artist Pino Daeni (artshopnc.com)
65	Beach break	Donald Zolan	http://www.saleoilpaintings.com/paintings/donald-zolan/beach-break.html
66	The Reader	Ferdinand Hodler	The Reader Painting by Ferdinand Hodler - Fine Art America
67	„What lies under"	Ferdiego Rizkiyanto	Siła przekazu artystycznego – plakaty społeczne Ferdiego Rizkiyanto | Poznaj To (wordpress.com)
68	Confession	Wlastimil Hofman	Confession – Wlastimil Hofman | #visual arts | Culture.pl
69	The Birches, Autumn	Małgorzata Rawicka	Małgorzata Rawicka, Brzozy, Jesień, Malarstwo (widoczki.com)
70	Madonna	Wlastimil Hofman	http://www.pinakoteka.zascianek.pl/Hofman/Index.htm
71	Winter, Mountains & Snow	Robert Norman "Bob" Ross	https://pl.pinterest.com/pin/655836764479129098/
72	Photo 4	Duma Leszek	https://liceumplastyczne.lublin.pl/nauczyciele/index.php?id=9
73	For the love it	Glen Tarnowski	https://www.paragonfineart.com/images/tarnowski/ForTheLoveOf.jpg
74	The Dance of the wine	Hélène Béland	Helene BELAND ✿ | Catherine La Rose ~ The Poet of Painting (catherinelarosepoesiaearte.com)
75	Mental Health in Immigration Detention Action Group Initial Report December 2013	Lucy Edkins	The national shame that is healthcare in UK immigration detention | openDemocracy
76	Touching the Sky	Donald Zolan	Donald Zolan - Touching The Sky (closer) (1280×1024) | Dipingere idee, Pittura carta da parati, Arte ombrello (pinterest.com)
77	Verdwaald	Sofie Van den Nest	http://sofievdn.weebly.com/schilderijen.html
78	La vieja de la Alberca	Vicente Giner	https://www.artelista.com/obra/9278957535268980-la-vieja-de-la-alberca.html
79	A bike	Joanna Rodowicz	https://artinfo.pl/dzielo/rower-2013
80	Por amor al arte	Alexandra Nedzvetskay	https://poramoralarte-exposito.blogspot.com/2015/11/alexandra-nedzvetskay.html
81	Selfie	Konstantin Sołowjow	https://t.me/FunkyFusion/707
82	The Secret Place	Magdalena Nahirny	https://magdalenanahirny.pl/sekretne-miejsce/
83	The Thinker – First Problems	Donald Zolan	Donald Zolan (1937 – 2009) « AMERICAN GALLERY (wordpress.com)
84	Tibetan girls	Ai Xuan	Tibet Girl Painting by Ai Xuan | Art and Design (cuded.com)
85	Forgiven	Thomas Blackshear II	Thomas Blackshear II Forgiven Print mounted on wood Inspirational Art (thecollectionshop.com)
86	The Girl with the Rose	Katarzyna Kurkowska	Katarzyna KURKOWSKA – "Dziewczyna z różą" - Obrazy, malarstwo współczesne, galeria sztuki Bielsko Biała (tadeo-art.pl)

(Continued)

	PICTURES	Artist	Link
87	Sherlock	Alice X. Zhang	alicexz - Professional, Digital Artist | DeviantArt
88	Contemplation	Gustav Rehberger	https://www.1stdibs.com/en-gb/art/paintings/figurative-paintings/gustav-rehberger-contemplation/id-a_118628/
89	Mother and Children	Marta Radziszewska	https://pl.pinterest.com/pin/308848486918846088/
90	Pittore figurativo, Napoli, 1953	Gianni STRINO	Gianni STRINO: Italian Master of the portrait | ART BLOG MarkovArt (wordpress.com)
91	Kanimbla Valley Dam	Graham Gercken	Kanimbla Valley Dam Painting by Graham Gercken - Fine Art America
92	Pedestrians	Aline E. Ordman	https://pl.pinterest.com/pin/294000681921648147/
93	Title: The card players	Paul Cézanne	https://encyklopedia.pwn.pl/haslo/Cezanne-Paul-Grajacy-w-karty;351203.html
94	The nature of Morta	Alexa Meade	Artists Turns People Into Living Paintings (earthlymission.com)
95	Florida-Lake Okeechobee	Leonid Afremov	FLORIDA-LAKE OKEECHOBEE (afremov.com)
96	Wood lake	dred2010	https://stock.adobe.com/images/Wood-lake/31192407?as_campaign=TinEye&as_content=tineye_match&clickref=1011lxPrwryX&mv=affiliate&mv2=pz&as_camptype=domain&as_channel=affiliate&as_source=partnerize&as_campaign=tineye
97	White card		
98	Home for Christmas	Robert Finale	Home for Christmas, by Robert Finale - Village Gallery
99	Hot Noon	Leonid Afremov	HOT NOON — PALETTE KNIFE Oil Painting On Canvas By Leonid Afremov - Size 24″×30″
100	Reach for the sky	Katarzyna Rutkowska	https://artinfo.pl/dzielo/siegnac-nieba-2013

Art dialogue methods: phronèsis and its potential for restoring an embodied moral authority in local communities

Heidi S. C. A. Muijen and René Brohm

ABSTRACT

We put forward Art-Dialogue-Methods (ADM) as an inquiry for practical wisdom within communities. It draws from a series of methodological traditions like artistic inquiry, participatory action research and narrative research. The practice of ADM could facilitate healing processes in fractured communities and organisations in today's world. ADM avoids a search from grand overarching solutions, but searches for outcomes as exemplars of the good life. We may find the relevance of this quest in the postmodern macro-context of the globalised world today with tendencies of individualization and neo-liberal markets. The authors explore the potential value of ADM for the development of practical wisdom within communities, by pointing out arguments in philosophical and sociological literature and by means of exemplary cases of ADM-programmes.

Introduction

As consumers in a postmodern globalised world we seem to have no trouble swallowing disturbing and "fake" news, unethical economic transactions, corrupt practices of political and corporate leaders, witnessing one crisis after another in almost every societal sector. We either stick to our routines in daily life, as easily to be manipulated consumers and professionals, reframing the shocking news, immoral acts and disturbing practices as "realistic" or "cynic" truths, or we waken up and take a stance. This is the choice that has to be made. The process of becoming conscious critical cosmopolitan citizens (Appiah, 2006) has its price though: the necessity to reflect on and criticise our own actions and routines, both personally as well as in the groups and teams in which we participate.

Reflecting on the post-modern situation of our globalised world many sociologists and philosophers notice a general fragmentation of moral authority in society. The recurrent critique, which focuses on our age of uncertainty, in *liquid* and *a-moral times* (Bakhtin, 1982; Bauman, 2006; Taylor, 2006), is that the ethos of communities is suppressed by instrumental rationality. Thus, the ethical question "what is good", is downplayed by the question what is efficient, and is answered in terms of economic rationality; not by means of ethical deliberation (DuGay, 2000).

If we are to legitimise authority, we must face the fact that we live in a world of multiple cultures and rationalities. We may choose to make the market logic dominant, so that whatever provides the greatest profits should define our actions. However, this instrumental "neoliberal spirit" makes, in the words of Paul du Gay, fragmented and anomic what should be organic and whole (DuGay, 2000, p. 67). In the light of the general fragmentation of moral authority in society we pose the question: How are we to address values and leadership when we do not have generally accepted and socially embodied narratives anymore that will have a binding power for people individually and in communities, as well as for society at large?

This special issue explores the potential of creative methods in counselling and guidance practices. We will contribute in particular to understand the aptness of creative methods for healing organisational rifts. Characteristic of our approach is the dismantling of daily routines and creatively evoking practical wisdom within communities, not as "human capital" to be managed, but as an emergent quality in and between people.

In the article we describe the importance of the contextual fine-tuning of explorative change processes and results of what we have called Art-Dialogue Methods (ADM).

The article shows in particular a case in which an ADM-programme helped to establish the right conditions for an interplay between participants, perspectives and modes of understanding and (inter-) acting in situations that involved values and practices within and between communities in a Dutch organisation of higher education. Smaller presented illustrative cases show how embodied, contextual knowledge can be articulated, not just individually, but as a community.

The next (second) paragraph starts by an exploration of characteristics of art and dialogue -, showing how ADM draws from existing methods of inquiry by embedding it in current methodological developments.

In the third paragraph we explore the interplay of different modes of "intelligence" in concrete ADM-practices, which have helped participants to explore existential, community and leadership issues, empowering professionals both individually and as a community. The core of this "methodos", we will argue, is the art of establishing an "in-between" space for co-creative interplay between people and between different voices and values, including subtle modes of understanding and inter-acting ("intelligences") to afford practical, contextual wisdom as a community ("phronèsis").

In the fourth paragraph we provide for a rich description and reconstruction of a case in which we show the interplay of the four discerned intelligences facilitated by an ADM-programme in the context of a department within an organisation of higher education.

In the concluding fifth paragraph the views and results presented in the article will be discussed in the light of tensions and contradictions characteristic of our postmodern condition and future developments of arts-based (educational) research.

Art-dialogue-method

Before going into the relevancy of ADM we start by explaining the distinctive qualities of Art Dialogue and Method as more serious than mere play and more comprehensive than rational reasoning.

Introducing ADM

Art is about the *invocation* of the senses by using multiple idioms or ways of sense-making at the same time. Invocation is by definition in the present and in the plural. Art invokes directly; it (re-)creates experience and consciousness to "dwell" in the moment. Therefore, art is quite different from generalising representations of reality, "transferring" these to future situations. It is about idiosyncracies and temptational imagining and sensing right here and now. The making of art interweaves with different traditions, such as mythical and religious texts in which music, rituals and symbols play an important role (Gadamer, 1975, 2010; Habermas, 1984). McNiff (1981) and Eisner (2008), the early advocates of arts-based research, elaborate on presentational aspects of knowledge to which the arts might contribute in qualitative research. Art addresses qualitative nuances in (social) situations; evokes empathy and compassion; generates new perspectives on old patterns of interaction and routines; helps create awareness of our feelings rather than cognitions. In other words, art does not provide just illustrations and subtitles for communication processes, but it does communicate in its own way. It creates.

Dialogue is a way of sensemaking through words, images, or any kind of symbolic interaction. We view these as different forms of media or "texts". Dialogue stems from the old-Greek "dia" (meaning "through an opening") and "logos", referring to the (natural) principle of ordering things. Dialogue refers both to a kind of internal understanding, a way of sense-making by reflecting on internal voices and experiences, as a way of voicing understanding ("logos") in-between ("dia") people, trying to come to a mutual understanding. In dialogue participants explore presuppositions, ideas, beliefs, images, recollections and feelings that subtly control their interactions, both individually and collectively (Bohm, 1996). It enables collaborative inquiry into the systems and processes that fragment and interfere with real communication between people and groups. Dialogue has the potential to heal social fissures by making new connections and revitalizing wholes in a fragmented world.

Art does not necessarily lead to a dialogue, it is *dialogic* in another "language" or medium: by means of images, tones, movements, etc. In order to understand the interweaving of artistic and verbal dialogue we need to explore this notion as being central to the narrative, existential and hermeneutic traditions of philosophers like Heidegger, Levinas, Buber, Habermas and Gadamer.

Method, according to the etymology of the old-Greek words "meta" and "hodos" – *methodos* – refers to an exploration (hodos = way) for insight (meta – what lies beyond).

Thus, ADM dwells in (between) people (Polanyi, 1966) by the invocational nature of art and the explorative power of dialogue. Dialogue and art are inherent to human nature, social interaction and community life as forms of symbolic communication (van den Berk, 2003; Cassirer, 2010; Langer, 1979; Jung, 1970).

Summarizing these constitutive elements we consider the "methodos" ADM by pointing out how co-creative explorations and multivocal perspectives may lead to new practices and changes in old routines which are *exemplary* for the issue at stake in (or between) communities in a particular cultural or organisational context.

The exemplar is more than just a solution to a problem and more vivid than just theoretical knowledge. We underline an important development in action research that argues for considering outcomes in terms of practical wisdom (Eikeland, 2006; Flyvbjerg, Landman, & Schram, 2012). We will argue that creative methods are particularly suitable for the development of contextual and practical wisdom in communities, which we refer to by its ancient Greek name – "phronèsis". We use this term to stress that "phronèsis" "is" not a psychological or cognitive characteristic of individuals and groups, but an emerging quality in (between) people and spaces – provoked through art and dialogue – manifested as an interplay between different voices, perspectives and modes of understanding and interacting with each other.

The methodological context

An exemplary case: "Man, Know Yourself!"

One ADM-based philosophical counselling programme is oriented on the dynamic game, "Man, Know Yourself" (Muijen, 2010), consisting of six rounds in which life themes are raised both by means of symbolic pictures, mythical stories and philosophical views and questions. How the game is played is described elsewhere (Muijen, 2009, 2011), here we will focus on the power of imagining an in-between (transitional) space (Winnicott, 2005). The game combines dialogue with arts (symbolic pictures, painting, music) into dramatic polylogues. In different rounds participants make associations and reflections on how they set goals, relate to others and make choices in life. Participants are invited to focus on moral and existential themes by using metaphors and play, dialogue and art. The game master/ counsellor may start by making an inventory among the participants: "How would you address your personal theme as a question or as a problem? Would you express it in an earthly (grounded), flowing, airy (light-hearted) or fiery (passionate) way?" (Figure 1)

In one round of the game the playful dialogical process is explicitly focusing on developing an inner (moral) compass for life orientation. For example, participants are invited to see the art of

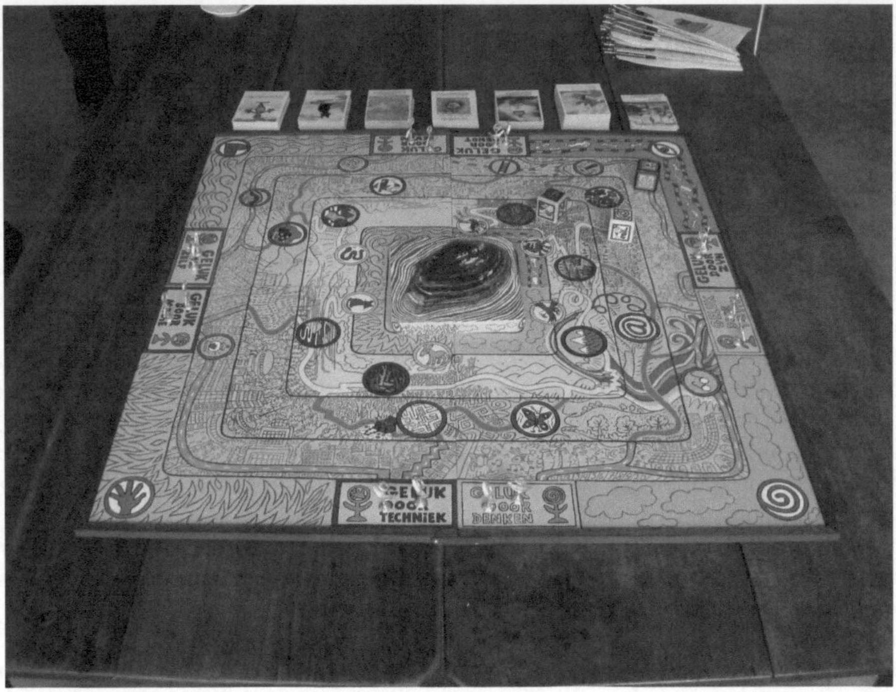

Figure 1. The dynamic game, "Man, Know Yourself".

making right choices in life as a quest in the labyrinth and will reflect their personal quest in the story about Theseus and the thread of Ariadne. Another round raises questions on how such a myth might contain a personal metaphor for their moral compass. The game cards suggest philosophical perspectives and mythical exploration. Similarly, crises are reflected upon metaphorically: both by symbolic images – for example a picture of a swamp – and by means of a provocative question on one's attitude when confronted with such a crisis: "would you prefer a helping hand or try to survive by yourself?"

A participant reflected on the metaphorizing process and her experience after a workshop with the game:

> The symbolic imagery allowed me as a player to feel the wild water literally rising to my lips. In imagining that situation, I visualised which roads I should take to get out of that situation. The surprising result was an intuitive feeling how to handle an issue I was facing in my actual life.

The reported experiences of participants of the game reflect what is called the senso-pathic (Mook, 2003) dimension in the context of play and art therapy: the game components (playing board, cards, dice, hourglass and rich objects) stimulate the senses and establish a creative tension between past and future, between cognition and feeling, between personal, private and social, cultural patterns, between moral and factual questions.

ADM in context

The methodological strength of ADM in philosophical counselling and community building is the interweaving of different "intelligences"; i.e. the ability to understand by discerning one thing or experience from another. By referring to different ways of being, or modalities, we stress the original connotation from Roman-Greek philosophy as opposed to cognitive, individualist orientations we find dominant in psychological discourse (Gardner, 2011). In the next paragraph we will introduce four "intelligences" in the sense of a multivocal, cocreative arrangement to explore human potential of becoming sensitive (pathos), invoking the imagination (mythos) through rich sensemaking (logos) by means of dialogues through art. The aim is not art for its own sake, but as a way to develop good ways in life (ethos). At the same time our positioning in the world (ethos) gives valuable input for the "methodos", as a way of questioning (lack of) taking a stance in professional practices, by exploring what our senses, experiences, imagination and other "intelligences" tell us.

We borrow from three important bodies of knowledge.

First, we relate the dynamics between the four intelligences to a narrative shift in dialogical and humanist traditions in the arts and the social sciences. The so-called death of the grand narratives does not have to result in a nihilism and (social and ethical) fragmentation of communities. We stress the importance of narratives by taking MacIntyre's words: "I can only answer the question, 'What am I to do?' if I can answer the prior question 'Of what story or stories do I find myself a part?'" (MacIntyre, 2007, p. 216). We are familiar with the way in which religions like Christianity, Judaism and Islam use the power of "story telling" to give an understanding of human nature, our destiny and the good way of living. Their stories relate truths that have a binding power to these communities, including rules for moral behaviour.

Being aware of its "political" and ethical power we emphasise that stories are composed of texts that are not limited to verbal narratives, but consist also of imagery (through paintings, thick descriptions), smell (incense, flowers, herbs), sounds (the way of telling, the timbre and use of voice, music), taste (ritual food and drinks), situations (the ritualistic environment such as a church, a theatre, a board room, etc.) as well as the rituals themselves which are part and parcel of the origin of narratives. Both smell and taste are fundamental in invoking memories and the sphere in which stories and narratives are told (Draaisma, 2010). Thus we position ADM as a narrative approach to social issues.

Secondly, ADM is related to the use of arts for individual, relational, social development and healing.

Creative methods (music, dance, art, and drama) enhance therapeutic possibilities for patients to recover from developmental problems, anxieties and traumas, in order to strengthen social and emotional competences (Dalley, 1994, 1996; Levine, 1995; Levine & Levine, 1996; Kuiper, 1988, 1989).

The invocational and explorative power of creative methods also enhances deep (existential) learning (Argyris, 1993; Argyris & Schön, 1978; Schön, 1991; Yuthas, Dillard, & Rogers, 2004). Following a narrative and dialogical perspective on developmental processes (Isaacs, 1999), we acknowledge the interconnectedness of individual and collective learning and empowerment processes. Therefore, creative methods (e.g. community art, folk art, story-telling) can foster both individual developmental processes and empower communities by taking collaborative action on social responsibilities.

Thirdly, there is the use of dialogue, in which the relational aspect of art-dialogues takes presidency over individualistic approaches.

Although we are aware of the differences between methods like career writing (Lengelle, Meijers, Poell, & Post, 2014), art based therapeutical and narrative approaches such as the self-confrontation method (Hermans & Hermans-Konopka, 2010) and Emerging Body Language (Bosman, 2012), we want to highlight a shared notion of dialogical enquiry and communication by creating a relational stage to invoke narratives and investigate meanings more than "truths" in a co-creative and dialogical way. In methodological research we witness a shift from representational to presentational forms of knowledge and the blurring of boundaries between researchers and practitioners (Barone & Eisner, 2012; Knowles & Cole, 2008; Levey, 2018; Levine, 1995; Liamputtong, 2007; Liamputtong & Rumbold, 2008; Rose, 2001). Both arts-based and collaborative methodologies (like action research) are helpful to study in-depth experiential forms of learning-by-doing. By qualitatively pointing out how thereby new practices and changes in old routines are developed the results are *exemplary* for the issue at stake in (or between) communities in a particular cultural or organisational context.

The significance of "phronèsis" to restore coherence in communities

The ancient philosophical question of "how to take care of ourselves?" has become particularly relevant in times of moral crisis. The socio-ethical configuration of contemporary times offers a striking similarity with Greek history: in both era's we witness a collapse of collective value systems. The art of living has been a substantial element in ancient Greek, Roman and even early Medieval culture. Since Socrates, practical philosophy contributed to societal coherence throughout more than nine centuries by affording a plurality of local and vital narratives on the good life. Care for ourselves is not a grand narrative of good and evil in the way some religious and secular "codes of conduct" demand. Rather, it is an appeal for the opposite: to find one's own answers to moral questions and to take responsibility to review moral answers throughout life. By responding to the appeal to live one's life accordingly, we may consider our life as "living art" (Foucault, 2005).

Following Nussbaum's analysis of Aristotelian ethics, we must be aware of the inherent vulnerability of everyone's striving for "the good life". Illustrative is her ethical analysis of the classical tragedy of Hekabe: even a moral outstanding character like Hekabe can morally erode given the circumstances of war and betrayal by her best friend. Just like a flower will wither when lacking the sun and rain needed to grow and to flourish (Nussbaum, 2001).

Realizing the dependency of ethics on social contexts, on ecological and cultural forces we use another metaphor, the moral compass, to address the question of "calibrating" plural value orientations of individuals, communities and of society at large. Especially artistic expression, dialogical exploration and sharing narratives are indispensible forms of symbolic communication and interaction to experience the moral compass as a *living* metaphor, by seeing wholes rather than fragmentation, fostering an eye for the "gestalt" (Langer, 1979) of the unifying parts. In our eyes this approach can give strong answers to postmodern tendencies of fragmentation and loss of meaningful activities and sense-making.

ADM as "methodos" for an incremental development of "phronèsis"

Our "methodos" is not oriented on implementing an overall value system but fosters an explorative dynamics of four intelligences. Therefore we don't offer a "model". ADM is about re-configuring social, emotional, cultural, moral, economic, ... patterns in individuals, groups and communities as *parallel processes*. The ancient philosophy on the art of living (Eikeland, 2008) established a tradition for the development of "phronèsis", understood as an enduring attempt for virtuous practices. Narratives offer a key how to take charge of our lives so that we learn to act wisely in and as a community.

Overviewing the history of ideas on the art of living, its ethical appeal demands more than merely rationality (logos), it requires emotional, social, rhetorical and moral intelligence. It demands us to be sensitive to the suffering of others and ourselves (pathos), daring to imagine what is utterly strange and to be able to tell stories about how we feel about tragic and unforeseeable events (mythos), as well as to explore the world courageously and to act in a dignified way (ethos).

To show how the interplay of these four intelligences contributes to restoring coherence in communities, we will reframe ADM as metaphoric communication (Muijen, 2001; Muijen & Van Marissing, 2011). Highlighting the importance of gaining insight in parallel processes between intra-, interpersonal and community levels we present ADM as an art of creating living metaphors, thereby widening the concept of metaphor (Cassirer, 2010; Langer, 1979; Ricoeur, 1975, 1984). In this manner an ADM-trainer needs to be capable of handling this (extra-)linguistic dynamics both as personal and group development, with cognitive and emotional dimensions of metaphorizing, evoking the imagination with the people involved. It is a playful, healing and dialogical process, evoking images of what could be real in-between actors and in-between reality and utopia. An increasing amount of studies provide the tools on how to use arts in (research and change) programmes, including literary forms, performance, visual art, narratives and folk art. The methodological strengths of these approaches in professional practices and research are, amongst others, the capacity to unsettle stereotypes, raising critical consciousness, forging micro-macro connections, being participative by its provocative-exploratory power and focussing on multiple meanings. Thereby arts-based methods enrich "the landscape of knowing" (Barone & Eisner, 2012; Eisner, 2008; McNiff, 1981).

Pathos: creating a symbolic in-between sphere invoking the senses.

In ADM, we understand the role of arts as of fundamental importance to the (de)construction of meanings and social practices. The famous quote of Michael Polanyi "we know more than we can tell", is to indicate that the tacit dimension to our knowledge is partly inexpressible. Yet at the same time the virtual opposite is true as well "we can express more, than we can (explicitly) know." Like this tacit dimension in knowledge we refer to tacit dimensions in communication and interaction, expanding this concept to analogical, symbolical non-discursive domains (Bouwman & Brohm, 2016; Brohm, 2005).

Nietzsche used a musical metaphor to point to "truth" as a primarily rhetorical quality of communication: "Mit tönen kann man die Menschen zu jedem Irrrtume und jede Warhheit verführen: wer vermöchte einen Ton zu widerlegen." (Nietzsche, 1984, p. 386) The way in which music touches the heart, conveys meaning and creates a sphere in which both listeners and musicians dwell, cannot be translated into words. Artistic expression embodies the quality of *showing and presenting* "truth" by means of in-dwelling and attunement between people. Dancing, music, the sculpturing process of making something in clay are based on a resonance. An in-between space is created by the sensing hands of the sculptor in the watery clay-substance through touching, feeling and forming. The boundaries between the subjective domain of the maker melts with the objective substance of clay into "flesh-clay", an in-between double skin (Muijen & Van Marissing, 2011, p. 67 ff). A similar resonance is obvious in dancing, seen as e-motion-al movements on the border between inside and outside (Brohm & Muijen, 2010). In this way art "is" pathos, as real as vitality affects (Stern, 2010), a power helping us to come to an understanding with the situation; and similar to the emotional way in which situations can be transformed all of a sudden from pleasant to anxious; according to Sartre's phenomenological view on emotions, not as states "in" subjects but as the way we dwell in situations. For this reason, we believe that ADM constitute open spaces in communication and interaction between people, in which imagining how the world could be, seems to be more powerful than analytical laws of logics.

Mythos: elaborating on living metaphors by co-creative dialogue.

The intelligence of "mythos" adds a dynamics (dialectics) between presentational and representational knowledge. In the playing field of the imagination the metaphorization process might be expanded by using different arts for *organizing* a musical, visual, theatrical or dance-metaphor. Here we give an example of how a musical metaphor facilitates a process of community building and leadership (Figure 2).

In the example described it is shown how the orchestrated musical metaphor stimulates an out-of-the-box inquiry of community building and leadership. The direct appeal of making music together allows the articulation of moral (existential) emotions, like bravery and cowardice; guilt and honour, resonating with the issues involved.

For example, feeling the significance of being afraid to sing solo and overcoming shyness to perform in front of the group may contribute in an experiential way to the development of leadership and empower both individuals and the community. Its strength is reflected in the context of the musical orchestration of the group dynamics: not as an abstract concept but as arts-based experiential learning how a certain style of leadership affects the group; how people can learn from the experience of playing solo and together (Willems, 2017). In the given example, the metaphorical power of verbal expressions – like "voicing", "creating harmony", "discordant tones", "operating solistically", "tuning in", "backing", "key-note player" etc. – is manifest in a follow up dialogue. Thus by enriching the musical metaphor with experiential narratives the participants add "mythos" to "pathos", explicating the significance of acting like an orchestra in their working life as well (Muijen, 2012).

A musical metaphor Voicework (Willems, M in Muijen, H. 2012) is used to stimulate both voicing personal feelings and the experimental exploration of different ways of how to create harmony in a group and how to handle conflicts; how to balance between dissensus and consensus.

Musical exercises might focus on keeping rhythm and melody (*being authentic, being in charge*) while at the same time you have to listen and adjust to other melodies and appreciate the differences between people.

A further complexity can be the development of the collaborative power by exercising the complexity and subtlety of the dynamics between *taking the lead* and the *need for backing*. A group of people using small instruments (e.g. percussion) might give more or less backing (or none at all) to a singer as soloist

Figure 2. A musical metaphor for community building and leadership.

Logos: installing a dialogical stage for existential learning processes

The in-depth explorative power of "logos", in the context of arts-based research and dialogues, is not to be understood as an abstract logical operation but as a relational process. Dialogical communication sets the stage for collaborative exploration of social and existential issues by means of learning processes, based on responsiveness, an open mind and a listening attitude. Lengelle and Meijers (2013, 2014, 2015) have shown extensively by research how deep learning processes are taking place in existential situations by means of a double hermeneutics in the sense of a dialogical attunement: internally, developing a feeling of identity by listening to different voices in and stories about oneself; and externally, with respect to others, to different social tasks and roles in the community. Thus dialogue presupposes ànd generates being tuned into other people's emotions, movements and voices as well as to inner voices and signals. At the same time participants and counsellor must be sensitive and responsive to the expressions and (body) language both of oneself and others.

In ADM-programmes the focus is on existential and relational themes by creative and explorative learning (as opposed to one-dimensional learning processes on a behavioural level). Illustrative is a research project in which therapists, consultants and trainers, using arts for personal and organisational change, were involved, investigating the transformative power of arts-based dialogue in their own field. In a follow up meeting they were invited to exchange narratives and experiences with each other about what could be the value of using arts in their professional work. In order to show the power of arts to facilitate developmental processes these professionals constructed images and metaphors themselves. The outcome pointed to the value of art-dialogues for (re-)uniting opposing forces and fragmented parts in the organisational context, within and between groups as well as between voices and "strivings" within themselves as professionals (Muijen, 2001, p. 204 ff).

Ethos: restoring ethical relations and reframing social issues by re-enactment and empowerment

As a starting point, we support the idea that we need to build moral communities rather than to look for a new universal ethical theory or a grand narrative, like Nussbaum (2001, 2014) argues. The before mentioned double hermeneutics, based on the confrontation of internal and external dialogues, is formative for the ability of calibrating the inner compass. This antique metaphor is more than just a competence for moral decision-making, it is referring to the "intelligence" of ethos. Poetical, musical, dramaturgical, ... metaphors function as a frame to give expression to existential feelings like loneliness, comradeship and responsibility, which involve both ethical and social questions (for example feeling guilty to resist group pressure).

It is known that the dynamics of a group fosters either authenticity or punishes deviation of the group norm by excluding outcasts, accepting bullying behaviour and condoning attitudes of bystanders, etc. Arts-based communication provokes the shifting of perspectives from judgemental (moral excuses and accusations) to explorative and empowers people to re-enact rather than acting out (Schaverien in: Dalley, 1994). By means of reframing social issues through metaphorical exploration ethical sensitivity is stimulated. The re-enactment of ethical dilemmas and social problems by means of dancing or visualising the situation, by means of dramaturgical dialogues between stakeholders is helpful not just to acknowledge or "solve" problems but to feel moral-emotional dimensions in relationships. In this way ethical voices and perspectives on the social issues at stake will evoke. Thereby ethical relationships can be restored in communities.

We argue that ADM allows for more than a restoration of traditional views: it has the potential to recover meaning and values in the complex contexts of late modern life, an era, in need of sense making and qualitative approaches to complex social issues. As we are facing the increasing power of large economic systems, while at the same time we are often less embedded in local communities, there is a general tendency towards a "self" that feels "atomatic", disempowered, alienated, purposeless. From the macro scale to the intrapersonal scale of keeping psychological health in existential frictions and the art of how to make good decisions in life, we are facing the loss of value systems and the inflation of meaning by the fragmentation of human life. When professionals, using creative methods in their counselling or supervision practices, do not take this larger dimension into account, we fear that these methods may become another fetish in the neo-liberal market system; an employability tool that produces conformity to company values

(Bloom, 2013) or an element of "fun" that is just another way for normative control (Fleming & Sturdy, 2009).

Therefore ADM needs careful framing in order to avoid this pitfall, by becoming aware of the multi-layered calibrating process between opposing values and by being sensitive to parallel patterns in personal development, community building and leadership.

The next session describes a case how the four "intelligences" are blended in an ADM-programme.

A case of developing phronèsis in a professional community

This case illustrates how the four intelligences, blended into an ADM-programme, might enhance the calibrating power of the moral compass and empower the ethos of a professional community (Muijen, Appel, & Cock Buning, 2004). In this programme about twenty lecturers and a manager of a department of Social Work were involved. The programme took place from 2002 to 2006 and its effects on collaborative action were monitored from 2006 to 2010.

The intake meeting resulted in a focus on the actual working conditions of the professionals. In an explorative dialogue, frictions were discovered between the value systems of different groups, especially between different generations of lecturers. More severe was the friction discovered between personal interests and educational values of the professionals on the one hand and the more economically and technically oriented team of managers on the other, which had caused incidents and conflicts. Thus, it was agreed that the five training sessions would be fine-tuned accordingly with three trainers, using creative methods to face the clash of values and interests.

Evoking mythos

The participants were responsible for different curricula on two professional levels. The programme started with an inventory by choosing pictures, symbolizing personal-professional values and attitudes. This resulted in several anecdotal stories about their shared history, which was followed by a dialogical process of collective sense-making by which the small narratives and anecdotal events became more meaningful within broader contexts, exemplifying relevant themes and moral issues in the community, such as pain resulting from conflicts between colleagues and between lecturers and managers. Then the metaphorization process started with questions such as: how do the different stories reflect community values? How do the issues affect them as a community? How do they want to act on them as a team?

Mobilizing logos

These questions were explored in-depth: The educational and social values – the sensed cohesion as a team by personal and social bonding; their humour and flexibility – were expressed by using a metaphor: the team felt as a "safe haven" for each other. A linked metaphor of "creating bridges" despite the differences within the (younger and older generation) group of professionals expressed their shared focus on values such as creativity, spirituality and educational flow with students, which was described as a flower garden.

The metaphorization processes resulted in a dialogue about ambivalences and emotional undertones in their shared values and feelings, referred to as "the secret of our school". At first glance this metaphor seemed to express their "powerful bonding". Further exploration of the (painted) metaphor revealed feelings of distrust towards the management, embedded in a longer history of incidents and organizational change from a traditional focus on educational values towards an instrumental way of "managing" education. This change was experienced and understood not just as a "neutral" new management approach, but as a cultural shift, which resulted in a gap between professionals and management.

Expressing pathos

The gap was most evident in a follow-up session, in which the participants were invited to visualise "the future of the school" by means of a "gardening metaphor". The three subgroups (containing four to six participants) characterised their paintings as:

"a blossoming flower garden underneath a midday sun with a garden house",

"a picture of a wild garden with real picked flowers on top of the painted garden" and

"The island garden" (Figure 3)

The last picture had a particular striking effect on the participants, confronting the group with an image of an "autarkic" community. The blossoming flowers referred in a metaphorical sense to a strong professional community, but living on an island in "splendid isolation". The image represented the "secret of our school": the strong personal and professional ties between the lecturers and the distance towards the management and "outside" world, symbolised by the water around the island. This metaphorical image resulted in some questions to be considered for further investigation: "Are we really working on an island? Who is part of 'our' community and who is excluded and belongs to the 'outside world'? How would it be possible to narrow the distance to 'the outside world'?"

Empowering their ethos

The confronting (pathos), visualizing (mythos) and reflective (logos) power of the metaphorizing- dia-logical process had helped the professionals to explore the historical roots and actual meaning of their professional values. A follow-up session was organised to empower them (ethos) by creating symbolical bridges between the professionals and the "outside world" (especially the management). These (2D and 3D) created living metaphors helped the professionals to develop their ethos as a

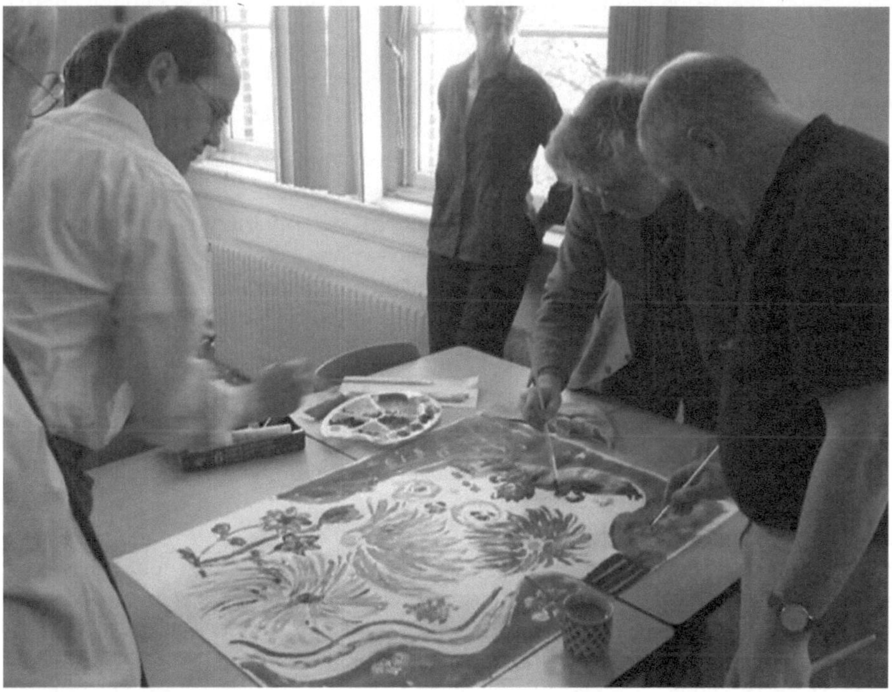

Figure 3. The island garden.

community. They now asked: "how are we able to change the policy making process from a 'bureaucratic obstacle' to something that is working for us by creating open communication channels with the management?"

Developing phronèsis as a community

We underline the limited scope of this arts-based intervention on the intermediate professional team level. It was not enough to change the on-going process of polarization and bureaucratization within the macro-organizational context. Still there was some longer-term impact of the mobilised phronèsis within the community. As a follow-up, several working groups were formed and an action plan was submitted to the management team. The fact that the different teams of lecturers were willing again to communicate and cooperate with the management turned out to be one first step in a reconciliation process in the years after the ADM-community building programme (2006–2010). It consisted in a setup of (in part inter-organisational) communities-of-practice. This resulted in a bottom-up process of professionalization and collaborative action. For example: they started writing a book on applied ethics for students and lecturers of the University of Applied Sciences.

The longer-term outcome of the reconciliation process took a different course though: despite the empowerment of the teams the managerial decision-making process was not changed accordingly. Economically driven pressure coming from the neo-liberal way in which education is organised in society at large, resulted in a harsher and no-nonsense output driven policy of managing education. Thus, the gap between the management and professional level was further deepened, undermining the thin layer of newly built trust and hope for possible change. Despite this fact the professional communities-of-practice continued to work collaboratively on their book on Human Recourses Management in Ethical Perspective, which was presented at a conference (Nijhoff & Wesseling, 2010).

However the overall case stands for a meaningful process of empowering and building bridges between students, professionals and management, creating an educational community despite conflicting forces.

Conclusion and discussion

In order to restore the ethos of a community in the face of fragmentary powers in society today, we have argued that ADM requires an incremental, embedded approach, exploring the development of contextual, practical wisdom (phronèsis). This "methodos" as an inquiry within communities was taken from (art) therapy, philosophical counselling, action and arts-based research and dialogical change approaches for collaborative action and community building. Crucial seems to be the fact that ADM is not externally designed as a "to-be-implemented-reform-plan", but as a contextually fine-tuned arrangement of arts-dialogue-methods.

We have argued that ADM has the potential for contributing to practical wisdom through an integration of multiple intelligences in a dialogical and creative way, so that it fits local contexts and cultural characteristics.

We demonstrated this potential within a professional community of lecturers. The context was characterised by a fragmentation in value systems between generations as well as a traditional conflict between the rationality of professional values, embodied by the lecturers, and the instrumental rationality represented by the managers. These social configurations reflect four decades of economic short-term rationality at the cost of sustainable value-driven processes of sense making (DuGay, 2000). The ADM-programme allowed for an enriched rationality as well as for a shared understanding of the significance of value orientation in educational practices. Thus, although on a small scale, ADM allows for viable exemplars that may have far-reaching consequences (Flyvbjerg et al., 2012).

A critical methodological reflection

ADM as "methodos" is more and less than another "mixed methods"-approach: it is "more" because the contextual, multi-layered blending of four "intelligences" is crucial to its success; it is "less" because it is disruptive of one-dimensional methodical devices such as protocols and focuses on parallel (dysfunctional) patterns at micro-, meso- and macro-levels.

The methodological power of ADM appears to transcend the level of psychological interventions, "personal growth" and "team spirit" by encountering existential questions and creating an in-between space (transitional area) in which metaphorization and deep learning (through art and symbolic play) contribute to healing processes reciprocally on individual and group levels.

We are well aware that the methodological principles, drawn from the literature and our own ADM-based programmes, have a limited empirical base in the sense of quantitative methods. Our claim is not contributing to an evidence-based model but rather to practice-based evidence, based on exemplary cases and philosophical analyses. Thus, instead of art-based inquiry in general we focussed on specifically designed small-scale philosophical counselling and community programmes.

This brings us to the importance of a narrative focus on ethical questions, meaning that our "moral sense" is shaped by the stories about "the good life" that are being told in communities. Stories about "the good life" encompass artistic expression in which we deliver clues that may tell the other more than we ever realise and are able to express verbally.

This might be the reason why ADM is helpful to foster reflection on values underlying conflicts and emotional disruptions; thus offering a valuable source for reconstructing the meaning of life stories and integrating the history of the (professional) community.

To develop ADM further to a next level would require in depth research of the processes described. We hope to have contributed a small step to this long-term goal: ADM as a way of lifelong value-learning (Brohm & Muijen, 2010; Muijen, 2004; Muijen, 2009, 2011).

Multiple intelligences

We have offered an outline of ADM as the art of mobilizing the dynamics between four "intelligences". The power of imagination as the intelligence of mythos helped to create small narratives by means of rhetorical metaphorization processes, counterbalancing the dominance of logos and its monopolistic reality claim. Our ADM-programmes stimulate emotional and ethical intelligence as well: by making the meaningfulness of moral emotions explicit and becoming aware of the necessity of polyvocal, multidimensional perspectives on situations.

To operationalise these aspects into narratives includes both story-telling as well as the apprehension of life events revealing an inherent quality of human life itself. Stories are valued as having a moral educational power: just like epics, legends and parables in narrative (religious) traditions. In the presented case the narratives on the professional community driven into "splendid isolation on the island garden" and exploring its future as a "blossoming garden" did have this impact. Crucial was the process of articulating their identity on the basis of shared professional values, which defined them as a community. Boosting the ethos of a community means the appropriation of the wicked problem (Conklin, 2006) together with the fragile reconciliation process with management by addressing conflicting issues, installing empowerment. Thereby emotional aspects and a cultural perspective on ethical questions and frictions are included (Kinni, 2003), taking all stakeholders into consideration (Abma, 2010).

To an integrated research program of artistic inquiry and dialogical change

A relevant question for further research would be how ADM could be extended by combining artistic-inquiry approaches and action research into a powerful tool for developing a learning organization (Bridges & Bridges, 2011; Wierdsma & Swieringa, 2011). To widen the concept of dialogue in this respect and to enclose art as a "third voice", we might refer to a Habermasian view on communication: "truth" is conveyed not just theoretically, but contains ethical (practical rationality) and expressive aspects (aesthetic rationality) as well.

Therefore we stress the fact that ADM-based programmes are not just a popular mix of creative methods but are embedded in expertise. Crucial is the contextual fine-tuning of ADM so that both our gut-feeling as trainers and counsellors and the "pathos" and tacit knowledge of professionals can be made constructive in dialogues. To accomplish this, we should become sensitive and responsive to ambivalent meanings, hidden plots, and what has not been said in the stories being told, thereby taking questions on authenticity and integrity into account. To capture ethical and aesthetic dimensions in sense-making ADM presents a powerful voice. Therefore, we stress the importance of an open atmosphere in which stories are being told.

In the context of ADM we have experienced that moral issues in communities and organizations can be addressed dialogically, not just by power-play. Crucial in this respect is the development of "phronèsis" by the "art of living": to make one's life meaningful both for oneself (authentic) as to other people in the organization and to broader contexts in society (polis, cosmopolis). This is what Foucault could mean by his phrase how to live one's life like living art: the human answer to the appeal of taking charge of one's life and sharing it with the community.

This implies an ontological claim of narratives in the sense of Ricoeurs analyses (1975, 1978). Dialogical philosophers like Levinas and Buber add another revealing implication concerning our identity, saying that we are, even when we understand ourselves as "individuals", in a very fundamental sense relational: that we are not so autonomous as we might think and that our "social and political nature" is not secondary but primal. We are in a very fundamental sense relative to (important) other persons, in the way Buber (1997) explicated: "in the beginning there was relationship".

Acknowledgments

Thanks to Victor Dobbin, CB MBE PhD DD, for his valuable suggestions on content and his editing of the text.

Disclosure statement

No potential conflict of interest was reported by the authors.

References

Abma, T. A. (2010). *Herinneringen en dromen van zeggenschap. Cliëntenparticipatie in de ouderenzorg*. Den Haag: Boom/ Lemma uitgevers.

Appiah, K. A. (2006). *Cosmopolitanism: Ethics in a world of strangers*. New York: W.W. Norton.

Argyris, C. (1993). *Knowledge for action. A guide to overcoming barriers to organizational change*. San Francisco: Jossey Bass.

Argyris, C., & Schön, D. (1978). *Organisational learning: A theory of action perspective*. Reading, MA: Addison Wesley.

Bakhtin, M. (1982). *The dialogic imagination: Four essay's*. (Paperback ed.). Austin: University of Texas Press.

Barone, T., & Eisner, E. (2012). *Arts-based research*. Thousand Oaks: Sage publications.
Bauman, Z. (2006). *Liquid modernity*. Cambridge Malden, MA: Polity Press, Blackwell.
van den Berk, T. (2003). *Mystagogie. Inwijding in het symbolisch bewustzijn*. Zoetermeer: Meinema.
Bloom, P. (2013). Fight for your alienation: The fantasy of employability and the ironic struggle for self-exploitation. *Ephemera, 13*(4), 785.
Bohm, D. (1996). *On dialogue*. London: Routledge.
Bosman. (2012). Downloaded 31 May 2017. Retrieved from http://annabosman.eu/EindrapportEBL.pdf
Bouwman, R., & Brohm, R. (2016). Phronetic judgement, an essential competence for a project manager in a complex project environment!. *International Journal of Business and Globalisation, 17*(4), 582–596.
Bridges, W., & Bridges, S. (2011). *Managing transitions: Making the most of change*. Cambridge, MA: Da Capo Press.
Brohm, R. (2005). *Polycentric order in organizations: A dialogue between Michael Polanyi and IT-consultants on knowledge, organization, and morality*. Rotterdam: Erasmus University Rotterdam.
Brohm, R. & Muijen, H. (2010) Leven in organisaties: een kunst! (3 parts). *Filosofie* 20 (1) 45–50; (2) 50–55; (3), 49–54.
Buber, M. (1997). *Ich und Du*. Gütersloh: Gütersloher Verlagshaus.
Cassirer, E. (2010). *Philosophie der Symbolischen Formen*. Hamburg: Meiner.
Conklin. (2006). *Dialogue mapping: Building shared understanding of wicked problems*. West Sussex: John Wiley & Sons.
Dalley, T. (1994). *Images of art therapy. New developments in theory and practice*. London & New York: Routledge.
Dalley, T. (1996). *Art as therapy. An introduction to the use of art as a therapeutic technique*. London: Routledge.
Draaisma, D. (2010). *Vergeetboek*. Groningen: Historische Uitgeverij.
DuGay, P. (2000). *In praise of bureaucracy: Weber - organization - ethics*. London: Sage.
Eikeland, O. (2006). Phronesis, Aristotle, and action research. *International Journal of Action Research, 2*(1), 5.
Eikeland, O. (2008). *The ways of Aristotle: Aristotelian phronèsis, Aristotelian philosophy of dialogue, and action research*. Bern: Peter Lang.
Eisner, E. (2008). Art and knowledge. In J. Gary Knowles, & A. L. Cole (Eds.), *Handbook of the arts in qualitative research: Perspectives, methodologies, examples, and issues* (pp. 3–12). London, Thousand Oaks, New Delhi: Sage Publications.
Fleming, P., & Sturdy, A. (2009). Just be yourself! Towards neo-normative control in organisations? *Employee Relations, 31* (6), 569–583.
Flyvbjerg, B., Landman, T., & Schram, S. (2012). *Real social science: Applied phronesis*. Cambridge: University Press.
Foucault, M. (2005). *The hermeneutics of the subject: Lectures at the Collège de France 1981–1982* (Vol. 6). New York: Picador.
Gadamer, H.-G. (1993/1975). *Wahrheit und Methode*. Tubingen: Mohr Siebeck Gardner.
Gadamer, H-G. (2010). *Het schone. Kunst als spel, symbool en feest*. (vert. Willem Dijkhuis). Amsterdam: Boom.
Gardner, H. (2011). *Frames of mind: The theory of multiple intelligences*. New York: Basic books.
Habermas, J. (1984). *The theory of communicative action*. Boston: Beacon Press.
Hermans, H. J. M., & Hermans-Konopka, A. (2010). *Dialogical self theory. Positioning and counter-positioning in a globalizing society*. Cambridge: Cambridge University Press.
Isaacs, W. (1999). *Dialogue and the art of thinking together*. New York: Currency and Doubleday.
Jung, C. G. (1970). *Collected works, volume 1*. London: Routledge and Kegan Paul.
Kinni, T. (2003). *The Art of appreciative inquiry. The harvard business school working knowledge for business leaders newsletter, September 22–2003*. The european business ethics network UK conference.
Knowles, G., & Cole, A. L. (Eds.) (2008). *Handbook of the arts in qualitative research: Perspectives, methodologies, examples, and issues*. London, Thousand Oaks, New Delhi: Sage Publications.
Kuiper, P. (1988). *Ver heen*. Den Haag: SDU.
Kuiper, P. (1989). *De mens en zijn verhaal*. Amsterdam: Athenaeum.
Langer, S. (1979). *Philosophy in a New Key. A study in the symbolism of reason, rite and Art*. London/Cambridge: Harvard University Press.
Lengelle, R., Meijers, F., Poell, R., & Post, M. (2014). Career writing: Creative, expressive and reflective approaches to narrative identity formation in students in higher education. *Journal of Vocational Behavior, 85*(1), 75–84.
Lengelle, R., & Meijers, F. (2013). Narrative identity: Writing the self in career learning. *British Journal of Guidance & Counseling*. doi:10.1080/03069885.2013.816837
Lengelle, R., & Meijers, F. (2014). Narrative identity: Writing the self in career learning. *British Journal of Guidance & Counseling, 42*(1), 52–72.
Lengelle, R., & Meijers, F. (2015). Career writing: A creative, expressive and reflective approach to qualitative assessment and guidance. In M. McMahon & M. Watson (Eds.), *Career assessment: Qualitative approaches* (pp. 145–153). Rotterdam/Boston/Taipei: Sense Publishers.
Levey, P. (Ed) (2018). *Handbook of art-based research*. New York: Guilford Press.
Levine, E. (1995). *Studies in art, therapy and creativity*. Toronto: Palmerston Press.
Levine, S., & Levine, E. (1996). *Foundations of expressive art therapy*. London: Jessica Kingsley Publishers.
Liamputtong, P. (2007). *Researching the vulnerable. A guide to sensitive research methods*. London, Thousand Oaks, New Delhi: Sage Publications.
Liamputtong, P., & Rumbold, J. (Eds.) (2008). *Knowing differently: Arts-based and collaborative research methods*. New York: Nova science Publishers.

MacIntyre, A. (2007). *After virtue: A study in moral theory* (3rd revised ed.). London: Duckworth.
McNiff, S. (1981). *The arts and psychotherapy. Springfield; Art-based research*. London: Jessica Kingsley Publishers.
Mook, B. (2003). Phenomenological play therapy. In C. E. Schaefer (Ed.), *Foundations of play therapy* (pp. 260–280). Hoboken: Wiley.
Muijen, A. S. C. A. (2001). *Metafoor tussen Magie en Methode*. Kampen: Kok Agora.
Muijen, A. S. C. A. (2004). Corporate social responsibility starts at college. *Journal of Business Ethics, 53*(I & 2), 253–246.
Muijen, A. S. C. A. (2009, 2011). Het innerlijk kompas. *Supervisie en Coaching*, 26, 2-2009, 65–88; Levenskunst als basis voor begeleiding. *Supervisie en Coaching*, 28, 3-2011, 103–121.
Muijen, A. S. C. A. (2010). *Mens, ken je zelf!* [game]. Weesp: Thymia.
Muijen, A. S. C. A. (2012). *Wat is de kwestie? Wat is de questie!*. Weesp: Thymia. [game].
Muijen, A. S. C. A., Appel, G., & Cock Buning, T. (2004). *Hoe word je wijzer als je ruim denkt?* Amsterdam: VU-uitgeverij.
Muijen, A. S. C. A., & Van Marissing, L. (2011). *Iets maken*. Antwerpen/Apeldoorn: Garant.
Nietzsche, F. (1984). *Jenseits von Gut und Bose; Zur Genealogie der Moral. Werke III*. Ulm: Ullstein Materialien.
Nijhoff, A., & Wesseling, H. (2010). *Human Recources in ethisch perspectief. De HR-professie in de Maatschappelijk Verantwoorde Organisatie*. Assen: Van Gorcum.
Nussbaum, M. C. (2001). *The fragility of goodness: Luck and ethics in Greek tragedy and philosophy*. Cambridge: Cambridge University Press.
Nussbaum, M. C. (2014). *Political emotions. Why love matters for justice*. Cambridge: Harvard University Press.
Polanyi, M. (1966). *The tacit dimension*. London: Routledge & Kegan Paul.
Ricoeur, P. (1975). *La metaphore vive*. Paris: Du Seuil.
Ricoeur, P. (1984). *Temps et Receit*. Paris: Du Seuil.
Rose, G. (2001). *Visual methodologies. An introduction to the interpretation of visual materials*. London, Thousand Oaks, New Delhi: Sage Publications.
Schön, D. (1991). *The reflective practitioner. How professionals think in action*. Aldershot, Brookfield USA, Singapore, Sydney: Ashgate Arena.
Stern, D. N. (2010). *Forms of vitality*. Oxford: Oxford University Press.
Taylor, C. (2006). *Sources of the self. The making of modern identity*. Cambridge, MA: Harvard University Press.
Wierdsma, A., & Swieringa, J. (2011). *Lerend organiseren. Als meer van hetzelfde niet helpt*. Groningen: Noordhoff uitgevers.
Willems, M. (2017). Downloaded. Retrieved from http://www.mauricewillems.com/
Winnicott, D. (2005). *Playing and reality*. Abdington: Routledge.
Yuthas, K., Dillard, J. F., & Rogers, R. K. (2004). Beyond agency and structure: Triple-loop earning. *Journal of Business Ethics, 51*, 229–243.

Arts for the blues: a new creative psychological therapy for depression

Ailsa Parsons, Joanna Omylinska-Thurston, Julianne Harlow, Shelly Haslam, Jessica Hobson, Kerry Nair, Linda Dubrow-Marshall, Scott Thurston, Julia Griffin and Vicky Karkou

ABSTRACT
Routinely prescribed psychological therapies for depression are not always effective. Arts therapies, particularly Dance Movement Psychotherapy, may offer additional therapeutic mechanisms for depression. Therefore, client-reported helpful factors from various therapy types, along with client preferences, are key in devising new therapeutic interventions. We present a framework for a new pluralistic "meta-approach" of therapy for depression, based on an interdisciplinary thematic synthesis (Thomas, J., & Harden, A. (2008). Methods for the thematic synthesis of qualitative research in systematic reviews. *BMC Medical Research Methodology*, *8*[1], 45) of active ingredients from both talking therapies and creative approaches. Lastly, we offer an illustrative group therapy workshop based on this approach, to be piloted with clients and practitioners within an NHS mental health service. Further research is required to evaluate this pilot and to devise a full treatment for trialling within the service.

Introduction

Depression affects 7.8% of the UK population (Mental Health Foundation, 2016). Although NICE (2018) recommends several psychological interventions, in practice a combination of Cognitive–Behavioural Therapy (CBT) along with anti-depressant medication is often offered as first line treatment for depression. Improving Access to Psychological Therapies (IAPT) service outcomes data shows that of those finishing treatments, people in less deprived areas were more likely to show improvement in their condition and move towards recovery (58%) when compared to those living in more deprived areas (39%) (Parliament, House of Commons, 2018). As CBT is the main therapeutic intervention for depression, it is possible to conclude that it may have a limited effect on clients' recovery, especially in deprived areas. Given the high levels of investment in IAPT, these findings have financial and ethical implications and require further investigation.

A survey undertaken by the charity Mind demonstrated that 70% of service users found arts psychotherapies (Art, Music, Drama and Dance Movement Psychotherapy [DMP]) beneficial and rated them in the top three treatments of choice (Dudley, 2006). A UK survey (Williams & Scott, 2009) also indicated that service users wanted more access to arts psychotherapies. However, while there is a marked increase in research in this area (Zubala & Karkou, 2018), there remains limited access to these creative interventions within IAPT. Arts psychotherapies are used for therapeutic change within an established therapeutic relationship, the process being facilitated by a qualified practitioner (Karkou & Sanderson, 2006). The development of a new evidence-based intervention for depression from arts and mainstream talking therapies has the potential to contribute to depression recovery for those clients who are functioning well enough to be able to engage with such treatment, as opposed to those in a catatonic or acutely distressed state.

DMP is an arts psychotherapy which through a movement or creative act, it is possible to express, explore, interact, understand and derive meaning (Meekums, 2002). It is possible that in addition to the value ascribed to the creative component, physical activity levels could be enhanced, leading to increased secretion of pain-relieving endorphins, reduced cortisol levels and increased production and release of monoamines in the brain, all of which contribute to a "feel-good" effect (Jola & Calmeiro, 2017). In the treatment of depression, Karkou, Aithal, Zubala, and Meekums (2019) suggest that active connection with the moving body leads to a sense of agency and vitality. Through mirroring and physical attunement and the use of props, rhythm and imagination, relationships can be fostered as an essential means of tackling social isolation and loneliness. Unearthing difficult feelings through imagery, communicating them through symbolic movement and creating links between new discoveries and one's experiences are important factors that operate at an intra-psychic level. Stern's (2010) vitality dynamics theory holds that humans experience affective states and life events physically through a variety of perception parameters such as; movement, time, force, space, and intention. Verbally, these states and events may be described imaginatively as; gliding, swinging, pushing or otherwise. By purposely engaging and interacting with dimensions of experience through physical and artistic representations, individuals can push out of habitual/default ways of processing personal material, deepening their self-awareness.

Prior to the commencement of this project three of the authors of this paper (JOT, ST and VK) began experimenting with expressive arts as a way of getting to know one another. This led to the development of a process, starting with a body scan and identifying body information. Subsequently, each author took turns to express their embodied material in one modality (e.g. writing, movement, drawing, talking), while the others witnessed this and expressed their feedback in different modalities. Reflecting on this process they discovered common themes as the group dynamic was activated. This helped to enrich and deepen the connection between them and led to the creation of this project.

These experimentations demonstrated the usefulness of diverse creative methods and their potential value for clients. The authors reflected that in practice psychotherapists engage with clients via these media in order to comprehend the full "Gestalt" of vitality dynamics surrounding the client's phenomenological reality, past and present (Geuter, 2012), allowing the client to choose the arts modality/ies most aptly representative of their experiences. They reflected, that having a range of co-constructive techniques available may help clients extend their agency, allowing them to make sense of their experiential story and find their "personal truth" (McLeod, 2013).

A variety of clinical experiences that highlight the utility of integrative and arts-based therapies have been brought together and reflected upon to inform this project. LDM – an integrative psychologist who uses hypnotherapy, EMDR and other non-verbal creative approaches – reflected on the helpfulness of being able to adapt psychological approaches to the needs and preferences of individual clients. Particularly moving reflections concerned the witnessing of survivors of physical and sexual abuse reclaiming a sense of personal agency and space around their bodies using dance and movement methods, while another client, a physicist, made a mobile of various objects representing traumatic experiences, balancing the weights according to the impact these had upon her.

A client of AP, who suffered with depression, anxiety and trauma, described the experience and benefits of DMP sessions:

> When I had to push the wall as hard as I could, I pictured ... all these bad things were like in this wall and I could just push it away and ... It was quite hard hitting because I'd never thought that I would be able to do something like that ... I was in control of those thoughts, and I could push it away ... it's hard to explain what I do but I change and I'm able to put my thoughts into like picturing them physically ... It was weird thinking about

> things in a whole different way ... I could decide what I was going to do with my body ... it felt really good to be in control because everything else in my life, I've got no control over.

While this client had previously received counselling-based talking therapy, it was only through DMP and the use of various modalities leading to the physical intervention referred to above, that she felt such a profound shift in her mind-set and lived experience.

Clients report helpful factors from disparate orientations of therapy, with common areas of overlap between the talking therapies (client factors, therapeutic alliance, model/technique, and placebo/ expectancy; Wampold, 2015) and arts psychotherapies (therapeutic alliance, insight, expression, interaction, interpretation and narrative integration; Karkou & Sanderson, 2006; Colbert & Bent, 2017). However, which therapeutic techniques, orientations or expressive modalities are most useful depends on the unique client-therapist-context and may change over time (McLeod & Sundet, 2015). Therefore, integrating creative methods in a client-led manner enables the therapist to offer the most appropriate and acceptable intervention at the right time, while adopting a pluralistic approach to the client journey.

Pluralism has been described as a meta-model of therapy integration, in which client and therapist collaborate in deciding which approach(es) would work best for the individual client, without the need for theoretical coherence, or adherence to one universally-valid theory (Cooper & McLeod, 2011; McLeod & Sundet, 2015). Central to this practice, as with other therapies, is the therapeutic alliance or relationship, typified by the person-centred ethos (Cooper, 2015) and a "non-expert" stance that allows for unfolding of mystery. Hence, the therapist "comes alongside" and allows the work to be led by the client, implementing and exploring techniques felt to be most salient.

Previous innovators have attempted to amalgamate creative therapies in a way that spans different arts modalities. Rogers (1993) *Creative Connection* builds upon client-centredness by listening for client language suggestive of a preferred arts modality as a basis for exploration, before developing less dominant modes, continually returning to the "expert-client", their senses and imagination, to determine the next direction. Knill, Levine and Levine's *Intermodal Expressive Arts Therapy* (2005) follows a similar order, using the client's dominant modality to begin exploration, subsequently centring on the client's internal sensation to determine how to amplify or use alternative art forms to enable client expression and exploration of other perspectives. Implementing the client's "felt sense", *Focusing-Oriented Art Therapy* (Rappaport, 2014) uses six steps of sensing and focusing (Gendlin, 1981) to structure therapy utilising any arts modality, returning to the client's felt sense to consider new knowledge, evaluate and direct activities. Lusebrink's (2015) *Expressive Therapies Continuum* arranges activities along a continuum from kinaesthetic/sensory (exploration), perceptual/affective imagery (engaging) to cognitive/symbolic integration (structuring). Other approaches involve connecting to spiritual aspects (Malchiodi, 2003).

Such integrative arts models show areas of overlap in their approaches, especially in returning to the client's own felt sense (Gendlin, 1981) and imagination as a guiding principle. However, they fall short in incorporating evidence-based research findings identifying which ingredients of therapy are felt by clients to have been most useful in depression recovery. A qualitative review of client-identified helpful events in therapy (Timulak, 2007) included just one study focusing on depressed clients, in which creative therapies were not taken into account. Another review did focus upon change processes in depressed adolescent clients (Webb, Auerbach, & DeRubeis, 2012), yet was limited to CBT treatment only. The authors are not aware of reviews of client-reported helpful factors for depression specifically, or any reviews incorporating a variety of talking and arts therapies.

Given that current IAPT treatments show limited effectiveness for clients with depression, it is necessary to find a way to offer a combination of evidence-based active ingredients from different traditions and orientations, reported to be helpful in clients' depression recovery. These should be integrated in a way that spans and extends beyond previous attempts to implement multiple approaches or modalities offered by previous integrative models. Hence, by incorporating findings from both mainstream therapies and arts-based approaches, the creation of a pluralistic and creative meta-approach may extend the "radical eclecticism" of pluralism beyond any current limits, in a way that engages and benefits clients with depression.

Aims

This paper presents an interdisciplinary synthesis of key active ingredients in psychological treatment for depression, from both talking therapies, and creative arts-based approaches. Further, we aim to incorporate these synthesised findings to construct and present an overarching framework for creative, pluralistic arts-based therapy for depression. Lastly, we offer an example of a group therapy workshop based on this new approach, to be piloted with clients and practitioners within an inner city IAPT service.

Methods

Orientation and design

Mirroring our therapeutic stance, a pluralistic research orientation (Barker & Pistrang, 2005; Easterby-Smith, Golden-Biddle, & Locke, 2008) informed our interdisciplinary approach to inductive data acquisition, exploration and synthesis. The main research method was a Thematic Synthesis of relevant research findings (Thomas & Harden, 2008). In tandem with this literature-based method, we posited the findings against our own ethnographic and experiential knowledge in a deepening and unfolding process of Crystallization (Ellingson, 2009), using some creative explorations of the topic to gain additional perspectives on the findings (Artistic Enquiry; Hervey, 2000).

Pluralistic sources of evidence for a pluralistic therapy

Our research design, as implied by "pluralistic", was not purely literature-based. Barker and Pistrang (2005) state the importance of using the best combination of methods to investigate the research question(s), rather than confining methodology to strict conventions, in accordance with the rationale of a mixed methods approach (Creswell, 2014). In this study, we have gone beyond the mixing of data from conventional research methods to add arts-based approaches influenced by ideas proposed by Hervey (2000) in *Artistic Inquiry*.

Valuable autoethnographic information situated within the researchers themselves provided knowledge and experience, grounded within real life and practice, to also take into consideration. Some researchers experimented creatively with the themes emerging from data analysis in order to understand them experientially through movement, creative wording, and performative material (Griffin & Thurston, 2018). Other researchers brought with them a wealth of experience working with both talking and non-verbal methods. Therefore, appropriately framed personal, professional and creative experiences enhanced our approach to interpretation. An additional rationale for incorporating more intuitive and non-linguistic perspectives was that our client-led treatment would involve a reliance on a certain level of intuition and non-verbal approaches, so it appeared fitting to take this approach as researchers in contemplating the evidence. This contextualised and embodied knowledge, removed from linguistic representations in the literature, crystallized and enriched the literature findings of what may work *in practice,* and was invaluable in creating a pilot experiential workshop to be delivered within the IAPT context.

Pluralism in thematic synthesis

For our thematic synthesis, we were particularly focused on published studies on retrospective client perspectives. However, as some quantitative findings contain aspects of qualitative data (Thomas & Harden, 2008), a range of other research data (therapists' perspectives, outcomes-based data) were reviewed concerning helpful factors for clients in treatment for depression, and incorporated if felt especially relevant with regards to client needs.

Search strategy

Researchers individually searched for papers on a range of therapy types: CBT, Cognitive Therapy, Behavioural Activation for Depression, Counselling for Depression, Psychodynamic, Pluralistic, Integrative, Arts (including DMP, Dramatherapy, Art Therapy and Music Therapy) and self-management/other individual strategies.

Inclusion criteria were as follows: published at any time, detailing client-reported helpful factors/ingredients which made their therapy effective (or not), written in English. The emphasis was on retrospective qualitative client reports, but also included were therapist reports of what clients found helpful, and to a lesser extent, quantitative outcomes-based studies of helpful factors and their effects, but only if they related to client evaluations of helpful therapy aspects. Only papers specific to depression were included.

Key words entered into electronic databases (including PsycINFO; Science Direct, SCOPUS and Google Scholar) included the name of the therapy itself (for example "CBT" or "cognitive behavioural therapy") and "helpful factors"; "helpful aspects"; "client-reported"; "client perspectives"; "client views"; "depression". Authors also hand-searched in journals for papers of interest, or presented research already possessed on the topic, including PhD theses or other grey literature that met the inclusion criteria.

Purposive sampling of papers was used, in order to reach an optimal level of conceptual saturation. Searching continued until either (a) further searching failed to add conceptually to the substantive array of data within each of the therapy types, or (b) no more studies could be found.

Quality assessment

In assessing papers for inclusion during the search, we were guided by Thomas and Harden's (2008) guidelines for assessing quality of studies in thematic synthesis. Briefly, these relate to the reporting of aims, context, rationale, methods and findings, establishing the reliability and validity of data collection, analysis and findings, and appropriateness of study methods for uncovering findings about client perspectives on what features are helpful in therapy for depression.

Data extraction

Based on their quality and appropriateness for answering the research question, a total of 14 suitable papers for CBT were analysed, six for Cognitive Therapy, seven for Behavioural Activation for Depression, nine for Counselling for Depression, 23 for integrative, pluralistic and psychodynamic, 17 for Arts therapies, and two for self-management/other. Key findings from these studies were collated verbatim into a table, before synthesising thematically.

Thematic synthesis

We used Thematic Synthesis (Thomas & Harden, 2008) to collate findings from the studies. This approach to analysing secondary qualitative data, follows the same basic steps as Thematic Analysis (Braun & Clarke, 2006), except the data is composed of previous authors' findings. These steps are as follows: (1) Free coding of the original extracted findings, (2) Grouping of similar free codes into descriptive categories, (3) Generating analytical themes that emerge from and step beyond the descriptive categories.

Individual researchers undertook duplicate and concurrent analysis of the data for each therapy type for the initial stages. Data were first-order coded for pertinent active ingredients of therapy, and these codes examined for similarities and differences, grouping them into second-order descriptive categories. Next, we as the researchers came together to compare codes, any relevant notes/contextual information and resolve any interpretive differences, before collaboratively agreeing on the overarching themes within the data for that therapy type. These themes were collated onto a master document, which was then added to after the analysis of each therapy type. All themes were then assimilated, resolving any overlaps, to arrive at a full list of themes across therapies.

Deepening understanding through crystallization

In their guide to Thematic Synthesis, Thomas and Harden (2008) have stated that in interpreting analytical themes, reviewers "go beyond" the initial data to generate new interpretive constructs and meanings. We interacted and experimented with the themes generated, thus deepening and refining our understanding of the data in a process of crystallization (Ellingson, 2009). Some researchers reflected upon how the themes related to their own experiences as both therapists and clients, and others engaged with multimodal artistic enquiry (Hervey, 2000) using movement, creative writing and verbalisation to identify how their own long-term creative explorations related to the developing framework, using the developing thematic framework as an impetus for artistic enquiry. The emerging material from these enquiries helped to validate and deepen understanding of the qualitative findings, enabling further emphasis and refinement of some subthemes.

Applied integration of helpful therapy features and arts modalities

After the synthesis of thematic findings, it was necessary to integrate the helpful factors in an applied way. In order to construct the basis of an evidence-based yet practical template for the new therapeutic treatment, we consulted other integrative models of multimodal therapies (those which use a mixture of creative modalities as well as verbal mechanisms). Features of these multimodal therapies – Rogers (1993) *Creative Connection,* Knill, Levine and Levine's *Intermodal Expressive Arts Therapy* (2005), *Focusing-Oriented Art Therapy* (Rappaport, 2014), Lusebrink's (2015) *Expressive Therapies Continuum* and multimodal *Expressive Therapies* (Malchiodi, 2003) – are described in the introduction. Similarities and differences between integrative models were evaluated: broadly, they present considerations around establishing space, safety and a client-led ethos, cultural and biological/inherited contexts, multilevel phenomenological experience, transitions between these levels (inter – or multimodal transfer, superimposition, amplification), and processes for exploring, expanding, deepening client awareness. We considered these features in light of our thematic findings as well as our practitioner-inherent experiences of creative therapy, informing the structure and material for the pilot experiential workshop.

Results

Table 1 presents themes and subthemes of helpful factors in psychotherapeutic treatment for depression, integrated from client-reported findings across different psychotherapies, crystallised by the researchers' experiential knowledge and creative explorations.

Findings revealed a hierarchy of seven themes and 30 subthemes, arranged by how "foundational" or primary they appear to be in the therapy approach. Theme 1, "Tailored structure and content to fit the client", is presented first because the planned structure and content of the therapy package is by necessity the initial consideration that a therapist or organisation must make. This leads to considering ways in which clients can focus on their "Client targets" as an important reference point to kick start the therapeutic process (theme 2). "Fundamental relational skills and features" (theme 3) sits at the core of *what the therapist does* in the session and the overall attitude of the therapist, in relation with the client(s). The active nature of the intervention and overall ethos of the approach is evident in "Encouraging vitality through active engagement" (theme 4), which stems from client-reported helpful factors relating to activation and empowerment through *doing*. Themes 5, 6 and 7 clarify ways of working in the here and now, in the past, and moving towards integration.

Table 1. Findings from thematic synthesis of client-reported helpful factors.

Theme/subtheme	Explanation
(1) Tailored structure and content to fit the client	The broad features and parameters of the therapy package and of each session
(a) Effective timing	Therapy commencement, schedule and number of sessions tailored to client/group
(b) Structured yet flexible variety	Well-organised, malleable content both in-session and out, e.g. homework; boundaried autonomy in tasks; unique sessions/activities
(c) Prompting	Reinforcing client behaviours/strategies where necessary to help keep 'on track', e.g. through text messaging
(d) Cultural adaptation	Appropriate and relatable group-specific content, e.g. tailored to different social groups
(e) Evolution of tasks	Smooth, appropriately paced transition between different ways of working (e.g. sensory levels, arts modalities, solo to group work, development of themes or expressive material)
(2) Client targets	Specific features or processes within the clients' inter/intra-personal repertoire that clients report have been helpful to target in therapy
(a) Increasing awareness and insight	Learning about self and depression; Self- and other-schemas/concepts and relationships; New understanding, conceptualising or reframing of problems
(b) Learning skills to manage self	Learning to manage and balance vitality, emotions, cognitions including rumination, and day-to-day behaviours
(c) Integrating personal material & narrative	Finding meaning through integrating a personal narrative, resolving past conflicts, bringing together personal story/motif/metaphor, revealing way(s) forwards
(d) Fostering social support & satisfaction	Developing positive personal relationships, network-building and frequent/regular purpose/reward in everyday life
(3) Fundamental relational skills and features	Fundamentals of the therapeutic space, process and relationship (therapist, client and/or group)
(a) Safe place	Comfort and containment in therapy space or organisation
(b) Coherent explanation of therapy	Building trust, confidence and hope through a clear explanation of process/mechanism(s)
(c) Warm, supportive alliance/group cohesion	Therapeutic and/or group relationship characterised by empathy, unconditional positive regard, full psychological 'contact', 'holding', comfort and reassurance, inclusivity
(d) Skilled, responsive balancing	Therapist's attunement with client needs in order to precisely negotiate and modulate different dynamics, challenges and boundaries as appropriate to foster client's development. Examples: Directing vs. non-directing, Affirming vs. challenging, Reassure vs. confront, Interpreting vs. holding, Guiding vs. exploring, Lead vs. follow, Depth vs. smoothness, Expert vs. 'friend', Distancing vs. disclosing
(e) Interpersonal collaboration – sharing with others	Through task-orientated group-work and observing relational dynamics within self (client) and responses to/from others in group.
(4) Encouraging vitality through active engagement	Maintaining a strong focus on activation and vitality, encouraging the client to take direct, independent action in own life and experience
(a) Nurturing autonomy and agency	E.g. making and carrying out decisions (such as the focus of, and which way to work in-session); devising and implementing strategies to confront challenges
(b) Engaging with the body	Avoiding inertia/increasing vitality dynamics by exploring and moving towards goals creatively and physically in own life and in-session
(c) Independent practice outside session	E.g. journaling, monitoring, cognitive restructuring, distraction/coping techniques, pleasant/mastery activities, creative and active pursuits, reading
(5) Working with the 'now'	Working with present capacities, issues and concerns
(a) Connecting body and mind	E.g. body scan, mindfulness, breathing; following impulse while 'switched off' from regular conscious cognition; responding to music; moving and mirroring
(b) Identifying, experiencing and expressing emotions	Building detailed perceptual awareness of emotion and experience in present moment; expressing emotions and catharsis of client material
(c) Structured improvisation	Experimenting solo or with others through structured improvisation based on a theme/idea, with some parameters

(Continued)

Table 1. Continued.

Theme/subtheme	Explanation
(d) Contemplating current self/other insights	Contemplating internal (self) and external (other) events, interactions, patterns and attachments in the present
(e) Experimenting with thoughts and actions	E.g. alternative thinking patterns, new actions/behaviours, 'trying on' ways of being
(f) Problem solving and planning	Helping the client to confront challenges logically and plan ahead
(6) Getting to the 'root'	Working with past experiences, issues and concerns
(a) Working with past self/other insights	Unearthing and reflecting on internal (self) and external (other) events, longitudinal patterns, emotions, interactions and attachments in past.
(b) Bridging the insight gap	Linking past events and current reality, reorganising their implications for personal 'narrative', capacities developed and coherent self-understanding.
(c) Nurturing self-regard	Normalising and accepting aspects of past self to enhance self-regard. Practicing helpful/positive self-reflection.
(7) Bringing it all together	Recognising, celebrating and integrating useful material back to one's life
(a) Identifying core values	Identifying personal values for future direction and action, towards a new narrative
(b) Constructing new self-concepts	Integrating new self-concepts that culminate the end point of the therapeutic journey through expressive narrative (story, choreography, artwork, poem etc)
(c) Practising new ways of being	Refining the self-concepts through reflection and/or repetition
(d) Sharing creative work with others	Exhibiting/performing this work to self and others if appropriate

Thus, clients are supported to bridge the gap between past events and current reality, while extending towards the future by capitalising on the lessons learned and capacities developed for coherent self-understanding.

The active and creative thread (theme 4) runs through many aspects of the model, featuring both in the evolving tasks in the structured content of therapy (theme 1e), and in the way in which the tasks and activities in-session are to be engaged – using client's preferred modality/ies, or combinations of talking/verbalising, writing, imagery, symbolism, movement, sound, story, other creative media (themes 5, 6 and 7). This approach also offers a helpful way to conclude the therapy journey creatively (theme 7 – Bringing it all together).

Unhelpful factors found in the thematic synthesis did not make the final edit because they all represented the opposite of some of the helpful factors featured. Therefore, by adhering to the recommended package of active ingredients, therapists would be avoiding these unhelpful factors. For example, one unhelpful factor "Not modulating the intensity of challenging aspects of therapy (lack of modulation causing distress/unsafety to client)" is neutralised by the helpful factor (3d) "Skilled, responsive balancing".

Although fairly complex and theoretical, these findings offer the key "building blocks" with which therapists and clinicians might devise a pluralistic psychotherapeutic treatment package for depression, appropriate to their specific client group and context. Based on these building blocks, the authors assembled a single-session pilot workshop to be trialled within an inner-city IAPT service with a small (<10) group of clients, and another of IAPT clinicians. Table 2 presents a chronological outline of this pilot intervention and highlights how it has been informed by the theoretical basis of Table 1's findings and/or potential active ingredients that may be operationalised by the activities (N.B. wording and features of the workshop should be adapted to suit the population and context).

The above outline comprises a number of activities and steps to undertake in facilitating a single 90-minute pilot workshop, as well as the rationale and/or potential active ingredients involved in the activities. The activities themselves will be by necessity of time limitation, very brief, and therefore the

Table 2. Outline and theoretical underpinnings of IAPT pilot intervention.

Task	Description	Theory/ 'active ingredients'
Preparation	Preparing room, materials, suitable language (wording to be appropriate to the population), and preparing and grounding self (facilitators)	1b, 1d, 3a, 3e
Introduction	Facilitators and clients introducing selves	3c
	Introducing time boundaries and any contingency plans (telephone/ email follow-up)	1a
	Introducing a brief chronological preview of workshop; normalising any client concerns about their competence	1e, 3b, 3c
Safety, ethical contracting and housekeeping	Outlining potential effects of workshop and safety precautions	3a, 3d
	Outlining participant responsibility for safety in activities, the right to withdraw and inviting clients to express any initial needs	3a, 3c, 4a
	Collaboratively establishing ground rules (i.e. confidentiality, respect, non-judgemental attitude)	1e, 3a, 3c, 3e, 4a
	Housekeeping	3a
Explain depression and intervention	Brief explanation of depression and intervention mechanisms	3b
Goal setting, sharing and rating	Inviting participants to set a small, manageable and immediate goal to work on during workshop, e.g. changing a feeling state or clarifying a problem or dilemma	1b, 4, 2a
	Participants sharing their goals in pairs. Facilitator(s) check goals are appropriate for workshop context	3e, 5
	Participants writing down their goal and rating it on the goal worksheet, according to how close they are to achieving this on the scale 0–10	5
	Inviting participants to share their goal and/or numerical rating with the group	3e, 4d, 5
Body scan and emotional check-in	Experiential mindfulness-based body scan (attending to body, breathing, sensation and affect)	5, 4b
	Sensing a connection to the goal: participants invited to sense how/ where the goal is perceived in the body (normalise any difficulties in doing this)	2c
	Inviting feedback on their experiences of this	1e, 3c, 2a, 5
Modelling expressive arts modalities	Briefly practice using the three different arts modalities[1] (making marks on paper, writing creatively on impulse, or movement) to respond to sensations and perceptions when focusing on different body parts.	1b, 1e, 5, 4a, 4b
	Inviting participants to share their experience of this, and to notice which modality/ies felt most natural to use for the next activity	1b, 1e, 2d, 5, 4a
Creative expression	Making participants aware that they will be sharing their creative expression in pairs. Normalising any potential challenges with this activity	1e, 3a, 3c
	Inviting participants to sense and focus in on bodily responses to their goal and allowing their imagination to evoke images, colours, words, textures, rhythms, sounds, movements, sensations etc in response to this experience	2a, 5
	Inviting participants to work with their preferred modality/ies in order to express and creatively extend this inner experience	1b, 1e, 5, 4a, 4b
Sharing in pairs	Inviting participants to share with another participant some or all of their creative expression and its personal meaning /how it links with their goal. Participants choose how much they want to reveal. Other partner in the pair witnesses non-judgmentally then mirrors or responds to the expression verbally/non-verbally without any interpretation. The pair then swap roles (expressing and witnessing)	1e, 3c, 3e, 2a, 2d, 4a, 5, 6
Reviewing goals and ratings	Inviting participants to review original goals and repeat rating, again using the 1–10 scale and writing this down	3b, 2a, 2e, 5
Whole group sharing and creating	Inviting participants to share their experiences of the workshop, uncertainties/questions, anything they have learned from the experience, and how they will apply this learning in their lives over the coming week	3e, 2, 4, 5, 6, 7
	Inviting all participants to creatively express their final responses to this group experience, by making marks or words on a large piece of paper (group drawing), or creating a collective movement	1e, 3e, 2d, 5, 7
Closure	Participants choosing whether to take their creative work or leave it behind	4a
	Providing participants with a list of resources in case of feeling upset after the session	3a

(*Continued*)

Table 2. Continued.

Task	Description	Theory/ 'active ingredients'
	Allowing extra time in the room in case participants want to stay and connect with each other or talk informally with facilitators after the session	3c, 2d

[1]For the purpose of this pilot workshop, participants are limited to a choice of three modalities – image making with pastels, creative writing, or creative movement. This is so as to provide some choice of widely-familiar modalities, without overwhelming with too many choices in the initial workshop. Longer-term interventions may use any number of arts modalities, e.g. sculpture, sound making, others.

workshop provides only a "taster" of the main tenets and activities of the approach, the order and transitions that might be followed, and the rationale for each.

Because of the brief activities and single-session nature of the workshop, deeper, longer-term therapeutic aims, features and outcomes (normally achievable in the context of a longstanding and therapeutic alliance) are unlikely to be met, such as prompting between sessions (1c), achieving full psychological "contact" (3c), integrating a personal narrative (2c), building a supportive social network and regular reward/enjoyment in life (2d), unearthing and reflecting on insight around the past (6a), positively integrating past events, strengths/achievements into self-narrative (6b) and unearthing core values (7a). These features and objectives are more likely to be developed and targeted over a series of therapy sessions.

Not explicitly stipulated within Table 2 are incidental considerations such as room size/features, adaptations for holding the workshop with the IAPT clinicians as opposed to clients, the optional use of music and how to deal with disruptions such as clients interpreting/dominating/chit-chat, although these matters broadly fall under the remit of *Safe place, Cultural adaptation, Structured yet flexible variety/Structured improvisation, and Skilled, responsive balancing,* respectively.

Discussion

We aimed to synthesise findings from both arts- and mainstream-therapeutic evidence with interdisciplinary collaboration, to present a set of key ingredients and helpful factors in the treatment of depression, structured into a coherent new pluralistic approach that extends beyond current integrative and arts models of therapy. Crystallised from the sum of published and experiential evidence, we established seven main themes which illuminate key tenets of the new approach: *Tailored structure and content to fit the client, Client targets, Fundamental relational skills and features, Encouraging vitality through active engagement, Working with the now, Getting to the root* and *Bringing it all together.* Within these seven themes, 30 subthemes detail the specific components which may be implemented in each of these areas. At the heart of the approach lies a client-led ethos within the safety of a strong and attuned therapeutic relationship, to ultimately encourage clients to become self-led in regaining their vitality and engagement with life.

Our secondary aim was to apply these findings in a real-world context, by devising an example workshop for a specific set of clients, using the new framework to guide our session plan. We found that the order of activities planned for the workshop naturally reflected the structure of the framework – beginning with the foundational and preliminary considerations, then to the safety of the therapeutic relationship(s), then to the clients' own target setting, followed by experiential activities and subsequent personally-reflective meaning-making, and finally concluding the experience in a shared expression. Throughout these activities, the thread of active engagement is built in by providing client choice and autonomy, inviting them to engage the whole self in "doing" and moving activities. Hence, the proposed workshop matches the theoretical model in a way that chronologically matches the layers (fundamental tenets, to specific tasks) of the framework.

The findings of our thematic synthesis support recent and ongoing DMP research findings, which propose that key processes involved in treating and alleviating depression include (i) connecting with the body, (ii) forming relationships (iii) unearthing and processing difficult emotions (iv) integrating emotional material (Karkou et al., 2019). Indeed, these facets are a close match with some of our active ingredients under the themes "client activation", the "therapeutic relationship" and working with "now", "getting to the root" and "bringing it all together". Further supporting the connection with the body, a recent Cochrane review (Meekums, Karkou, & Nelson, 2015) proposed some similarly body-oriented theoretical mechanisms: non-verbal communication, kinaesthetic responding and embodied empathy. In addition, the review highlights the potential "unblocking" of *vitality* – energy, stamina, and physical or mental vigour, reflecting physical and emotional components of wellbeing (Deng, Guyer, & Ware, 2015) – through movement and creative processes. This aligns somewhat with our "Encouraging vitality through active engagement" theme, which proposes a strong focus on client agency and physical engagement to support vitality and overcome inertia. It also strongly ties in with Stern's (2010) theories on vitality dynamics arising from physical and creative actions and interactions, as opposed to more passive, inert experiences and speaks to research on physiological and neurological research in dance (see Jola & Calmeiro, 2017).

Furthermore, the centrality of symbolism and metaphor in movement and imagination (Karkou et al., 2019) – to increase client-therapist closeness, safely process distressing content and creatively apprehend change. Our framework features the use of arts modalities to engage metaphor throughout themes five through seven. Finally, the inclusion of physically creative acts in these themes and especially 5a) *Connecting body and mind*, are supported by empirical findings on embodied affectivity (Fuchs & Koch, 2014) – that is, the circular effects of "moving" (action, expression, movement and sensation) and "being moved" (perceptions of affective stimuli in the external environment) – to progress understanding and promote vitality.

Extending beyond DMP research, the framework features key ingredients which are derived from other evidence-based approaches, for example active engagement strongly aligns with principles of Behavioural Activation (a behavioural therapy focused on breaking the cycle of inertia seen in depression; Veale, 2008). The centrality of the therapeutic relationship echoes common factors research (e.g. Wampold, 2015) and Humanistic/Rogerian orientations, yet beyond this, evidence-based techniques have been incorporated such as negotiating client targets and goals, planning, problem solving, setting homework and skills training, which are more affiliated with CBT (Beck, 2011). Nevertheless, the means by which the targets are engaged – through sensory, embodied and creative processes – are shared with arts-based, body and mindfulness orientations (Rappaport, 2013).

Within our framework, we do not see the methods involved (from supposedly opposing approaches) as being mutually-exclusive. Schmid (2005) has defined creativity as:

> An innate capacity to think and act in original ways, to be inventive, to be imaginative and to find new and original solutions to needs, problems and forms of expression. It can be used in all activities. Its processes and outcomes are meaningful to its user and generate positive feelings. (p. 6)

Therefore, the more reason-based "problem solving" (e.g. of more cognitive/rational therapies) and the depth-based illumination of material outside of conscious awareness (e.g. through the creative act) are seen as mutually augmentative – one may inspire, enrich and extend the other within our pluralistic framework.

While the use of spontaneous creative acts and an embodied locus of attention have the potential to transcend the limits of talking therapies, these aspects nevertheless pose a challenge for many and may invoke feelings of anxiety in some clients. Clients may lack the confidence to engage with the inherently unpredictable nature of the creative act and may fear "putting themselves out there" (Parsons & Dubrow-Marshall, 2018) through creative expression. Hence, it is necessary to "scaffold" a clear, secure and reliable structure within sessions, and to evolve tasks gradually and at a client-led pace, as set out in our framework (1e – *Evolution of tasks*). The therapist must use their competencies of *Skilled, responsive balancing* (theme 3d) to sensitively and precisely negotiate and modulate levels of directive versus non-directive elements, and the depth (impact) and smoothness (client-perceived safety) of the work (Stiles et al., 1994). Particularly in the group context, a more directive approach to structure activities is necessary, and setting of parameters for depth/difficulty of individual client material, to contain the process of multiple clients simultaneously. Our pilot workshop implements this structure and parameters, while offering client-led options within these limits as appropriate for the population and setting. Finally, bearing in mind our client-led, pluralistic ethos, it is important to note that ultimately there are some individuals who are simply averse to the use of arts generally or therapeutically, and for these individuals no amount of structuring or negotiating will overcome their aversion to creative methods. This intervention might not be appropriate for them.

Throughout our approach, clients' active engagement is encouraged (theme 4) – instilling an overarching ethos of agency, autonomy, physical action and skill building throughout the other ingredients; in other words, developing clients' capacity to be self-led. This self-determination begins with the choosing of an immediate goal to work with in-session. The list of *Client targets* (theme 2) is based on changes reported by clients to have been helpful in the treatment of depression. However, the list is not exhaustive, and the immediate goals chosen by clients may, at face value, bear little relation to these overall *Client targets*. Nevertheless, the client-led approach supports a view of the client as "expert" and therefore we do not impose preconceived ideas about what they need to work on in a particular session.

As clinicians and researchers, we allowed our own creativity to guide our collaborative approach to the project – thus "practising what we preach" in terms of modulating challenges, integrating perspectives, following creative interests and valuing imagination. We worked alongside a performance team who composed a movement and spoken word composition based on emergent findings of our research (Griffin & Thurston, 2018). In this crystallisation of approaches, four elements stand out as beneficial to the overall process and worthy of mention here. Firstly, the centrality of a trusting relationship that is needed when working performatively, especially within the context of interdisciplinary collaboration where neither participant was an expert in the other's discipline. Notions of sharing internal phenomena expressively and co-constructing meaning lie at the heart of both the compositional/performative process, and of our therapeutic approach.

Secondly, the performance team experimented with different arts modalities, combining movement, spoken word and music to arrive at a complete composition that enabled and mobilised the full expression of inner experience, enacting movement metaphor across different disciplines to develop a shared movement and verbal language. Thirdly, the performance team contemplated the emergent themes, finding a high level of recognition in support of their own experiential findings. They were able to recognise the common practices of structured improvisation, relational dynamics and reflection across artistic and therapeutic practice, reporting that outcomes from the creative collaboration were comparable to those of therapy, i.e. a sense of extending one's repertoire, developing an aptitude for embodied action, and accepting the wholeness of one's experience. Lastly, the experience of working "holistically" – combining both empirically supported and subjective, experiential types of evidence – has highlighted the overall value of working pluralistically.

It is important to note, reflexively, that although the review of published literature was undertaken collaboratively by a group of Psychologists, Dance Movement Psychotherapists and Counsellors, the therapists' background and preferences may have impacted the way data were sought and presented (Haynes, 2012). In interpreting, analysing and synthesising evidence, we may have perceived things that resonated with our personal and professional (therapeutic or research) experiences to date. This innate tendency has been acknowledged and mitigated as far as possible through checking in and dialoguing as a (diverse) team about the rationale for different decisions in the research process, and holding each decision up to the scrutiny of both tacitly-developed knowledge, and the rationally-selected research methodology we adopted from the beginning.

Regarding the implications of the findings themselves, our creative treatment framework is not "manualised" and therefore does not offer a step-by-step set of instructions to clinicians, rather it is an assemblage of principles and active ingredients, to be used with therapist and client discretion according to individuals and context. Whereas, the outline of a pilot workshop provides a limited, context-specific example only. The workshop is not intended to be a therapy or to work at great depth – indeed, it would be unsafe to do so under the circumstances of a single instance of experimental research. Hence, not all of the active ingredients have been explicitly operationalised within this workshop, and a longer-term intervention will be needed to demonstrate the full range of active ingredients as appropriate to the client/group. To this end, a manual for longer-term application of the approach should be developed and trialled.

Conclusions

Our thematic synthesis of helpful factors in therapy for clients with depression generated a framework of seven themes and 30 subthemes, which clinicians may implement using multimodal artistic and verbal methods with their clients. The findings align with previous purported mechanisms in Dance Movement Psychotherapy, while also extending beyond previous work to incorporate client views from all therapies, in a new meta-approach not previously attempted by other integrative models. At the heart of this new approach lies both the therapeutic relationship, and clients' active engagement, in order to enable both safety and vitality.

Our innovative research process has highlighted the value of interdisciplinary work, marrying the science and art of the researchers' psychological, psychotherapeutic, health and arts-based professional disciplines, perspectives and methods, enabling a multidimensional understanding of the findings and their application within both performance and therapy. Furthermore, we provide an example of how the blueprint of this meta-approach has been used to devise a specific pilot workshop to be trialled in an inner-city IAPT setting. However, neither the theoretical framework nor the pilot intervention constitutes a standardised treatment package, and therefore testing for efficacy or effectiveness is not yet possible. Further research is anticipated to evaluate the IAPT workshop and future objectives should be to conduct studies testing a more standardised version of the approach. Nevertheless, therapists of all orientations may find value in this embryonic creation by using their professional judgement as to which overarching tenets – or specific active ingredients – of the approach are felt to be appropriate to implement with their clients.

Disclosure statement

No potential conflict of interest was reported by the authors.

ORCID

Ailsa Parsons http://orcid.org/0000-0002-3540-5660
Joanna Omylinska-Thurston http://orcid.org/0000-0001-8329-171X
Vicky Karkou http://orcid.org/0000-0001-8986-956X
Shelly Haslam http://orcid.org/0000-0003-2023-6734
Scott Thurston http://orcid.org/0000-0002-5326-593X

References

Barker, C., & Pistrang, N. (2005). Quality criteria under methodological pluralism: Implications for conducting and evaluating research. *American Journal of Community Psychology, 35*(3-4), 201–212.

Beck, J. S. (2011). *Cognitive behavior therapy: Basics and beyond.* New York: Guilford press.

Braun, V., & Clarke, V. (2006). Using thematic analysis in psychology. *Qualitative Research in Psychology, 3*(2), 77–101.

Colbert, T., & Bent, C. (Eds.). (2017). *Working across modalities in the arts therapies: Creative collaborations.* Oxon: Routledge.

Cooper, M. (2015). Core counselling methods for pluralistic practice. In M. Cooper, & W. Dryden (Eds.), *The handbook of pluralistic counselling and psychotherapy* (pp. 80–93). London: Sage.

Cooper, M., & McLeod, J. (2011). *Pluralistic counselling and psychotherapy.* London: Sage.

Creswell, J. W. (2014). *A concise introduction to mixed methods research.* Thousand Oaks, CA: Sage.

Deng, N., Guyer, R., & Ware, J. E. (2015). Energy, fatigue, or both? A bifactor modeling approach to the conceptualization and measurement of vitality. *Quality of Life Research, 24*(1), 81–93.

Dudley, J. (2006). *Service users and carers: Arts therapies available in the trust; South West London and St George's Mental Health NHS Trust.* Retrieved from http://www.swlstg-tr.nhs.uk/service_users/arts_therapies_available_in_the_trust.asp

Easterby-Smith, M., Golden-Biddle, K., & Locke, K. (2008). Working with pluralism: Determining quality in qualitative research. *Organizational Research Methods, 11*(3), 419–429.

Ellingson, L. L. (2009). *Engaging crystallization in qualitative research: An introduction.* Thousand Oaks, CA: Sage.

Fuchs, T., & Koch, S. C. (2014). Embodied affectivity: On moving and being moved. *Frontiers in Psychology, 5*, 508.

Gendlin, E. T. (1981). *Focusing* (2nd ed.). New York, NY: Bentam Books.

Geuter, U. (2012). Forms of vitality. Exploring dynamic experience in psychology, arts, psychotherapy, and development, by Daniel N. Stern. *Body, Movement and Dance in Psychotherapy, 7*(3), 235–239. doi:10.1080/17432979.2012.674062

Griffin, J., & Thurston, S. (2018). *'Getting out of your own way'* (dance and poetry performance), performed at Edge Hill University on 23 February 2018 and 13 June 2018, University of Bedfordshire 14 June 2018, Starptelpa: Riga Performance Festival, Riseba, Riga, Latvia 17 June 2018.

Haynes, R. B. (2012). *Clinical epidemiology: How to do clinical practice research.* Philadelphia: Lippincott Williams & Wilkins.

Hervey, L. W. (2000). *Artistic inquiry in dance/movement therapy: Creative research alternatives.* Springfield, IL: Charles C Thomas Publisher.

Jola, C., & Calmeiro, L. (2017). The dancing queen: Explanatory mechanisms of the 'feel-good effect' in dance. In V. Karkou, S. Oliver, & S. Lycouris (Eds.), *The Oxford handbook of dance and wellbeing* (pp. 13–41). Oxford: Oxford University Press.

Karkou, V., Aithal, S., Zubala, A., & Meekums, B. (2019). Effectiveness of dance movement therapy in the treatment of adults with depression: A systematic review with meta-analyses. *Frontiers in Psychology.* doi:10.3389/fpsyg.2019.00936

Karkou, V., & Sanderson, P. (2006). *Arts therapies: A research-based map of the field.* Edinburgh: Elsevier Health Sciences.

Knill, P. J., Levine, E. G., & Levine, S. K. (2005). *Principles and practice of expressive arts therapy: Toward a therapeutic aesthetics.* London: Jessica Kingsley Publishers.

Lusebrink, V. B. (2015). Expressive therapies continuum. In D. Gussak, & M. L. Rosal (Eds.), *The Wiley handbook of art therapy* (pp. 57–68). Sussex: Wiley Blackwell.

Malchiodi, C. A. (2003). Expressive arts therapy and multimodal approaches. In C. A. Malchiodi (Ed.), *Handbook of art therapy* (pp. 106–117). New York, NY: Guilford Press.

McLeod, J. (2013). Developing pluralistic practice in counselling and psychotherapy: Using what the client knows. *The European Journal of Counselling Psychology, 2*(1), 51–64.

McLeod, J., & Sundet, R. (2015). Integrative and eclectic approaches and pluralism. In M. Cooper, & W. Dryden (Eds.), *The handbook of pluralistic counselling and psychotherapy* (pp. 158–171). London: Sage.

Meekums, B. (2002). *Dance movement therapy: A creative psychotherapeutic approach.* London: Sage.

Meekums, B., Karkou, V., & Nelson, A. (2015). Dance movement therapy for depression. *Cochrane Database of Systematic Reviews, 2*, 1–54.

Mental Health Foundation. (2016). *Fundamental facts about mental health.* Retrieved from https://www.mentalhealth.org.uk/sites/default/files/fundamental-facts-about-mental-health-2016.pdf

NICE. (2018). *Depression in adults: Treatment and management. NICE guideline: short version. Draft for second consultation, May 2018.* Retrieved from https://www.nice.org.uk/guidance/GID-CGWAVE0725/documents/short-version-of-draft-guideline

Parliament, House of Commons. (2018). *Mental health statistics for England: Prevalence, services and funding.* (HC 6988 2018) [Online] London: The Stationary Office. Retrieved from https://researchbriefings.parliament.uk/ResearchBriefing/Summary/SN06988

Parsons, A. S., & Dubrow-Marshall, L. (2018). 'Putting themselves out there' into the unknown: Dance movement psychotherapy as perceived by five educators and three pupils. *Body, Movement and Dance in Psychotherapy, 13*(4), 251–267.

Rappaport, L. (2013). *Mindfulness and the arts therapies: Theory and practice.* London: Jessica Kingsley Publishers.

Rappaport, L. (2014). Focusing-oriented expressive arts therapy. In G. Madison (Ed.), *Theory and practice of focusing-oriented psychotherapy: Beyond the talking cure* (pp. 204–218). London: Jessica Kingsley Publishers.

Rogers, N. (1993). *The creative connection: Expressive arts as healing.* Monmouth: PCCS Books.

Schmid, T. (2005). *Promoting health through creativity for professionals in healthcare arts and education*. London: Whurr.

Stern, D. N. (2010). *Forms of vitality: Exploring dynamic experience in psychology, the arts, psychotherapy, and development*. Oxford: Oxford University Press.

Stiles, W. B., Reynolds, S., Hardy, G. E., Rees, A., Barkham, M., & Shapiro, D. A. (1994). Evaluation and description of psychotherapy sessions by clients using the session evaluation questionnaire and the session Impacts scale. *Journal of Counselling Psychology, 41*(2), 175–185.

Thomas, J., & Harden, A. (2008). Methods for the thematic synthesis of qualitative research in systematic reviews. *BMC Medical Research Methodology, 8*(1), 45.

Timulak, L. (2007). Identifying core categories of client-identified impact of helpful events in psychotherapy: A qualitative meta-analysis. *Psychotherapy Research, 17*(3), 305–314.

Veale, D. (2008). Behavioural activation for depression. *Advances in Psychiatric Treatment, 14*(1), 29–36.

Wampold, B. E. (2015). How important are the common factors in psychotherapy? An update. *World Psychiatry, 14*(3), 270–277.

Webb, C. A., Auerbach, R. P., & DeRubeis, R. J. (2012). Processes of change in CBT of adolescent depression: Review and recommendations. *Journal of Clinical Child & Adolescent Psychology, 41*(5), 654–665.

Williams, J., & Scott, S. (2009). Service responses to women with mental health needs. *Mental Health Review Journal, 7*(1), 6–14.

Zubala, A., & Karkou, V. (Eds.). (2018). *Arts therapies in the treatment of depression*. Oxon: Routledge.

Towards a deeper integration of creative methods in counselling: some thoughts about frameworks for practice

Valerie Thomas

ABSTRACT
Creative methods in counselling are generally regarded as adjunctive techniques and procedures. In this paper I advocate for a deeper integration of creative methods within counselling and propose that one way forward would be to develop more inclusive frameworks for this practice. To this end, I consider some of the ways clinicians and theorists, particularly from the creative/expressive arts therapies, have sought to develop integrative approaches for imagination-based therapeutic practices. This overview also pays attention to attempts within talking therapies to develop more descriptive/functional models for the use of mental imagery that allow an integration across theoretical orientations. Some of the most relevant models and theoretical positions are then discussed in the light of their potential to inform frameworks for the use of creative methods in counselling.

Introduction

Given that creativity is so fundamental to human life, evident from infancy onwards (Winnicott, 1971), it is perhaps surprising that creative methods in counselling continue to be viewed predominantly as adjunctive techniques. There are encouraging indications of a change in attitude particularly in North America with the recent establishment (2004) of The Association for Creativity in Counseling (a division of the American Counseling Association), and the publishing of the *Journal for Creativity in Mental Health*. However, despite these recent developments, it would appear, certainly in the UK, that creative methods are employed, often in an ad hoc way, dependent on the counsellor's therapeutic approach or personal preferences. The lack of evident commitment within counselling to the significant contribution that creative interventions can make to the therapeutic process is underscored by the British Association of Counselling and Psychotherapy criteria for accredited counselling courses (BACP, 2012). These criteria do not require specific competency in creative or imagination-based procedures; instead the assumption is that such methods are school-based and can be included within a general criterion, that is, B4.8 (iii) 'Apply and monitor a range of therapeutic interventions consistent with the rationale and philosophy of the course' (p. 4). Meanwhile, as creative methods remain somewhat marginalised in counselling, elsewhere very significant developments are occurring in the theory and practice of the therapeutic application of imagination (Malchiodi, 2006). In this paper I advocate for a deeper integration of creative methods in talking therapies and suggest that the creation of more inclusive frameworks for these practices would support this move. I consider how the therapeutic disciplines have approached the challenge of finding ways to integrate the different modalities, theoretical orientations and range of expressive media involved in imagination-based methods. I discuss these attempts in the light of the contributions they could make to developing more inclusive frameworks for the utilisation of creative methods in counselling.

Background

For the purposes of this paper, creative methods in the counselling context are defined as the purposive use of the client's creative imagination for therapeutic ends. This is a broad church and includes a very wide range of creative activities, procedures and techniques. A broader understanding of creativity in talking therapies, such as the creative dimensions of the therapeutic relationship and creative thinking more generally in therapy (Carson & Becker, 2003), lies outside the scope of this discussion. In this section I will briefly attend to the history of these therapeutic methods before attempting to make some sense of their contemporary use in counselling particularly within the UK.

Right from the beginning, talking therapies have made use of the imagination to access and work with aspects of the self hidden from conscious awareness. In the very early days of developing his psychoanalytic method, Freud (Breuer & Freud, 1955) would elicit his patients' imagery by tapping their foreheads. However, as he developed his views on the defensive nature of mental images, he soon shifted his attention to verbal association methods for gaining insights into the unconscious inner dynamics of his patients. It fell to Jung (1968), with his commitment to the inherently creative nature of the psyche, to lay the ground for imagination-based methods. His emphasis on the primacy of the image and his development of 'active imagination', a method that facilitates the amplification and unfolding of imagery – often further developed in the form of paintings and drawings – continues to exercise a powerful influence on the theory and practice of creative/expressive arts therapies (McNiff, 2004) and talking therapies (Sawyer, 2002).

Meanwhile, alongside the early development of verbal psychotherapy, individual pioneers were experimenting with different arts modalities as a means of therapy, examples would be: Moreno's (1889–1974) use of dramatic enactments with his patients; and the use of music to reach patients traumatised by their experiences in the first world war (Malchiodi, 2006). More collaborative work happened during the 1930s and 1940s as clinicians working in long-term psychiatric hospitals were becoming more aware of the limitations of using a highly verbal psychoanalytic approach with very disturbed individuals. Some psychotherapists and artists began to work together in order to incorporate art, music making and other expressive arts in the patients' treatment. The foundations were being laid for professional creative arts therapies.

Not long afterwards, the 1970s was a pivotal time for the therapeutic use of the imagination. The advent of humanistic therapies and the human potential movement saw an explosion of interest in creative ways of working therapeutically. Fritz Perls (1893–1970), in particular, made a significant contribution to expanding the repertoire of creative interventions in counselling (Lobb & Amendt-Lyon, 2003). His legacy includes procedures that are now regarded as classics in the field such as the empty chair technique – (see Schimmel & Jacobs [2013] for a discussion of contemporary developments in its application). The 1970s also saw the rapid diversification of creative arts therapies modalities, each one becoming established with its own professional organisation, body of theory and therapeutic procedures. The creative arts therapy field developed and expanded over the following decades running in parallel with talking therapies. And, as the field evolved, it mirrored some of the debates taking place within the disciplines of counselling and psychotherapy, in particular, the tension between individual modalities and a push towards integration (Estrella, 2006). During the 1980s pioneering clinician-theorists (McNiff, 1987) began to articulate a move towards an integrated arts approach to therapy. In this approach (now commonly termed expressive arts therapies), founded on the inter-relatedness of the arts, the therapist draws on different art modalities dependent on therapeutic requirements (Knill, Barba, & Fuchs, 1995). It would be fair to say that over the last three decades it has been the field of creative/expressive arts therapies which has provided the main container for research and theorising in the use of the client's imagination for therapeutic ends.

Returning to the current state of the use of creative methods in counselling, the overall picture is a less than coherent patchwork of practices. A detailed discussion of the creative techniques used within different schools lies outside the scope of this paper, instead I will be referring to the methods that have become more generic to the field. These include some of the most commonly-used methods (drawn from a range of sources) such as: guided imagery (Hall, Hall, Stradling, & Young, 2006); the use of drawings to concretise presenting issues, (art therapy), (Oster & Crone, 2004); diagrams such as time-lines, (Neuro-Linguistic-Programming), (James, 1989); using objects (miniatures or pebbles) to symbolise intra or interpersonal dynamics, (sandtray therapy), (Pearson & Wilson, 2001); using photos to elicit insights (Ginicola, Smith, & Trzaska, 2012); creative writing experiments such as imaginary letters (Kress, Hoffman, & Thomas, 2008); using published literature to explore issues (bibliotherapy) (Detrixhe, 2010); and creative roleplay (dramatherapy and psycho-drama) (Landy, 2006). Mostly, these methods will be incorporated into integrative/pluralist and humanistic approaches. It is important to note that, historically, Cognitive Behavioural Therapy (CBT) has made significant use of imagination-based techniques but these have been used in a more instrumental way. Although there are indications that some contemporary CBT approaches are moving in a more creative direction, such as by adapting Perls' and Jung's methods with clients' imagery and drawings to illuminate hidden cognitions (Hackmann, Bennett-Levy, & Holmes, 2011).

Alongside the use of stand-alone techniques, there have been some advances in particular practices which have begun to emerge as distinct approaches in their own right. A particularly important one is therapeutic writing pioneered by Pennebaker (1997) who researched the health and psychological benefits of writing about traumatic experience. Writing therapy is becoming established as a particular approach that employs a range of reflective, creative and expressive processes with the written word to enhance therapeutic processes (Bolton, Howlett, Lago, & Wright, 2004). Another different example is an approach that arose within experientially-focused psychotherapy, that is, Expressive Arts Focusing (EAF) therapy (Rappaport, 2014). In EAF, clients have the opportunity to amplify their 'felt sense' (unclear, preverbal sense of something held in physical body) further through using different arts and expressive media.

However, despite the advances in the theory and practice of creative methods represented by these new approaches, there is hardly any literature on developing frameworks that would encompass different expressive media and apply across the counselling orientations. It is noteworthy that even recent scholarly work on the theory and practice of integrating expressive arts into counselling practice (Degges-White & Davis, 2011) does not present any significant discussion of integrating across different approaches.

Developing a more integrative position

How can the use of creative methods become more deeply integrated in talking therapies? One avenue worthy of exploration could be the development of more inclusive frameworks for their practice. At a pragmatic level, such frameworks would be helpful as they would allow integrative and pluralistic practitioners a means of drawing more coherently from the wealth of techniques, procedures and methods developed across the different schools. Some moves in the direction of more inclusive theory and practice in imagination-based practices can be seen particularly within creative/expressive arts therapies. The following section identifies and discusses some of the more relevant ones.

Historically, the creative arts therapies have drawn on the paradigms informing talking therapies (Johnson, 2009). The field continues to be very open to assimilating theoretical innovations taken from counselling and psychotherapy, – a good example is the way that some arts therapists are beginning to integrate schema therapy into their practice as it provides a useful conceptual framework (Van den Broek, Keulen-de Vos, & Bernstein, 2011). Talking therapies, however, have not demonstrated a reciprocal receptivity to the disclosures of the creative/expressive arts therapies. This lack of openness and awareness may be attributed to the fact that talking therapies have been viewed as having more professional status. The consequences for creative and expressive arts therapies are eloquently expressed by Johnson,

> 'We are a field perpetually at the margin; not only are we placed there by the dominant forces holding sway at the center, but we place ourselves there, between art and health, in the liminal, transcendent, and transitional, spaces between body and mind, observation and action, containment and expression' (2009, p. 114).

However, whatever the cause of this imbalance, it is important to recognise that expressive and creative arts therapies are now established as the site of significant theoretical innovations in the applications of imagination to practice and that these advances are impacting on other disciplines. A good example is arts-based research, a new qualitative research approach, whereby art-making is used as the primary means of inquiry (McNiff, 1998). The following section focuses on how this field has risen to the challenge of developing more inclusive theory and practice.

Creative arts therapists have needed to justify their focus on using arts modalities as the main means of therapy. Initially, they drew on a basic creative/expressive paradigm, which, 'proposes that the expression of deeply held thoughts and feelings within a trusting therapeutic relationship can alleviate mental suffering caused by fear, shame, and anxiety' (Johnson, 2009, p. 115). However, general propositions such as these have limited currency in a wider health and social care context that values evidence-based practice. Arts therapies have not been immune to the explanatory potential of neuroscience (Berrol, 2006; Lusebrink, 2004). 'The argument appears to be that if processes central to the creative arts therapies can be located in the brain (regardless of location), then their legitimacy is established' (Johnson, 2009, p. 116). More recently, McGilchrist's (2009) seminal thesis on neural lateralisation has provided compelling new ground for the old idea that imagination-based interventions facilitate communication from the right to the left brain hemisphere and thereby promote therapeutic processes (Afford, 2014).

Of particular relevance to this paper is the approach taken in the creative arts therapies field to generating models to inform more integrative practice. In the main, these developments have been driven by the need for expressive arts therapy to provide a framework for the integration of different arts modalities within therapeutic work (McNiff, 1987). Knill helped to lay the ground for integrative model-building with his influential theory of intermodal expressive therapy (Knill et al., 1995). According to this theory, the use of a combination of different expressive art media amplifies the therapeutic effect. An example of an intermodal arts model would be the psychokinetic imagery process (Halprin, 2002) where expressive movement is linked with both drawing and also with poetic dialogues. The rationale for this model is that a more systematic use of different expressive arts facilitates a deeper integration across different dimensions of the self.

Outside the particular discipline of expressive arts therapies, there are examples of arts therapy models that can be applied across the modalities. One that has achieved prominence in the field is the Expressive Therapies Continuum, (ETC) originally developed within art therapy by Kagin and Lusebrink (Lusebrink, 1991). This framework organises interactions with media into a three stage developmental sequence from simple to complex cognitive processing. ETC presents 'a unifying theoretical construct that cuts across therapeutic orientations to describe how qualities of the media, or the experiences chosen, interact with each person's preferred style of image formation and information processing to convey content or meaning' (Hinz, 2009, p. 36). The usefulness of this model is based on the way it can be applied to clinical assessments: that is, identifying a poorly functioning level of processing and pointing to suitable expressive arts interventions. Another example is Mazza's (2003) tripartite model for poetry therapy. Mazza identifies the three components as: receptive/prescriptive where literature is introduced for validating/exploring feelings; expressive/creative where therapeutic expression is encouraged through various writing methods; and symbolic/ceremonial where metaphor, storytelling and performance are used to deal with life transitions. This model (termed the RES model) has the potential to be applied to not only linguistically-based arts therapies but also visual arts and performance based ones (Mazza & Hayton, 2013).

New theories in other disciplines, particularly the cognitive sciences which have embraced theories of embodied cognition, have also informed some of the integrative perspectives in the creative arts therapy field. Cognitive linguists, Lakoff and Johnson's (2003) influential work on conceptual metaphor was recognised early on as having significant potential as a locus of integration for expressive arts therapies (Meekums, 2000). Lakoff and Johnson argue that metaphor shapes the way we think. Conceptual metaphors (nonverbal experiential gestalts) emerge directly out of embodied experience and are theorised as the foundations of higher order cognitive processes. At higher levels of cognition these gestalts can be perceived as images before finally arising as linguistic metaphors (Gibbs & Berg, 2002). As conceptual metaphor has somatic, visual and linguistic aspects, this theory can operate as a unifying construct for all the therapeutic arts modalities. As Meekums (2000) has explained, metaphor can be used to explore alternative ways of thinking and behaving:

> 'So, an image of help can be imported into a picture, a gesture can change from pushing to reaching, relationships can be redefined by using space differently, and a drama or poem can be reconstructed to bring hope into present reality' (p. 57).

However, in an important recent paper, Koch and Fuchs (2011) argued that embodied cognition has limitations as a unifying construct: it does not take into account that the body is a special category because we can perceive it from both the outside and also from the inside. They argue that embodiment rather than embodied cognition provides a more genuine approach to the interface between arts therapies and cognitive sciences because "(t)he body is the unifying base of the constant first person perspective that we 'carry with us'" (p. 278). Although, as yet undeveloped as an integrative model for the practice of expressive arts therapies, Koch and Fuchs explain how embodiment provides greater scope as a locus of integration because it is not limited to the psychological self. They identify three levels of embodiment and put very simply these comprise: the embodied self, that is, the individual mind-body system; the enactive self, that is, the individual embodied self in relation to other embodied selves and interacting with the environment; and the extended self, that is, the individual embodied self in relation to external culture and this includes symbolisations of the self expressed in artworks. In terms of its capacity for inclusiveness, Koch and Fuchs's three level embodiment framework represents a significant advance as it encompasses not only psychologically-informed approaches but also postmodern orientations which emphasise intersubjectivity and the socially-constructed self. Before I discuss its potential (along with the other models and theories described here) to inform inclusive frameworks for the use of creative methods in counselling, it is important to return to the field of talking therapies to consider if there are any equivalent developments.

Out of all the disparate creative methods used in talking therapies, there is one particular practice that has been extensively employed over a long period of time: that is, mental imagery techniques and approaches. Despite the longevity of this practice, it is either harnessed to particular paradigms of different schools or developed as a stand alone therapy (Thomas, 2016). Some clinicians and theorists (Faranda, 2014) (similarly to those previously mentioned within the expressive arts fields) have noted the potential for conceptual metaphor theory to provide a locus of integration. Gibbs and Berg (2002) make the case that representing a conceptual metaphor as an image will reveal not only the person's sense of self but it will also disclose their experience of their embodiment. Apart from this, there have been a couple of attempts to develop models that integrate different approaches to the therapeutic use of mental imagery: that is, the Image Somatic Meaning (ISM) model (Ahsen, 1984) and the Interactive Communicative (IC) model (Thomas, 2016).

Ahsen's ISM model links image representation with somatic and cognitive aspects of the self. The basic premise of his model is that every important experience is impressed in memory in the form of a semi-permanent representation which he termed an 'eidetic'. Furthermore the mental image operates as a container for all the elements involved in this eidetic. When the mental image surfaces, the memory contained within it is available for instantaneous playback and this will include the somatic aspect and the associated meaning. In Ahsen's approach to psychotherapy, presenting issues are theorised as eidetics that require surfacing and re-experiencing in order to transform dysfunctional ways of being (Sheikh, 2002). Eidetic image therapy has been developed for working with different clinical populations e.g. adults with intellectual disabilities (Syed, 2012) and a range of presenting issues such as phobias (Dolan, 1997).

Thomas's IC model steps outside an explicitly psychologically-informed paradigm and offers another means of bridging the radically different approaches within the main counselling and psychotherapy orientations to the practice of mental imagery. The IC model emerged out of the findings produced by a grounded theory study of the commonalities in practice across different talking therapy orientations (Thomas, 2015, 2016). The research findings supported the generally accepted clinical distinction made between directive (consciously and purposively produced) and receptive (spontaneously arising) imagery. More significantly, the findings indicated that it was possible to differentiate out this basic distinction into a range of generic therapeutic operations. The directive set contains the reparative, process management and framing functions. The receptive set contains the diagnostic, monitoring and processing functions. Different functions come to the fore dependent on therapeutic need and in this regard the model resembles Clarkson's (2003) Five Relationship framework. The IC model of mental imagery captures some of the complexity inherent in the way that mental imagery is used as a means of intra-psychic communication for therapeutic purposes and offers a means of integration across different orientations.

Discussion

How useful are the models and theoretical positions described above for supporting a deeper integration of creative methods in talking therapies? They are all attempts to identify some common ground that can inform the various imagination-based therapeutic practices. In the following brief discussion, some tentative thoughts are offered regarding their potential as starting points for developing frameworks for the use of creative methods in counselling.

Beginning on a pragmatic level, there is potential for using the intermodal approach as the basis for models that can integrate imagination-based and verbal processes in talking therapies. In particular, Kagin and Lusebrink's Expressive Therapies Continuum (ETC) could provide a basis for developing a framework that delivers a coherent rationale for creative interventions in counselling. Although its scope is limited because it is informed by a psychological developmental model, it could allow counsellors a means of incorporating creative methods more systematically into their practice. An ETC-based framework would provide a way for these methods to be informed by an initial and ongoing clinical assessment of the client's developmental issues. For example, if a client's presenting issue is linked to very early formative experiences, an ETC-informed approach to creative methods would prescribe activities that support learning through the senses such as finger painting (Hinz, 2009).

Models that are grounded in common therapeutic functions offer other possible starting points. Maza's tripartite model for poetry therapy (RES) could be adapted to counselling because the three dimensions of practice identified within it apply generally to therapy. An RES-informed framework would allow counsellors a way of selecting the best type of creative method for general therapeutic functions. For example, writing a letter to express feelings (expressive-creative dimension) or using movement/performance to deal with transitions (symbolic/ceremonial dimension).

The potential for the models developed within talking therapies for the practice of mental imagery are perhaps more limited than the ones emerging in the field of creative/expressive arts therapies. This limitation is predicated on the fact that, although these models bridge orientations, they focus on only one particular type of imagination-based practice. The basic principle informing Thomas's IC model, i.e. common therapeutic functions, may have potential to be expanded beyond mental imagery to include other creative interventions. However, identifying commonalities across the different creative methods would involve a significant research programme. Ahsen's ISM model appears superficially to have more potential as a model for creative methods because it explicitly links imagination, body and meaning-making together. However, on deeper examination, its limitations are evident: it is a psychological model that attributes a particular function to the mental image, i.e. as the container of the therapeutic process. It is difficult to see how the ISM model could be developed further to encompass imagination-based procedures utilising different expressive media.

At a more theoretical level, conceptual metaphor stands out as having the potential to bridge across the different expressive arts modalities used in creative methods as well as most counselling orientations. As discussed earlier, It offers a persuasive theoretically and research-informed account of how body and mind are interlinked in therapeutic imagination-based practices. Indeed, Gorelick (1989) asserts that metaphor provides the link between expressive arts and talking therapies. However, it is important to take on board Koch and Fuchs' view of the limitations of embodied cognition as the locus of integration. Their championing of embodiment as a wider, more inclusive construct is particularly relevant to talking therapies. As the three levels of embodiment that they outline (as discussed earlier) encompass both modern and postmodern perspectives on the self, it can encompass all of the therapeutic orientations. Because it explicitly addresses intersubjectivity, this unifying principle is the one that is most likely to be welcomed, particularly in psychotherapy. However, the challenge will be to operationalise embodiment into a workable framework for counselling practice with creative methods.

Conclusion

Until the late 1970s, counselling and psychotherapy were at the cutting edge of developments in use of creative interventions. Since then, most of the main advances in the therapeutic use of imagination have been happening outside talking therapies, particularly within the field of the creative/expressive arts therapies. Although there are promising signs of renewed interest, such as the emergence of therapeutic writing as a distinct approach in its own right (Bolton et al., 2004), creative methods in talking therapies tend to be viewed merely as adjunctive techniques and procedures. Along with other clinicians and theorists, (Carson & Becker, 2004; Gladding, 2005) this paper advocates for the importance of developing the use of creative methods in talking therapies. One way of supporting a deeper integration of creative methods in counselling is to develop more inclusive frameworks for this practice. Starting points for such an endeavour can be discovered in the field of expressive and creative arts therapies and in allied practices of mental imagery in counselling and psychotherapy. Some of these already extant models have the potential to be adapted to talking therapies, e.g. as discussed earlier, Kagin and Lusebrinks Expressive Continuum Therapies (Hinz, 2009) could be a helpful assessment tool for counsellors wanting to integrate creative techniques into their practice.

It is to be hoped that clinicians and theorists will rise to the challenge of creating more inclusive frameworks for the use of creative methods in counselling – ones that can bridge across the different expressive media, modalities and theoretical orientations. These frameworks could pave the way for a time when all counsellors would be expected to have a set of generic competencies in the use of imagination-based (linguistic and nonverbal) means of facilitating therapeutic processes. A move towards a deeper integration of creative methods in counselling practice is long overdue.

Disclosure statement

No potential conflict of interest was reported by the author.

References

Afford, P. (2014). Neuroscience and psychological change in focusing. In E. Madison (Ed.), *Theory and practice of focusing-oriented psychotherapy: Beyond the talking cure* (p. 248). London: Jessica Kingsley.

Ahsen, A. (1984). ISM: The Triple Code model for imagery and psychophysiology. *Journal of Mental Imagery, 8*(4), 15–42.

BACP. (2012). *Accreditation of training courses: Criteria for course accreditation 2009 scheme* (Revised 5th ed.). Lutterworth: BACP.

Berrol, C. (2006). Neuroscience meets dance/movement therapy: Mirror neurons, the therapeutic process and empathy. *The Arts in Psychotherapy, 33*(4), 302–315.

Bolton, G., Howlett, S., Lago, C., & Wright, J. K. (Eds.). (2004). *Writing cures: An introductory handbook of writing in counselling and psychotherapy.* Hove Brunner-Routledge.

Breuer, J., & Freud, S. (1955). Studies on hysteria. In J. Strachey (Ed.), *The standard edition* (Vol. 2, pp. 135–181). London: Hogarth.

Carson, D. K., & Becker, K. W. (2003). *Creativity in psychotherapy: Reaching new heights with individuals, couples and families.* Binghamton, NY: Haworth Clinical Practice Press.

Carson, D. K., & Becker, K. (2004). *Creativity in psychotherapy: Reaching new heights with individuals, couples and families.* Hove: Routledge.

Clarkson, P. (2003). *The therapeutic relationship* (2nd ed.). Hoboken, NJ: Wiley-Blackwell.

Degges-White, S., & Davis, N. L. (Eds.). (2011). *Integrating the expressive arts into counselling practice: Theory-based intervention.* New York, NY: Springer.

Detrixhe, J. J. (2010). Souls in jeopardy: Questions and innovations for bibliotherapy with fiction. *The Journal of Humanistic Counseling, Education and Development, 49*(1), 58–72.

Dolan, A. T. (1997). *Imagery treatment of phobias, anxiety states and other symptom complexes in Akhter Ahsen's image psychology.* New York, NY: Brandon House.

Estrella, K. (2006). Expressive therapy: An integrated arts approach. In C. A. Malchiodi (Ed.), *Expressive therapies* (pp. 183–209). New York, NY: Guilford.

Faranda, F. (2014). Working with images in psychotherapy: An embodied experience of play and metaphor. *Journal of Psychotherapy Integration, 24*(1), 65–77.

Gibbs, R. W., & Berg, E. A. (2002). Mental imagery and embodied activity. *Journal of Mental Imagery, 26*(1–2), 1–30.

Ginicola, M. M., Smith, S., & Trzaska, J. (2012). Counseling through images: Using photography to guide the counseling process and achieve treatment goals. *Journal of Creativity in Mental Health, 7*(4), 310–329.

Gladding, S. (2005). *Counseling as an art: The creative arts in counseling* (3rd ed.). Alexandria, VA: American Counseling Association.

Gorelick, K. (1989). Perspective: Rapprochement between the arts and psychotherapies: Metaphor the mediator. *The Arts in Psychotherapy, 16*, 149–155.

Hackmann, A., Bennett-Levy, J., & Holmes, E. A. (2011). *Oxford guide to imagery in cognitive therapy.* Oxford: Oxford University Press.

Hall, E., Hall, C., Stradling, P., & Young, D. (2006). *Guided imagery: Creative interventions in counselling and psychotherapy.* London: Sage.

Halprin, D. (2002). *The expressive body in life, art and therapy: Working with movement, metaphor and meaning.* London and New York, NY: Jessica Kingsley.

Hinz, L. (2009). *Expressive therapies continuum: A framework for using art in therapy.* New York, NY: Routledge.

James, T. (1989). *Timeline therapy and the basis of personality.* Capitola, CA: Meta Publications.

Johnson, D. R. (2009). Commentary: Examining underlying paradigms in the creative arts therapies of trauma. *The Arts in Psychotherapy, 36*, 114–120.

Jung, C. G. (Ed.). (1968). *Man and his symbols.* New York, NY: Dell Publishing.

Knill, P. J., Barba, H. N., & Fuchs, M. N. (1995). *Minstrels of soul: Intermodal expressive therapy.* Toronto, Ontario: Palmerston Press.

Koch, S. C., & Fuchs, T. (2011). Embodied arts therapies. *The Arts in Psychotherapy, 38*, 276–280.

Kress, V. E., Hoffman, R., & Thomas, A. M. (2008). Letters from the future: The use of therapeutic letter writing in counseling sexual abuse survivors. *Journal of Creativity in Mental Health, 3*(2), 105–118.

Lakoff, G., & Johnson, M. (2003). *Metaphors we live by* (2nd ed.). Chicago, IL: University of Chicago Press.

Landy, R. (2006). Dramatherapy and psychodrama. In C. A. Malchiodi (Ed.), *Expressive therapies* (pp. 90–116). New York, NY: Guilford.

Lobb, M. S., & Amendt-Lyon, N. (Eds.). (2003). *Creative license: The art of Gestalt therapy.* New York, NY and Vienna, Austria: Springer.

Lusebrink, V. B. (1991). A systems oriented approach to the expressive therapies: The expressive therapies continuum. *The Arts in Psychotherapy, 18*(5), 395–403.

Lusebrink, V. B. (2004). Art therapy and the brain: An attempt to understand the underlying processes of art expression in therapy. *Art Therapy, 21*(3), 125–135.

Malchiodi, C. A. (2006). Expressive therapies: History, theory and practice. In C. A. Malchiodi (Ed.), *Expressive therapies* (pp. 1–15). New York, NY: Guilford.

Mazza, N. E. (2003). *Poetry therapy: Theory and practice.* New York, NY: Routledge.

Mazza, N. E., & Hayton, C. J. (2013). Poetry therapy: An investigation of a multidimensional clinical model. *The Arts in Psychotherapy, 40,* 53–60.

McGilchrist, I. (2009). *The master and his emissary.* London: Yale University Press.

McNiff, S. (1987). Pantheon of creative arts therapies: An integrative perspective. *Journal of Integrative and Eclectic Psychotherapy, 61*(3), 259–281.

McNiff, S. (1998). *Art-based research.* London: Jessica Kingsley.

McNiff, S. (2004). *Art heals: How creativity cures the soul.* Boston, MA: Shambala.

Meekums, B. (2000). *Creative group therapy for women survivors of child sexual abuse.* London: Jessica Kingsley.

Oster, G. D., & Crone, P. G. (2004). *Using drawings in assessment and therapy: A guide for mental health professionals.* New York, NY: Brunner-Routledge.

Pearson, M., & Wilson, H. (2001). *Sandplay and symbol work: Emotional healing and personal development with children, adolescents and adults.* Camberwell, Victoria: ACER Press.

Pennebaker, J. W. (1997). *Opening up: The healing power of expressing emotions.* New York, NY: Guilford.

Rappaport, L. (2014). Focusing-oriented expressive arts therapy. In E. Madison (Ed.), *Theory and Practice of focusing-oriented psychotherapy: Beyond the talking cure* (pp. 204–218). London: Jessica Kingsley.

Sawyer, D. (2002). Images and depth psychology: The legacy of Carl Jung. In A. A. Sheikh (Ed.), *Therapeutic imagery techniques* (pp. 253–268). Amityville, NY: Baywood.

Schimmel, C. J., & Jacobs, E. E. (2013). Creative interventions using chairs: Going beyond Gestalt. *Journal of Creativity in Mental Health, 8*(4), 428–443.

Sheikh, A. A. (2002). Eidetic psychotherapy techniques. In A. A. Sheikh (Ed.), *Therapeutic imagery techniques.* Amityville, NY: Baywood, 145–154.

Syed, A. A. (2012). "A way to grow": An eidetic model of growth for intellectual disability. *Journal of Mental Imagery, 36*(3), 1–32.

Thomas, V. (2015). The therapeutic functions of mental imagery in psychotherapy: Constructing a theoretical model. In S. Goss, & C. Stevens (Eds.), *Making research matter: Researching for change in the theory and practice of counselling and psychotherapy* (pp. 106–120). Oxon: Routledge.

Thomas, V. (2016). *Using mental imagery in counselling and psychotherapy: A guide to more inclusive theory and practice.* Oxon: Routledge.

Van den Broek, E., Keulen-de Vos, M., & Bernstein, D. P. (2011). Arts therapies and schema focused therapy: A pilot study. *The Arts in Psychotherapy, 38,* 325–332.

Winnicott, D. W. (1971). *Playing and reality.* London: Routledge.

Inter-professional learning: initial observations of the art psychotherapy tools used in the post-qualifying postgraduate training in counselling children and young people

Blanka Hubena and Judith Mulcahy

ABSTRACT

Children and young people (C&YP) counselling training and art psychotherapy training lead to two distinctive psychological therapy approaches; one is informed by British Association for Counselling and Psychotherapy's Competences for work with children and young people (4–18 years) [BACP. (2019a). *Competences for work with children and young people (4–18 years)*. Retrieved from https://www.bacp.co.uk/media/5863/bacp-cyp-competence-framework.pdf], the other by Health and Care Professions Council's Standards of Proficiency for Arts Therapists [HCPC. (2013). *Standards of proficiency - Arts therapists*. Retrieved from http://www.hpc-uk.org/publications/index.asp?id=39#publicationSearchResults]. In this article we outline the training methods utilised on the Postgraduate Diploma in Counselling C&YP at a British University and share initial observations of how creative and arts-based therapeutic tools form an important part of the curriculum delivery. The aim of this paper is also to outline the role of intentionality application in the use of creative interventions in therapeutic practice.

Background and history

Since 2010, we have been delivering Level 7[1] postgraduate (PG) and post-qualifying counselling training for practitioners from, or with an interest in, the field of children and young people (C&YP) therapy. This collaborative partnership of two different professions (BACP-accredited integrative counsellor and an HCPC-registered art psychotherapist) enabled the PG Diploma in Counselling C&YP to benefit from the specialists' adaptation of the use of arts therapeutically. The art psychotherapy (APT) practitioner's knowledge and first-hand experience of personal process induced using creative therapeutic tools helped support students' reflective process, which was previously not fully considered as essential for the course. In this paper we explore how the arts can be used in C&YP counselling practice and the emerging issues around ethics, boundaries and safety in the use of such therapeutic tools. The paper focuses on the best conditions for safe training in C&YP counselling in reference to the use of arts-based therapeutic techniques. It also gives an insight into the emergence of the concept of "intentionality" in APT practice, as observed by us.

Increasingly, C&YP counselling services have been gaining prominence in the preventative and non-specialist settings, such as education, youth service and the third sector since the

1990s (Polat & Jenkins, 2005). Significant changes in the way CAMHS[2] deliver C&YP therapy in the UK (HM Government, 2008), and the developments taking place in the field of school-based counselling in Wales, for example (WG, 2008, 2013), have resulted in the need to rethink how young people's mental health and emotional well-being needs are addressed and met. To facilitate effective therapeutic processes in C&YP counselling, counsellors need to be able to incorporate specialist skills and tools which may not be used widely in adult counselling (Williams & Jenkins, 2016). This was recognised in the BACP's (2019b) Counsellors' Guide: The competences for humanistic counselling with children and young people (4–18 years), with one specific competence being linked directly to counsellors' ability to use creative methods in C&YP counselling.

The attractiveness of using arts-based methods and therapeutic approaches in counselling service delivery may at times minimise the challenges that practitioners and clients may experience by engaging with such C&YP therapy tools. The impact of the use of arts and creative methods in therapy on both clients and practitioners may present itself in a powerful way, bringing strong and potentially disturbing personal material to the surface quickly, cutting through layers of clients' defences and their cognitive processing (Case, 2014). There is no doubt that working this way can be highly effective and helpful; however, we have found that students in C&YP therapy training courses should learn in a more experiential way to meet their professional competences in C&YP counselling practice.

Specific competencies for counselling with young people

It would be impossible to fully outline how practitioners should acquire an "(a)bility to use creative methods and resources to help young people express, reflect upon, and make sense of their experiences" (BACP, 2019a, pp. 18, 27) as each counsellor brings a different set of professional skills, experience and knowledge that will shape their counselling practice. The counsellor's objective to phenomenologically follow the client's narrative and reality, however, requires the counsellor to apply therapeutic tool adaptations and fine-tune each counselling session (Geldard & Geldard, 2009) due to the frequently changing personal landscapes of C&YP needs. BACP's (2019b) guide to humanistic competences in C&YP counselling is generic enough to enable creativity, and, hopefully, specific enough to avoid causing harm to young people. Nevertheless, further exploration of how these competences are achieved may be needed to support effective training for such specialist practice.

We found it crucial that every student C&YP counsellor asks themselves the question if the use of the arts therapeutically could cause harm to their clients. We explored the safe creative methods use within a C&YP counselling training programme offered at a University[3] level in the UK, by adapting and modifying our teaching tools to ensure students' reflexivity and applied sensitivity to clients' needs and safety.

Effective assessment of C&YP needs and ability to work non-verbally

Sensory experiences are invaluable in accessing C&YP's pre-verbal selves and early childhood memories, which may need to be addressed or explored in therapy (Geldard & Geldard, 2009). Additionally, as many young people do not yet possess fully developed cognitive skills to process experiences through thinking (Erikson, 1959), it is imperative that C&YP counsellors offer therapeutic techniques "when young person may not have highly developed verbal skills" or "when young person demonstrates a preference for visual/symbolic rather than verbal forms of communication" (BACP, 2019a, p. 97). The therapeutic use of play, humour, symbolism and metaphor can provide the necessary tools for C&YP counsellors to effectively engage hard-to-reach children and young people.

The BACP suggests that,

> ... the use of creative resources such as art materials, play materials, sand tray and life-story techniques can be helpful when working with younger clients as these often represent natural ways of communicating for this age group. Such methods can help express experiences that young people may otherwise struggle to verbalise. They can also provide a working distance or reflective space between a young person and their problems as well as providing opportunities for them to project their inner experience into the perceptual field they share with the counsellor. When using such methods, a non-interpretative stance is often most useful, helping clients explore the personal meanings that emerge in creative work. (BACP, 2019b, p. 27)

However, this stance may present a lack of acknowledgement that C&YP counsellors must be adequately equipped to practise safely and ethically in the suggested use of creative tools and resources. Assessment of C&YP's creative needs, under the outlined "preference" in working non-verbally, is not an easy task to undertake. In an APT's practice this would require drawing upon several theoretical concepts (e.g. attachment theory – Bowlby, 1969; cognitive and psychosocial development – Erikson, 1959; Piaget, 1972), as well as taking "account of psychological, social, cultural, economic and other factors when collecting case histories and other appropriate information" (HCPC, 2013, p. 8). It would also include the consideration of a client's expressive preference, and the adverse impact of engaging in the arts on a person's well-being. To ensure that such competences are embedded in the C&YP counselling practice, the professional associations of C&YP counsellors in the UK may need to work together across the therapeutic modalities spectrum to develop a minimum standard in training programmes to meet the necessary competences. As they currently stand, the competences may be interpreted in ways that could lead to an unsafe C&YP counselling practice.

Springham (2008) has critically explored an act of negligence which was centred around a practitioner's failure to recognise and assess effectively a client's vulnerability and to appropriately manage it in the context of making art. He evidences clearly how "not knowing" or not having "trained to recognise" is not acceptable in offering creative or arts-based therapeutic interventions in the eyes of the law. He claims that the issue of safety while engaging in the arts is often minimised and it is clear to us that it is not addressed fully by BACP who focus instead on the practitioners' "(a)bility to maintain standards of competence" and "knowledge of policies and legislation" (BACP, 2019a, pp. 13, 15). The omission of the necessity for specialist training in this area as discussed later in this paper, could lead to client complaints and expensive litigation by those perceiving their C&YP counsellor's practice as damaging or harmful.

Art psychotherapy-based approach to safe practice

In contrast to C&YP counselling training, arts therapists[4] in the UK benefit from standardised and regulated education and training, outlined in the Standards of Proficiency: Arts Therapists[5] (HCPC, 2013) and Standards of Education (2014).

Much debate has taken place among psychological therapists and counselling professionals in the UK since the regulation of arts therapies in 2003 (Boseley, 2010; DoH, 2011; HCPC, 2011; HM Government, 2007) regarding the benefits of all psychological therapies following the same path. Arts therapies have benefitted from clear guidance and practice standards relating to safety, the recognition of personal limitations, and duty of care to service users while using specialist arts-based therapeutic skills (HCPC, 2013); which has resulted in almost eliminating client complaints (0.21% of all registrants, only 2 cases upheld, HCPC, 2017).

It is clear that understanding of and approach to using creative therapeutic methods are essentially different in two key documents relating to professional practice (BACP, 2019a; HCPC, 2013), each outlining how therapeutic interventions should be carried out from a distinctive professional perspective (Table 1).

Table 1. Overview of similarities and differences in training CYP counsellors and APT practitioners from our perspective.

C&YP Counselling training[a]	APT training
Post-qualifying counselling training	Initial practitioner training
Building upon existing knowledge, experience and skills in counselling practice	Building upon and developing knowledge and experience in arts-based practice fields and related disciplines
Based on and developed from a range of therapeutic approaches and modalities	Mainly psychodynamic, attachment-focused
Explorative in clients' experience/frame of reference, sometimes through creative means	Explorative in clients' experience/frame of reference, almost always through creative means
Directive and solution-focused in the use of creative tools	Providing a space for expression and exploration through client-led choice of creative means, directive and non-directive
Safety- and ethics-driven, based on specific competences	Scope of practice, standards of proficiency, safety- and ethics-driven
Experiential learning employed in practical aspects of the curriculum delivery	Highly experiential in all elements of the curriculum delivery
Informed by BACP (2018) Ethical Framework for the Counselling Professions & BACP (2019a) Competences for work with children and young people (4–18 years)	Informed by HCPC (2013) Standards of Proficiency: Arts Therapists; HCPC (2014) Standards of Education and Training; and by HCPC (2016) Guidance on conduct and ethics for students
One Specific Competence (8 sections) informing practice	Practice regulated by 12 standards of proficiency

[a]As experienced at our home University; the training may differ in other educational institutions that do not follow the BACP Competences for work with children and young people (4–18 years) and Counselling Young People (11–18 years) Training Curriculum.

Bringing two perspectives on the use of creative methods into C&YP counselling training

Working to incorporate the two perspectives on professional use of creativity in training practice, we found that in preparing counsellors for therapeutic work with C&YP, modifications of widely available creative tools and techniques were needed to ensure safe practice and to avoid causing harm. In order to feel confident in making such modifications, students had to understand how creative tools may impact on a client's experience of counselling. As students did not respond well to purely theoretical or didactic teaching, we found that experiential learning (Kolb, 1984) was the most effective, enabling counsellors to "try things out" and experience the impact of creativity on the self in a safe and containing environment.

It was our experience that experiential learning was difficult for some counsellors as it presented a different paradigm of learning compared to their initial practitioner training. The counsellors' knowledge of techniques such as role play and the use of timelines, in different contexts for example, were often the only previously experienced non-verbal tools in training. We became aware of the fundamental differences between the two distinctive professions, one skilling practitioners in the use of creative methods, as required, the other utilising the students' existing creativity and arts-based practice in all elements of therapy training.

Most APTs complete a first degree in a creative arts discipline, which provides an opportunity to become absorbed in personal art-making for a substantial amount of time. They also gain, amongst others, social, theoretical, anthropological and cultural insights into how art can be created, and how people engage in creativity in different settings and cultures. This knowledge forms an important foundation for art psychotherapy training, enabling practitioners "to use a range of art and art-making materials and techniques competently and be able to help a service user to work with these" (HCPC, 2013, p. 13). Furthermore, the HCPC Standards of Proficiency require trainees to

> understand that while art therapy has a number of frames of reference, they must adopt a coherent approach to their therapy, including the relationship between theory, research and practice and the relevant aspects of connected disciplines including visual arts, aesthetics, anthropology, psychology, psychiatry, sociology, psychotherapy and medicine. (HCPC, 2013, p. 16)

The C&YP counselling trainees often arrived with preconceived and deeply embedded ideas about creativity, some of which have been explored extensively by contemporary authors in areas of the often-shaming experiences in compulsory arts education (Robinson, 1998, 2001, 2013), fear of creativity in organisations (Huet, 2011, 2012), and the impact of social standing on creativity (Löwenfeld & Brittain, 1987; Ogletree & Uljaki, 1973). Any such preconceptions were challenged through practical exercises, which enabled students to consider how their arts-based experiences during childhood and youth may influence their future success in using creative therapeutic tools in C&YP counselling practice.

We found that our students often lacked an insight into experiential self-exploration through creative means, which was then expected to be applied in their future C&YP practice. An opportunity to connect with their own inner child and inner adolescent (Berne, 2010) was often experienced for the first time while using creative tools during the Counselling C&YP course – a repeated phenomenon present in each cohort since the course's commencement in 2010.

As it is important to improve practitioners' awareness of their unconscious and transferential processes,[6] the training focuses on experiential learning to enable C&YP counsellors to tackle their own personal blind spots (Geldard & Geldard, 2009). Repeatedly, with each new cohort, students highly valued the opportunity to have practical, experience-based opportunity to try the therapeutic use of arts in classroom. Such practical learning often led to personal childhood-based material emerging in the classroom. Many students felt that their ability to empathise effectively with their clients could be impaired should they not have had the chance to explore their personal constructs and self-concepts (Kelly, 1991) before commencing C&YP counselling work.

So how is it done? What works? What helps C&YP counsellors to work effectively and safely in their therapeutic work with young people? The answers are not simple, but we noticed some emerging themes concerning the best methods of preparing trainees for an effective C&YP counselling practice.

Connecting with and using creatively own inner child/inner adolescent

C&YP counselling training must involve creative tools and arts-based opportunities for personal and professional development and insight, and using own personal experiences and life events in the classroom. Not all counsellors undertake personal therapy in their initial counselling training (Robson & Robson, 2008; Wiseman & Shefler, 2001) to process effectively any such personal experiences. This could lead to counsellors' entanglement with clients' emptions and their loss of focus on how to best help their clients in effectively engaging creative tools in their practice.

The facilitation of the use of creative methods is delivered by an art psychotherapist, to ensure a safe environment and containment of the varied responses to both working with creative tools and the personal material evoked by such work. Modelling of professional skills, focus on the development of critical reflection in the use of creative methods and resources, and containing of unprocessed personal material creatively enables a first-hand experience of how C&YP may respond to these in therapy.

C&YP counselling trainees may feel overwhelmed (McGoldrick, Gerson, & Petry, 2008) by, for example, the use of miniatures in personal genograms, an effective tool in assessing a child's familial and other significant relationships. The power of visual representation of those engaged relationally with us is a tool that provides much insight into C&YP personal constructs and the sense of self. It is also used in art psychotherapy through the House/Tree/Person (H-T-P) drawing assessment (Burns, 1987). Being able to engage in such activities with an APT practitioner-trainer may be invaluable in keeping students safe while they are exposed to transferential processes, and in considering the ethical and professional responsibility for another when using creative techniques in practice. HCPC makes a reference to this element of a practitioner's ability to "understand the role and use of visual symbols in art that communicate conscious and unconscious processes" in Standard 13.21 (HCPC, 2013, p. 14).

Experiential group learning

Hands-on learning experiences were valued by trainees as more effective and more meaningful than attaining knowledge theoretically. One of the aims of the C&YP counselling training therefore should be experiential learning and the adaptation of the Adult Experiential Learning Cycle (Kolb, 1984) for such purposes. This presents a practical challenge in how such a training could be delivered; however, it is in line with the in-situ experiential training for APTs in the UK (HCPC, 2014) and BACP's own position in their requirement that counsellors should possess "(a)n ability to help a young person make sense of the meanings and experiences that emerge from using creative methods and resources" and "(a)n ability to adopt a non-intrusive and non-interpretative stance when helping a child/young person explore the personal meanings which emerge from using creative methods and resources" (BACP, 2019a, p. 97). Experiential groups (also known as training groups) could provide a safe learning environment to enable art making in the presence of other trainees, where such experiences are reflected upon through group discussions and the exploration of interpersonal processes. Group dynamics (Bion, 1961) may be utilised in learning about each other's creative expression in C&YP counselling training, which otherwise form a fundamental element of APT training, thus enabling trainees to reflect on transferential processes.

The other important element of experiential learning is recognising the harm that could be experienced by clients when they are exploring their personal difficulties creatively. Counsellors should be able to establish the safe limits of the therapeutic techniques they use (BACP, 2018). It could be argued that without trying creative tools themselves, counsellors cannot use them safely in their C&YP counselling practice. If not having experienced creative tools "first hand", counsellors may run a risk of not being able to determine how art as a process is likely to interact with a client's mental state. The potential harm is so likely, that it led authors such as Sandford (2007) and Springham (2008) to advocate careful consideration of the use of arts in general health and well-being services, outside of counselling and psychotherapy.

Modification of practical creative therapeutic techniques

There are many APT processes that can be used effectively in C&YP counselling training, as long as they are carefully adapted to the students' recognised and accepted limitations. Reciprocally, art psychotherapy could benefit from the practical application of certain creative therapeutic methods as used by, for example, cognitive behavioural counsellors (vicious cycles, guided visualisation) (Leahy, 2017), to support a more coherent approach to using practical arts-based exercises.

The APT tools offered to C&YP counsellors may include directive exercises, such as making a YaYa box as part of a therapeutic intervention designed to "represent a person's innermost self on the inside of the box and the person's outward self on the outside of the box" (Janesick, 2004, p. 145). This intervention is often utilised successfully by students to make sense of their own defence mechanisms, personal scripts and ego states (Berne, 2010). We found that with careful experiential exploration of specific techniques in a classroom setting, C&YP counsellors were "able to practice safely and effectively within their own scope of practice" (HCPC, 2013, p. 7).

As there are countless opportunities to translate APT techniques and tools into a C&YP counselling practice, the main focus should be on the facilitation of the creative methods' use in training. Careful introduction, an outline of potential risks and benefits, use of self-care tools and a permission to work at one's own pace, if the experience becomes too intense, must be included in all teaching. The need for group reflection on and discussion of the experience is also key in enabling the development of understanding of one's scope of practice. It could be argued that these are skills many counsellor-trainers may have. However, the inclusion of an art psychotherapist on a C&YP counsellor training allowed participants to explore their blind spots and provided them with an opportunity to be creatively challenged in the areas of personal arts-based assumptions and fears.

Intentionality of creative methods use in art psychotherapy

Schmidt (1984) developed the concept of therapeutic "intention" as part of his focus on counselling micro-skills and establishing a purpose and direction in therapy. The concept of practitioner's intentionality could be described as a cognitive intention to select the type of intervention suitable for client work at hand (Hill & O'Grady, 1985). The terminology is also informed by Geldard, Geldard, and Yin Foo's (2015) proactive approach to counselling young people, which fittingly incorporates the critically informed reflexive process in counselling by using creative tools fit for purpose, and not just because they are available.

We found that the exposure to each other's teaching and learning strategies enabled a deep sense of the importance of intention in the use of arts-based methods in practice. The APT lecturer developed an effective approach to identifying and communicating to students the intentions for the use of specific tools. As a second-nature skill stemming from an in-depth study of, and an experience in, an arts-based subject, it came to be a focus and a fundamental element of developing a C&YP counsellors' practice and the APT lecturer's teaching methods.

It is our view that APTs could benefit from considering intentionality further within their initial training. As many APTs use the arts as a form of expressive language, they might find it difficult to recognise that others do not speak it or understand it the same way. Such improved awareness could lead to a development of a more effective approach of therapy delivery in art psychotherapy, with the practitioners' ownership of all they offer therapeutically being formulated better.

This would also be in line with the call for evidence-based approaches in therapy, the consideration of practitioner and practice-setting resources and their limitations, and the diversity of client needs and systems (Cooper & McLeod, 2011; NICE guidelines).

Conclusion

There are many advantages to using creative methods in C&YP counselling and in C&YP counsellors' training. Increasingly, as the public and service users become better informed about the available types of psychological therapies and therapeutic intervention, they may gradually demand better quality from the practitioners delivering them.

It is exciting to see the development of arts-based techniques for the use of C&YP counsellors (Geldard & Geldard, 2009). However, by comparing the BACP competences and HCPC standards documents, it became clear that one profession may have a better grasp of the impact of arts-based therapeutic interventions on their clients, and that in-depth collaboration might be needed between the professional and regulatory bodies and practitioners in the UK to harness the different types of expertise from the many psychotherapeutic fields of practice.

This would provide a fertile ground for professional learning and making sure clients experience no harm when engaging in therapy. C&YP are particularly vulnerable and often unable to make an informed choice of therapy. Fundamentally, the practitioner is professionally and ethically responsible for making an appropriate assessment of the client's mental state, the suitability of any creative intervention used, and of his or her own scope of practice and the professional capacity to employ such interventions with each C&YP client.

As part of our teaching practice, we encountered strong personal responses to the use of arts-based methods in counsellors' training for C&YP therapy work. These responses often took place as class-based creative activities funnelled unprocessed personal material to their full awareness. It was surprising to find that the counsellors in training often reflected on the strength of these experiences and how the arts-based techniques resulted in an impact not experienced before.

The second-nature approach to using creative methods in therapy by art psychotherapists makes them more susceptible to not having clear intentions and justification for introducing and/or offering such tools. The profession could benefit from improving practitioners' intentionality in its requirements for safe practice, and the subsequent effectiveness of creative interventions.

There seems to be much potential in the joining of forces between C&YP counsellors and APTs (and those involved in their training and curriculum development) that could enrich each other's established practices in C&YP therapy. We have experienced in-depth learning from each other while working alongside in a classroom. Furthermore, recognising each other's differences in the inclusion of intentionality in the use of creative tools, and the subsequent modification of the course's teaching methods has contributed to several improvements in the learning and teaching strategies across other programmes.

Ultimately, it will be the C&YP clients who benefit from counsellors' better insight and preparedness to provide a wider range of creative tools in C&YP therapy, as well as being supported safely and ethically in an effective therapeutic relationship.

Notes

1. Level 7 qualifications in the UK are postgraduate diploma, postgraduate certificate in education (PGCE), postgraduate certificate, master's degree, for example master of arts (MA), master of science (MSc) and others; full list is available at https://www.gov.uk/what-different-qualification-levels-mean/list-of-qualification-levels.
2. Child and Adolescent Mental Health Services, NHS.
3. http://courses.southwales.ac.uk/courses/1649-pg-dip-in-counselling-children-and-young-people.
4. Art psychotherapy, Music therapy, Dramatherapy, HCPC regulated arts therapies professions in the UK.
5. For the purposes of this article, only standards relevant to art psychotherapists are included, excluding those specific to dramatherapy and music therapy.
6. First described by Freud (1915) as a process of projection of client's unconscious thoughts onto their therapist and the therapist's response to them, potentially in an emotionally entangled way.

Disclosure statement

No potential conflict of interest was reported by the authors.

References

BACP. (2018). *Ethical framework for the counselling professions*. Lutterworth: BACP.

BACP. (2019a). *Competences for work with children and young people (4–18 years)*. Retrieved from https://www.bacp.co.uk/media/5863/bacp-cyp-competence-framework.pdf

BACP. (2019b). *Counsellors' Guide: The competences for humanistic counselling with children and young people (4–18 years)*. Retrieved from https://www.bacp.co.uk/media/5864/bacp-counsellors-guide-cyp-competence-framework.pdf

Berne, E. (2010). *Games people play: The psychology of human relationships*. New York: Penguin.

Bion, W. R. (1961). *Experiences in groups*. London: Tavistock.

Boseley, S. (2010, May 2). Psychotherapy rebels consider rebranding to avoid state regulation. *The Guardian Sunday*. Retrieved from https://www.theguardian.com/society/2010/may/02/psychotherapy-rebrand-avoid-state-regulation

Bowlby, J. (1969). *Attachment. Attachment and loss: Vol. 1. Loss*. New York: Basic Books.

Burns, R. C. (1987). *Kinetic-house-tree-person drawings: An interpretive manual*. London: Brunner-Routledge.

Case, C. (2014). *The handbook of art therapy*. London: Routledge.

Cooper, M., & McLeod, J. (2011). *Pluralistic counselling and psychotherapy*. London: Sage.

DoH. (2011). *Enabling excellence: Autonomy and accountability for health and social care staff.* London: Department of Health. Retrieved from https://www.gov.uk/government/publications/enabling-excellence-autonomy-and-accountability-for-health-and-social-care-staff

Erikson, E. H. (1959). *Identity and the life cycle.* New York: International Universities Press.

Freud, S. (1915). The unconscious. *SE, 14*, 159–204.

Geldard, K., & Geldard, D. (2009). *Counselling adolescents: The proactive approach for young people.* London: Sage.

Geldard, K., Geldard, D., & Yin Foo, R. (2015). *Counselling adolescents: The proactive approach for young people.* London: Sage.

HCPC. (2011). *Psychotherapists and counsellors. Regulation of further groups: An update.* Retrieved from http://www.hpc-uk.org/aboutregistration/aspirantgroups/psychotherapistscounsellors/

HCPC. (2013). *Standards of proficiency - Arts therapists.* Retrieved from http://www.hpc-uk.org/publications/index.asp?id=39#publicationSearchResults

HCPC. (2014). *Standards of education and training.* Retrieved from http://www.hcpc-uk.org/publications/standards/index.asp?id=183

HCPC. (2016). *Guidance on conduct and ethics for students.* Retrieved from https://www.hcpc-uk.org/globalassets/resources/guidance/guidance-on-conduct-and-ethics-for-students.pdf

HCPC. (2017). *Fitness to practise annual report.* Retrieved from http://www.hpc-uk.org/assets/documents/100055BAFitnesstopractiseannualreport2017.pdf

Hill, C. E., & O'Grady, K. E. (1985). List of therapist intentions illustrated in a case study and with therapists of varying theoretical orientations. *Journal of Counseling Psychology, 32*, 3–22.

HM Government. (2007). *Trust assurance and safety - the regulation of health professionals in the 21st century* (White Paper). Retrieved from https://www.gov.uk/government/uploads/system/uploads/attachment_data/file/228847/7013.pdf

HM Government. (2008). *Children and young people in mind: The final report of the national CAMHS review.* Retrieved from http://webarchive.nationalarchives.gov.uk/20081230004520/publications.dcsf.gov.uk/eorderingdownload/camhs-review.pdf

Huet, V. (2011). Art therapy-based organisational consultancy: A session at Tate Britain. *International Journal of Art Therapy: Inscape, 16*(1), 313.

Huet, V. (2012). Creativity in a cold climate: Art therapy-based organisational consultancy within public healthcare. *International Journal of Art Therapy, 17*(1), 25–33.

Janesick, V. J. (2004). *"Stretching" exercises for qualitative researchers.* Thousand Oaks: Sage.

Kelly, G. (1991). *The psychology of personal constructs.* London: Routledge in association with the Centre for Personal Construct Psychology.

Kolb, D. A. (1984). *Experiential learning.* Englewood Cliffs, NJ: Prentice Hall.

Leahy, R. L. (2017). *Cognitive therapy techniques: A practitioner's guide.* 2nd ed. London: Guildford Press.

Löwenfeld, V., & Brittain, W. (1987). *Creative and mental growth.* New York: MacMillan.

McGoldrick, M., Gerson, R., & Petry, S. S. (2008). *Genograms: Assessment and intervention.* New York: WW Norton & Company.

Ogletree, E. J., & Uljaki, W. (1973). Effects of social class status on tests of creative behaviour. *The Journal of Educational Research, 67*(4), 149–152.

Piaget, J. (1972). *The psychology of intelligence.* Totowa, NJ: Littlefield.

Polat, F., & Jenkins, P. (2005). Provision of counselling services in secondary schools: A survey of local education authorities in England and Wales. *Pastoral Care in Education, 23*(4), 17–24.

Robinson, K. (1998). *All our futures: Creativity, culture, and education (The Robinson report).* Retrieved from http://sirkenrobinson.com/pdf/allourfutures.pdf

Robinson, K. (2001). *Out of our minds: Learning to be creative.* Chichester: Capstone.

Robinson, K. (2013). *Finding your element: How to discover your talents and passions and transform your life (with Lou Aronica).* London: Penguin.

Robson, M., & Robson, J. (2008). Explorations of participants' experiences of a personal development group held as part of a counselling psychology training group: Is it safe in here? *Counselling Psychology Quarterly, 21*(4), 371–382.

Sandford, S. (2007). Patient and staff safety. In *A prospectus for arts and health* (p. 87). London Arts Council/Department of Health. Retrieved from http://www.emergenceplus.org.uk/images/Documents/prospectus%20for%20arts%20and%20health.pdf

Schmidt, J. J. (1984). Counselor intentionality: An emerging view of process and performance. *Journal of Counseling Psychology, 31*, 383–386.

Springham, N. (2008). Through the eyes of the law: What is it about art that can harm people? *International Journal of Art Therapy (Inscape), 13*(2), 65–73.

Welsh Assembly Government. (2008). *School-based counselling services in Wales: A national strategy.* Retrieved from http://gov.wales/dcells/publications/publications/guidanceandinformation/counsellingstrategy/counsellingstrategy-e.pdf?lang=en

Welsh Government. (2013). *Statutory guidance to Welsh local authorities on the provision of independent counselling services*. Retrieved from http://gov.wales/docs/dcells/publications/130611-independent-counselling-services-en.pdf

Williams, A., & Jenkins, P. (2016). Key differences between counselling adults and children/young people. *MindEd*. Retrieved from https://www.minded.org.uk/Catalogue/Index?HierarchyId=0_39474_39480_39482&programmeId=39474

Wiseman, H., & Shefler, G. (2001). Experienced psychoanalytically oriented therapists' narrative accounts of their personal therapy: Impacts on professional and personal development. *Psychotherapy*, *38*(2), 129–141.

Career assessment and creativity: potential complementarity or a contradiction in terms?

Mark Watson and Mary McMahon

ABSTRACT
In this research we investigated whether creativity and career assessment are a contradiction in terms or whether, through creative thinking, their potential complementarity in career guidance and counselling can be realised. The research demonstrates the creative application of the systemic Integrative Structured Interview (ISI) for the Self-Directed Search (SDS) with a South African female mid-life career changer. Results indicated that the ISI positions clients as storytellers who create rich systemic stories about their quantitative SDS scores. The constructs of story telling are evident throughout an interview about quantitative scores; the scores become unifying themes across the stories. In sum, the ISI can assist mid-life career changers to make meaning of their career transition; and by embedding career assessment in a systemic story telling process creativity is evidenced as a multilayered process.

Counselling has long been regarded as a creative activity (Frey, 1975) in which clients and counsellors collaborate to generate plans, develop new perspectives, and formulate strategies and courses of action towards preferred futures. Creativity concerns finding appropriate solutions or courses of action to problems or issues (Moran, 2010). In today's rapidly changing world, the constant adaptation required to live and survive necessitates that individuals are creative (Gabora & Kaufman, 2010). A contemporary example of such adaptation is career change. Individuals can reasonably expect to change careers several times during their lives.

Donald Super (1980, 1990) was the first theorist to recognise that careers develop across the lifespan; since that time, the term mid-life career change has become widely recognised in career guidance and counselling. Developing a clear sense of direction in relation to such mid-life career change is best achieved by engaging in self-reflectivity through which individuals learn about becoming (Bimrose, Barabasch, Brown, & Mulvey, 2015). Mid-life career change may originate from external influences (e.g. factory closure or forced redundancy) or from personal choice. Thus a systemic view of mid-life career change positions it as a complex process in which individuals may experience a range of personal, economic, social, and learning challenges, positive and negative emotions such as hope, concern, anticipation, self-doubt, depression and stress (Sharf, 2013).

Career guidance and counselling can provide support to adults experiencing mid-life career change and assist them to successfully manage their transitions (Barabasch, Merrill, & Zanazzi, 2015); indeed, career guidance and counselling has the "potential to foster and facilitate the process of self-reflexivity" (Bimrose et al., 2015, p. 257) needed by individuals to develop a sense of future career direction. In the face of more diverse client groups and more complex client needs, career guidance and counselling has itself entered a period of transition and change as it seeks to adapt to survive in a changing world. Even though career guidance and counselling is seeking to develop new perspectives and find appropriate solutions to career concerns, it has seldom been associated with creativity throughout its history, a situation that has been criticised and considered a negative influence on graduate students' interest and training in career counselling (Heppner, O'Brien, Hinkelman, & Humphrey, 1994). This unfortunate situation may be largely a result of the dominance of quantitative career assessment and its associated linear, objective, and rational models of career counselling which deemphasised creativity and led to labelling, stereotyping or "black and white" thinking (Peavy, 1998).

A quality dialogue between career counsellors and clients underpins the emerging narrative approaches to career counselling which are more accepting of creativity because they are founded on storytelling, reflection, meaning making and creative thinking in order to "construct" or "design" future stories (Amundson, 2009; McMahon, 2017a; Savickas et al., 2009). Complementing such narrative approaches to career counselling are the creative, flexible, meaning-making processes of qualitative career assessment (McMahon & Watson, 2015a, 2015b). Valuing emotion, subjectivity and intuition, qualitative career assessment differs from quantitative career assessment with its emphasis on objectivity, logic and rationality. Finding creative ways of valuing and utilising both quantitative career assessment and narrative approaches to career counselling in the best interests of clients warrant consideration and provide the focus of this article.

In response to the major challenge identified by this symposium's theme — that is, to use more creative methods to confront situations in novel, open and different ways — in this article, we consider career assessment in career guidance and counselling. We explore whether creativity and career assessment are a contradiction in terms or whether, through creative thinking, their potential complementarity can be realised in new and novel approaches. Accepting the invitation to facilitate a "shift to more meaning-oriented modes of learning" (Lengelle, Hambly, & Hughes, 2018, p. 269), in this paper we focus on the career assessment process and how storytelling has the potential to make meaning of quantitative career scores in creative ways.

Drawing on our research and experience with career assessment and career counselling, in this article we demonstrate the creative application of assessment in career guidance and counselling in research with a South African Caucasian female mid-life career changer. Beginning with a review of literature related to mid-life career change and career assessment, the Integrative Structured Interview (ISI; McMahon & Watson, 2012; Watson, 2017; Watson & McMahon, 2014) for the Self-Directed Search (Holland, 1985) is then described as a creative response to the vexed question about how to combine storytelling and quantitative career assessment to elicit their complementarity. In addition, the ISI process offers a creative approach to changing the dynamic of the career counselling relationship by positioning clients as storytellers who create context rich personal stories about their quantitative scores.

Mid-life career change and transition

Mid-life career change is a contemporary reality for many people as labour markets shift towards greater use of part-time, casual, and contract work at the expense of permanent fulltime jobs, and the traditional "job for life". There is increasing consensus in the career literature that most adults will need to continually adapt their career choices to meet the realities of a fluid world of work and their own changing developmental tasks and needs (Jain, 2014). Similarly, the goals of career guidance and counselling also need to shift, particularly those concerning helping adult clients to develop transition skills and the adaptability to identify and respond to both barriers and opportunities in their career development, and to engage in continuous lifelong learning. Indeed, lifelong learning is a core aspect of mid-career development (Bimrose & Brown, 2014).

This article illustrates a mid-life career changer who has committed to lifelong learning through tertiary study in a university. There is an international trend of adult students transitioning into some form of lifelong education, with Schaefer (2010) stating that adult learners are a significant research issue. Research has established that adult students have less linear, more unpredictable transitions into tertiary education than traditional entry students (Stevenson & Clegg, 2013). This increasing cohort of mature students is an emerging and growing client group for career guidance and counselling practitioners and creative ways of understanding and supporting them are needed.

Assessment in career guidance and counselling

Career assessment can be used to assist individuals in their career transitions. While career test scores have always been interpretable, their quantitative nature has invariably dominated how and by whom they have been interpreted in career guidance and counselling. Indeed, career practitioners may struggle to incorporate the dominant and didactic role of interpreting quantitative career assessment within the broader narrative of career practice, reflecting a challenge concerning the relationship between quantitative career assessment and narrative forms of career counselling. Indeed, over three decades ago Goldman (1972) questioned the relationship between "tests and counseling" (p. 213) because quantitative career assessment and narrative career counselling are based on different philosophical assumptions (Sampson, Peterson, Osborn, & Hayden, 2015) which could be viewed as "seemingly incompatible viewpoints" (Hartung, 2007, p. 103). Taking an either/or approach however, is neither desirable nor necessary (Sampson, 2009) as Super (1954) recognised over half a century ago when he urged career counsellors to "use both methods, sometimes emphasizing one, sometimes the other" (p. 16). Similarly, more recently, several authors have called for a multistoried approach to career assessment (e.g. Arulmani, 2015; McMahon & Watson, 2015a; Pryor & Bright, 2015; Sampson et al., 2015) and the need for creative approaches to qualitatively storying quantitative scores (McMahon & Watson, 2012), that is to craft stories from scores (McMahon & Watson, 2015b). Finding a creative way to address the longstanding challenge of integrating quantitative career assessment with career counselling provided a rationale for the present research.

There are several issues that need to be considered in the encouragement of more creative use of career assessment in career counselling. One issue is that the career literature has remained more conceptual than practical in its consideration of assessment within narrative approaches (McMahon, Watson, Chetty, & Hoelson, 2012b). Another issue is the inherent danger of creating interventions that are not theoretically underpinned (McMahon, 2006); there seems to be an emphasis on describing creative activities as qualitative career assessment rather than as theoretically driven instruments intentionally used within career counselling (McMahon & Watson, 2015b).

There has been little available in the way of models to creatively convert quantitative scores into qualitative interpretation. Creative qualitative interpretation of quantitative career assessment would encourage intuitive thinking in addition to the present dominant emphasis on analytic thinking (Banks, 2014). The former thinking would allow clients to emotionally respond to test scores as well as to take a more holistic perspective of what those scores could mean within the context of their present lives. Encouraging intuitive thinking requires creative approaches to career counselling that can stimulate a qualitative narrative of a quantitative score, and that can integrate assessment. The Integrative Structured Interview (ISI; McMahon & Watson, 2012; Watson, 2017; Watson & McMahon, 2014) is presented as a creative theoretically-driven method that can use quantitative career scores to stimulate a qualitative and narrative career counselling process.

Integrative structured interview

The Integrative Structured Interview (McMahon & Watson, 2012; Watson, 2017; Watson & McMahon, 2014) has been applied to the quantitative Self-Directed Search (SDS; Holland, 1985) and also to Super's Work Values Inventory-Revised (SWVI-R; Zytowski, 2006). Concomitant with the trait-factor dominance of career assessment is the view that "career counselling has not been viewed as a creative discipline" (McMahon, 2006, p. 153). McMahon (2017b) has captured the motivation for the creation of the ISI well when she stated that: "There is nothing inherently creative about facts and matching. However, there may be something inherently creative about how 'the facts' are interpreted or the meaning they are ascribed by clients and counsellors" (p. 225). The creative interpretation of quantitative scores is at the heart of the ISI which is underpinned by three principles. First, it enables quantitative career assessment, in the case of this article, the SDS (Holland, 1985), to be qualitatively storied through a reflective learning process. Second, the ISI story crafting questions stimulate the telling of rich systemic stories reflective of the ISI's theoretical foundation in the Systems Theory Framework of career development (STF: Patton & McMahon, 2021) and its career counselling application, story telling. Story telling is the term that refers to this specific narrative approach, as opposed to the term storytelling which refers to generic narrative career counselling approaches. Third, clients systemically contextualise their quantitative scores in the multiple contexts of their lives.

While the SDS can be self-administered, self-scored and self-interpreted (Holland & Messer, 2015), the career counsellor scored and psychometrically interpreted the SDS in the present research. The ISI, however, enables clients rather than career counsellors to "interpret" their SDS by reflecting on their scores, making meaning of them in the context of their personal systems of influence, and learning from their reflection in order to construct a future career story. This creative meaning making process differs considerably from previous examples where practitioners had the primary responsibility for the interpretation of interest inventories (see Savickas, 1998) including the SDS (Rayman, 1998). Previous research (McMahon, Bimrose, Watson, & Abkhezr, 2020) has shown that, because the career counsellor assumes the role of facilitator, almost 70% of an ISI is spoken by the client unlike many career counselling interviews that are dominated by the career counsellor. Prior to outlining the method employed in this research, which includes a description of the ISI and the SDS, a brief overview of the ISI's theoretical and practice foundations is warranted.

Theoretical foundation

The ISI is theoretically grounded in the Systems Theory Framework of career development (STF; Patton & McMahon, 2021). The STF is the first direct application of systems theory in career development and it depicts individuals in a complex and dynamic system of influences with which they are in constant recursive interaction. At the outset, individuals themselves are systems comprising intrapersonal influences such as personality, beliefs, abilities, values, gender and self-concept. In general, individuals are influenced by social systems such as family, peers, and media. More broadly, individuals are influenced by environmental-societal systems such as geographic location, socioeconomic circumstances, historical trends, globalisation and political decisions. These systems of influence are depicted within the context of past, present and future time. Patton and McMahon regard these influences as the content of career development and proffer recursive interaction within and between influences, change over time and chance as the processes of career development. A strength of the STF is its ready application in practice as demonstrated by the story telling approach to career counselling.

Practice foundation

Systemic thinking is fundamental to the story telling approach to narrative career counselling (McMahon & Watson, 2012). By taking a "person in context" (McMahon, Watson, & Patton, 2014, p. 35) view, career counsellors can encourage clients to tell stories of experiences from paid and unpaid work and non-work roles and diverse settings across their lifespan. The quality of the client-counsellor relationship is critical in order to facilitate an environment where clients feel "safe" and supported to tell their stories. Rich dialogue is a feature of the story telling approach. Essentially the story telling approach to career counselling is a process in which clients construct and tell rich systemic stories and, guided by the career counsellor, reflect on their thoughts and feelings about and their reactions and responses to those stories. Together, clients and career counsellors engage in a creative process of identifying connections which may not have been previously evident to the client, i.e. themes and patterns within and between stories from which clues to future stories may be elicited. Underpinning the story telling approach are the five core process constructs of reflection, connectedness, meaning making, learning and agency which have been described in detail previously (see McMahon, Watson, Chetty, & Hoelson, 2012a). McMahon et al. (2012a) also describe the recursiveness that can occur between the five core constructs, i.e. their potential interrelatedness. A summary of the definitions and key elements of the process constructs is provided in Table 1.

Method

The aims of the present research were to investigate (a) the use of the ISI in career guidance and counselling with a mid-life career changer, specifically an older university student in transition, and (b) the potential complementarity of story telling guided by the ISI and a quantitative career instrument, the SDS. A qualitative design was chosen given the exploratory aim of the research. A single case is presented in this article because it enables a detailed interrogation of the use (Gay, Mills, & Airasian, 2009) of the ISI and its creative assessment process. Single cases have previously been reported to evaluate career counselling (e.g. Cardoso, Goncalves, Duarte, Silva, & Alves, 2016; Hartung & Vess, 2016).

Recruitment and participant

Subsequent to obtaining ethical clearance, potential participants were recruited using non-probability purposive sampling. A final year social services class was approached and the research was explained to them. Potential participants were provided with a Participant Information Sheet and Consent Form. The interview reported here was conducted in South Africa with the first volunteer from the potential participants, a 43-year-old middle class Caucasian woman who was married with two children. She had previously worked in business and finance and was studying a postgraduate diploma in a social services profession. Her SDS Code was SCI, i.e. Social, Conventional and Investigative.

Table 1. Process constructs of the story telling approach.

Process construct	Definition	Key elements
Reflection	"transform a situation in which there is experienced obscurity, doubt, conflict, disturbance of some sort, into a situation that is clear, coherent, settled, harmonious" (Dewey, 1933, p. 195)	transformation; a different end point; the same end point understood differently; considering an idea/concept from different angles; a thought process
Connectedness	"the term is understood in terms of concepts such as belongingness, relatedness, attachment or affiliation to something bigger than oneself, such as the family, the community, and the spiritual domain. The term is also used to refer to a subjective sense of belongingness or closeness to others" (Townsend & McWhirter, 2005).	an "other"; a relationship, connection, recursiveness
Meaning making	Meaning making enables people to better understand who they are and co-exists with action and context (Chen, 2001); "meaning making and interpretation helps individuals make sense of what has happened in their past and present, and more importantly, project their future life career course" (Chen, 2001, p. 328).	awareness, insight, sense making, understanding, interpretation, subjective process
Learning	"the process of individuals constructing and transforming experience into knowledge, skills, attitudes, values, beliefs, emotions" (Holmes, 2002)	transformation, new understanding, and knowledge creation
Agency	the capacity for individuals to "act for themselves and speak on their own behalf" (Monk, Winslade, Crocket, & Epston, 1997, p. 301); a combination of intention and action that makes things happen (Chen, 2006)	'I' statements, intention and commitment, action

Instruments

A semi-structured interview was conducted after the participant had completed the SDS independently. The interview comprised four parts. Part 1 comprised five questions seeking demographic information such as age, marital status, dependents, and previous and future employment. Part 2 comprised seven questions seeking information about the participant's programme of study and career aspirations. Part 3 comprised the ISI for the Self-Directed Search (see McMahon & Watson, 2012). Part 4 comprised eight questions about transitioning from university. The present research reports on Part 1 demographic detail and Part 3 in order to illustrative a qualitative approach to the use of quantitative career scores.

Integrative structured interview

Consisting of 13 questions in an interview structure of six sections, the ISI (McMahon & Watson, 2012; Watson, 2017; Watson & McMahon, 2014) enables clients to creatively construct stories about their scores and connect disparate and fragmented stories from their different life contexts to discern themes that can guide their career decisions. *Crafting a story about the quantitative scores* is the first section of the ISI and comprises three story crafting questions about the client's understanding of their quantitative results. *Crafting a story about the relative value of the quantitative scores* is the second section and comprises two questions about the relative value of scores and differences in scores. *Crafting a story about the quantitative scores in life contexts* is the third section and comprises four story crafting questions that contextualise the quantitative scores in relation to clients' life roles. *Crafting a story about the quantitative scores in work contexts* is the fourth section and comprises two story crafting questions that contextualise the quantitative scores by exploring clients' past, present and future work roles (i.e. both paid and unpaid work). *Crafting a story about the quantitative scores through personal reflection* is the fifth section and comprises one question designed to facilitate deep reflection on and contextualisation of the scores in relation to personal qualities. *Crafting an integrative future story using the quantitative scores and past and present experience* is the sixth and final section and comprises one question relating to crafting a future story based on the meaning and learning derived from the previous five sections. Across all sections of the ISI, story telling's core constructs of meaning making, connectedness, reflection, learning and agency are evident in the ISI's questions.

In addition to the 13 specific ISI questions, interviewers may use further probes, questions and reflections to encourage clients to fully elaborate their stories.

Self-directed search

The Self-Directed Search (Holland, 1985) is a quantitative career instrument based on Holland's (1997) theory which proposes that a good career choice reflects a good match between individuals' personality types and the work environment of their choice. Personality types are defined by the SDS in six categories or types represented by the acronym RIASEC (i.e. Realistic, Investigative, Artistic, Social, Enterprising and Conventional). The Realistic type shows an interest in working with objects, tools and machinery, and this often leads to the mastery of manual skills, and the development of practical and physical interests. The Investigative type indicates a preference for the systematic investigation of physical, biological and cultural matters, which can lead to the mastery of scientific and mathematical skills. The Artistic type prefers using creative and artistic skills, and this often leads to the mastery of artistic skills, irrespective of whether they relate to language, art, music or drama. The Social type shows a preference for working with people, by training or caring for them. This often leads to the mastery of interpersonal and educational skills. The Enterprising type shows a preference for persuading people, for taking the lead, and for acting in an enterprising way in the business world or in public life. This often leads to the mastery of leadership skills, good interpersonal abilities and persuasive abilities. The Conventional type shows a preference for ordered activity that includes the manipulation of data, and this often leads to the mastery of clerical and computational skills. Ideally, the SDS provides an individual with a three letter code which can then be matched to occupations that are classified with the same three letter code. According to Holland's secondary constructs, individuals ideally should choose work environments that are congruent with their personality type and that such congruence is enhanced when the individual's three letter code is well-differentiated (Holland & Messer, 2015). Holland (1997) believed that the SDS was amenable to both quantitative and qualitative interpretation.

Procedure

Prior to the semi-structured interview, the SDS was explained to the participant who then completed it in her own time. The interview was conducted for the researchers by a trained career counsellor in a room on the university campus at a time convenient to the participant. The interview duration was approximately 60 min. The psychometric scores were explained to the participant at the start of the interview but over two-thirds of the interview was related to the ISI questions. The interview was audiorecorded, and the career counsellor transcribed the transcript and then showed it to the participant for verification.

Data analysis

Data were analysed in a three stage coding process by us; both of us practice and teach career narrative approaches. Given that we reside in different countries there was a need for electronic means of communication (both Skype and email). First, the ISI section of the transcript was independently coded by us using deductive coding based on the five systemic process constructs of the storytelling approach, specifically reflection, connectedness, meaning making, learning, and agency, as well as for recursiveness (see Table 1). Second, the coded transcripts were compared and agreement and differences in the coding identified. Third, following discussion between us, agreement on the coding was reached (there were only three coding responses that required clarification) and the codes refined. We were aware of the subjective nature of the data analysis and reporting, and applied the four criteria of credibility, dependability, transferability and confirmability to ensure the trustworthiness of the research (Lincoln & Guba, 1985).

Results

The results report on the core constructs of the story telling approach as reflected in the client's responses to the ISI questions. The data analysis indicated discrete examples of the five process constructs of reflection, connectedness, meaning making, learning and agency, as well as examples of recursiveness between these constructs (see Table 1 for construct definitions). The constructs are also tallied numerically in order to demonstrate their embeddedness in the participant's narrative. Reflection was coded 30 times in the transcript. Reflection was evident as a discrete construct in the participant's frustrated response to her Conventional Holland code being higher than she had anticipated:

> Then I had more work history related to that in the industry before I realised it is not what I wanted to do, in fact even in my second year of studying I knew it isn't what I wanted to do but I didn't know what I wanted to do.

Connectedness was coded 26 times in the transcript and was evident as a discrete construct in the participant's relating her Social Holland code to her previous work experience: "In … business I am dealing with a lot of people – artists, employees, clients and so forth. So I think I relied a lot on those abilities". Meaning making was coded 28 times in the transcript and is reflected as a discrete construct in the participant's response to how she understood the order of her Social Holland code in her three letter code:

> I am not a very chatty-chatty person. I am not someone who will be a life and the soul of a party but I am social in the sense that I will want to get on well with everyone and help others to reach goals.

Learning was coded 17 times in the transcript and is evident as a discrete construct in the participant's response to what she found least satisfying and rewarding in her previous work responsibilities: "Well that is the conventional part and I am still frustrated why it came up so high in terms of Holland's systems … But I can understand why". Agency was coded 13 times in the transcript and is evident as a discrete construct in the participant responding to why she had an Investigative Holland code: "Yes, I believe it was inherent [the Investigative code] but I had to work on it, it didn't come naturally".

Recursiveness between constructs was coded 37 times. An example of recursiveness between the constructs of reflection and learning is the participant's exploration of how her Holland Conventional code may impact on a career in the social service:

> So that could be that, yes, that I will have to accept that I can only do what I can in that time frame and you really have to trust a person's inner resources, coping mechanisms and their strengths, that they are going to be able to do that on their own.

An example of recursiveness between the three constructs of reflection, connectedness and meaning making was the attempt by the participant to relate the Holland code of Conventional to facets of her life:

> I wouldn't say I am orderly but when I need to be I can organise myself and I can organise my environment. It is not how my house, for example, is not very orderly and I have to set notes to remind myself. I wouldn't say that I am the kind of person who would be a strictly conventional person but I do have access to those skills.

Finally, there are results that indicate the verbal contribution of both the career practitioner and the participant within an ISI interview structure. The transcript was 311 lines, of which the career practitioner spoke for 92 lines (29.6% of the total dialogue) and the participant spoke for the remaining 219 transcript lines, i.e. 70.4% of the total dialogue.

Discussion

Contemporary career counselling faces the complex challenge of reinventing itself so that it can better cater for increasingly diverse client groups and accommodate complexity. In the first symposium issue on creative methods in guidance and counselling, Lengelle et al. (2018) identified many reasons why creative methods are necessary for guidance and counselling: "Creative methods … let us break rank with the rational linear thinking, planning, efficiency and goal-orientation that has dominated policy and some practice discourses" (p. 269). In the context of this article, the challenge that provided a rationale for the research was that of improving practice by finding creative ways of integrating quantitative career assessment and career counselling. Creativity was evidenced through combining storytelling and quantitative career assessment which, on the surface, seem like a contradiction in terms given their underpinning philosophies (e.g. Sampson, 2009; Sampson et al., 2015).

In relation to the first aim of the research the ISI provided a meaningful experience for a mid-life career changer, in this case an older university student. Moreover, it showed how the compartmentalised stories of the participant's life could be integrated through the SDS scores which became integrative themes across the stories. This suggests that, although such scores are not inherently creative, they can be used in creative ways in career counselling by combining them with story telling processes (McMahon, 2006, 2017b). In particular, the meaning of scores is determined by test developers, whereas clients can invest them with personal meaning through the stories they create and tell.

Although, the results reported in this article are based on a sample of only one participant, it seems therefore in relation to the second aim, that career assessment and creativity can indeed be viewed as complementary. Specifically, the scores of a quantitative career instrument are invested with meaning through the creative construction and telling of stories about those scores in a story telling process that revealed the process constructs as well as recursive relationships between them. This creative process of constructing stories about scores ensures that assessment rather than testing is the focus of career counselling because of the emphasis on critical reflection and meaning making about psychometric scores (de Bruin & de Bruin, 2017; Peavy, 1998). Future research could explore the use of the ISI with a diversity of clients. In addition, there is a need to investigate other creative ways of combining quantitative assessment with narrative career approaches.

Positioning the client as the storyteller shifts some of the responsibility for interpreting the SDS scores from the career counsellor unlike other examples found in the literature (e.g. Rayman, 1998). This effectively invests the client with a greater degree of agency for the conduct and outcome of the interview and positions the career counsellor as a facilitator rather than as an expert. Despite this different role for career counsellors, it remains incumbent on them to administer the SDS in accordance with the test manual and to use their counselling skills throughout the ISI process. Moreover, the need to assume a facilitative role suggests an expanded role for career counsellors that may require additional training in counsellor preparation programmes and professional development programmes. Although the ISI provides a set of guided questions, the counselling skills of probes, questions and reflections may elicit greater detail about stories. Positioned as storytellers, clients can create rich systemic stories about their quantitative SDS scores (McMahon & Watson, 2012; Watson, 2017; Watson & McMahon, 2014, 2015) as reflected in this research. Moreover, the systemic stories evidence the theoretical foundation of the ISI in the Systems Theory Framework (Patton & McMahon, 2014). Also evident in the stories of the participant were subjectivity and emotions that illustrate how intuitive thinking as well as analytic thinking (Banks, 2014) were being used by the participant.

Throughout the interview reported in this research, the process constructs of the story telling approach to career counselling were evidenced. The five process constructs of reflection, connectedness, meaning making, learning and agency were coded discretely and also in recursive relationships with other constructs. The number of times each construct was coded provides evidence of their relevance in storytelling in general, and to the story telling approach to career counselling in particular. While these constructs have been described in the narrative career counselling literature, exactly how they manifest in storytelling has received little attention. Moreover, while the process constructs are invariably presented in the literature as discrete constructs, this research shows how they may also exist in interconnection with other constructs. As in previous research (McMahon et al., 2020), reflection was coded recursively several times with other constructs suggesting that it provides an overarching function. Moreover, its regular occurrence throughout the interview suggests the importance of providing a safe reflective space for clients. Agency and learning were coded less frequently which may be a function of the ISI as a reflective interview rather than as an exercise in action planning. Both were the last constructs to first be coded and the final codes of the transcript which suggests that the earlier reflective meaning making process of connecting previously disparate stories may provide a foundation on which learning and agency can be built. Further, the recursive coding of learning and agency towards the end of the transcript suggests that gaining new insight may be facilitative of individuals assuming greater agency.

The results indicated that by embedding career assessment in a systemic story telling process creativity is evidenced as a multilayered process that is a product of recursiveness between the SDS, the ISI and the participant and between the participant's own systems of influence. For example, the participant identified new connections between previously disparate stories as the SDS codes became themes of integration. A further recursive process is also evident through the creative use of probes, questions and reflections by the interviewer to encourage more rich and in-depth stories to be told.

Conclusion

While the present research reports the results of a single participant, the ISI encouraged this client to create a rich systemic story about her quantitative SDS scores. Rather than compartmentalise individual SDS scores, the ISI provided the client with an opportunity to integrate these scores into recursive themes within the rich and complex story she created and told. The research demonstrates that career assessment and creativity can complement each other to the advantage of clients. In particular, the Integrative Structured Interview (ISI) is a creative means of uniting the potentially contradictory practices of career assessment and career counselling, especially narrative career counselling. Moreover, the ISI represents a creative way of assisting midlife career changers to reflect systemically on their career change and make meaning of their past, present and future stories by using scores as unifying themes across their stories.

Disclosure statement

No potential conflict of interest was reported by the authors.

References

Amundson, N. E. (2009). *Active engagement: The being and doing of career counselling*. Richmond, BC: Ergon Communications.
Arulmani, G. (2015). The cultural preparedness approach to assessment: The question is the answer. In M. McMahon & M. Watson (Eds.), *Career assessment: Qualitative approaches* (pp. 207–218). Rotterdam, The Netherlands: Sense.
Banks, A. (2014). *Fresh thinking in learning and development part 2 of 3: Cognition, decision and expertise*. London: CPID (Chartered Institute of Personnel and Development) Research insight.
Barabasch, A., Merrill, B., & Zanazzi, S. (2015). Structural support, networking and individual survival: Career changes in Italy and Spain. *British Journal of Guidance & Counselling, 43*, 323–336.
Bimrose, J., Barabasch, A., Brown, A., & Mulvey, R. (2015). Editorial: Midcareer changes symposium. *British Journal of Guidance & Counselling, 43*, 255–262.
Bimrose, J., & Brown, A. (2014). Mid-career progression and development: The role for career guidance and counseling. In G. Arulmani, A. J. Bakshi, F. T. L. Leong, & A. G. Watts (Eds.), *Handbook of career development: International perspectives* (pp. 203–222). New York, NY: Springer.
Cardoso, P., Goncalves, M. M., Duarte, M. E., Silva, J. R., & Alves, D. (2016). Life design counseling outcome and process: A case study with an adolescent. *Journal of Vocational Behavior, 93*, 58–66.
Chen, C. P. (2001). On exploring meanings: Combining humanistic and career psychology theories in counselling. *Counselling Psychology Quarterly, 14*, 317–330.
Chen, C. P. (2006). Strengthening career human agency. *Journal of Counseling and Development, 84*, 131–138.
de Bruin, K., & de Bruin, G. P. (2017). Career assessment. In G. B. Stead & M. B. Watson (Eds.), *Career psychology in the South African context* (3rd ed., pp. 185–193). Pretoria, South Africa: Van Schaik.
Dewey, J. (1933). *How we think: A restatement of the relation of reflective thinking to the educative process*. Boston, MA: Heath.
Frey, D. H. (1975). The anatomy of an idea: Creativity in counseling. *The Personnel and Guidance Journal, 54*(1), 22–27.
Gabora, L., & Kaufman, J. C. (2010). Evolutionary approaches to creativity. In J. C. Kaufman & R. J. Sternberg (Eds.), *Cambridge handbook of creativity* (pp. 279–300). New York, NY: Cambridge University Press.
Gay, L., Mills, G., & Airasian, P. (2009). *Educational research: Competencies for analysis and applications* (9th ed.). Upper Saddle River, NJ: Pearson Educational International.
Goldman, L. (1972). Tests and counseling: The marriage that failed. *Measurement & Evaluation in Guidance, 4*(4), 213–220.

Hartung, P. J. (2007). Career construction: Principles and practice. In K. Maree (Ed.), *Shaping the story: A guide to facilitating narrative career counselling* (pp. 103–110). Pretoria, South Africa: Van Schaik Publishers.

Hartung, P. J., & Vess, L. (2016). Critical moments in career construction counseling. *Journal of Vocational Behavior, 97*, 31–39.

Heppner, M. J., O'Brien, K. M., Hinkelman, J. M., & Humphrey, C. F. (1994). Shifting the paradigm: The use of creativity in career counseling. *Journal of Career Development, 21*, 77–86.

Holland, J. L. (1985). *The self-directed search: A guide to educational and vocational planning*. Odessa, FL: Psychological Assessment Resources.

Holland, J. L. (1997). *Making vocational choices: A theory of vocational personalities and work environments* (3rd ed.). Odessa, FL: Psychological Assessment Resources.

Holland, J. L., & Messer, M. A. (2015). *The self-directed search* (5th ed.). Lutz, FL: Psychological Assessment Resources.

Holmes, A. (2002). *Lifelong learning*. Oxford: Capstone Publishing.

Jain, A. (2014). Second career: An eventual need in today's world. In G. Arulmani, A. J. Bakshi, F. T. L. Leong, & A. G. Watts (Eds.), *Handbook of career development: International perspectives* (pp. 291–305). New York, NY: Springer.

Lengelle, R., Hambly, L., & Hughes, D. (2018). Connecting to the muses. *British Journal of Guidance and Counselling, 46*, 269–271.

Lincoln, Y., & Guba, E. (1985). *Naturalistic inquiry*. London: Sage.

McMahon, M. (2006). Creativity and career counselling: A story still to be narrated. In M. McMahon & W. Patton (Eds.), *Career counselling: Constructivist approaches* (pp. 150–160). Abingdon: Routledge.

McMahon, M. (Ed.). (2017a). *Career counselling: Constructivist approaches* (2nd ed.). London: Routledge.

McMahon, M. (2017b). Creativity and constructivist career counselling. In M. McMahon (Ed.), *Career counselling: Constructivist approaches* (pp. 222–232). Abingdon: Routledge.

McMahon, M., Bimrose, J., Watson, M., & Abkhezr, P. (2020). Storytelling and quantitative career assessment: An integra tive process. *International Journal for Educational and Vocational Guidance*, 20, 523–542.

McMahon, M., & Watson, M. (2012). Telling stories of career assessment. *Journal of Career Assessment, 20*, 440–451.

McMahon, M., & Watson, M. (Eds.). (2015a). *Career assessment: Constructivist approaches*. Rotterdam, The Netherlands: Sense.

McMahon, M., & Watson, M. (2015b). Qualitative career assessment: Future directions. In M. McMahon & M. Watson (Eds.), *Career assessment: Qualitative approaches* (pp. 257–262). Rotterdam, The Netherlands: Sense.

McMahon, M., Watson, M. B., & Patton, W. (2014). Context-resonant systems perspectives in career theory. In G. Arulmani, A. J. Bakshi, F. T. L. Leong, & A. G. Watts (Eds.), *Handbook of career development: International perspectives* (pp. 29–41). New York, NY: Springer.

McMahon, M., Watson, M., Chetty, C., & Hoelson, C. (2012a). Examining process constructs of narrative career counselling: An exploratory case study. *British Journal of Guidance and Counselling, 40*, 127–141.

McMahon, M., Watson, M., Chetty, C., & Hoelson, C. (2012b). Story telling, career assessment and career counselling. *South African Journal of Higher Education, 26*, 729–741.

Monk, G., Winslade, J., Crocket, K., & Epston, D. (1997). *Narrative therapy in practice: The archaeology of hope*. San Francisco, CA: Jossey-Bass.

Moran, S. (2010). The roles of creativity in society. In J. C. Kaufman & R. J. Sternberg (Eds.), *Cambridge handbook of creativity* (pp. 74–91). New York, NY: Cambridge University Press.

Patton, W., & McMahon, M. (2021). *Career development and systems theory: Connecting theory and practice* (4th ed.). Brill.

Peavy, R. V. (1998). *Sociodynamic counselling: A constructivist perspective*. Victoria, Canada: Trafford.

Pryor, R. G. L., & Bright, J. E. H. (2015). Chaotic career assessment. In M. McMahon & M. Watson (Eds.), *Career assessment: Qualitative approaches* (pp. 191–198). Rotterdam, The Netherlands: Sense.

Rayman, J. R. (1998). Interpreting Ellenore flood's self-directed search. *The Career Development Quarterly, 46*, 330–338.

Sampson, J. P., Jr. (2009). Modern and postmodern career theories: The unnecessary divorce. *The Career Development Quarterly, 58*, 91–96.

Sampson, J. P., Peterson, G. W., Osborn, D. S., & Hayden, S. C. W. (2015). Using career theory to integrate qualitative and quantitative career assessment. In M. McMahon & M. Watson (Eds.), *Career assessment: Qualitative approaches* (pp. 181–190). Rotterdam, The Netherlands: Sense.

Savickas, M. L. (1998). Interpreting interest inventories: A case example. *The Career Development Quarterly, 46*, 307–310.

Savickas, M. L., Nota, L., Rossier, J., Dauwalder, J.-P., Duarte, M. E., Guichard, J., … van Vianen, A. E. M. (2009). Life designing: A paradigm for career construction in the 21st century. *Journal of Vocational Behavior, 75*, 239–250.

Schaefer, J. L. (2010). Voices of older baby boomer students: Supporting their transitions back into college. *Educational Gerontology, 36*, 67–90.

Sharf, R. S. (2013). *Applying career development theory to counseling* (6th ed.). Pacific Grove, CA: Brooks/Cole.

Stevenson, J., & Clegg, S. (2013). 'My past is a double edge sword': Temporality and reflexivity in mature learners. *Studies in Continuing Education, 35*(1), 17–29.

Super, D. E. (1954). Career patterns as a basis for vocational counseling. *Journal of Counseling Psychology, 1*, 12–20.

Super, D. E. (1980). A life-span, life-space approach to career development. *Journal of Vocational Behavior, 16*, 282–298.

Super, D. E. (1990). A life-span, life-space approach to career development. In D. Brown & L. Brooks (Eds.), *Career choice and development: Applying contemporary theory to practice* (2nd ed., pp. 197–261). San Francisco, CA: Jossey-Bass.

Townsend, K. C., & McWhirter, B. T. (2005). Connectedness: A review of the literature with implications for counseling, assessment and research. *Journal of Counseling and Development, 83*, 191–201.

Watson, M. (2017). Bridging quantitative and qualitative career assessment: The integrative structured interview process. In M. McMahon (Ed.), *Career counselling: Constructivist approaches* (pp. 260–269). London: Routledge.

Watson, M., & McMahon, M. (2014). Making meaning of quantitative assessment in career counseling through a storytelling approach. In G. Arulmani, A. J. Bakshi, F. T. L. Leong, & A. G. Watts (Eds.), *Handbook of career development: International perspectives* (pp. 631–644). New York, NY: Springer.

Watson, M., & McMahon, M. (2015). Integrative structured interview process. In M. McMahon & M. Watson (Eds.), *Career assessment: Qualitative approaches* (pp. 199–205). Rotterdam, The Netherlands: Sense.

Zytowski, D. G. (2006). *Super's work value inventory revised. Technical manual*. Adel, IA: Kuder. Retrieved from http://www.kuder.com/downloads/SWV-Tech-Manual.pdf

The vocational ID: connecting life design counselling and personality systems interaction theory

Marc Schreiber, Adrian Gschwend and Marie-Louise Susanne Iller

ABSTRACT

We introduce the Vocational ID that integrates linguistic and visual representations of a career counselling client's self. Based upon findings from the Life Design paradigm [Savickas, M. L., Nota, L., Rossier, J., Dauwalder, J.-P., Duarte, M. E., Guichard, J., … van Vianen, A. E. M. (2009). Life designing: A paradigm for career construction in the twenty-first century. *Journal of Vocational Behavior, 75*(3), 239–250. doi:10.1016/j.jvb.2009.04.004] and the Personality Systems Interaction theory [Kuhl, J. (2000b). The volitional basis of personality systems interaction theory: Applications in learning and treatment contexts. *International Journal of Educational Research, 33*(7–8), 665–703. doi:10.1016/S0883-0355(00)00045-8], the Vocational ID facilitates working on clients' vocational identity. In this article, we present the theoretical framework, its practical applications, and a case study.

Introduction

We developed the Vocational ID as a counselling tool and framework that integrates linguistic and visual representations of a career counselling client's self and vocational identity. The Vocational ID serves primarily to facilitate career counselling from the Life Design perspective, especially for working with the Career Construction Interview (CCI; Savickas, 1989, 2015b), a method derived from the Career Construction Theory (Savickas, 2011a, 2013, 2015b). However, it also easily connects to many other theoretical approaches and counselling methods. In presenting the Vocational ID, we especially refer to and combine two approaches that both focus on career counselling clients' self and identity: (1) The Life Design perspective (Savickas, 2011c, 2012a; Savickas et al., 2009) and (2) Kuhl's (Kuhl, 2000a, 2000b, 2001) Personality Systems Interaction (PSI) theory.

The Life Design perspective includes reviewing and revising a client's identity narrative. In following Kuhl's theory for integrating motivational and volitional aspects, we focus on the interplay of clients' cognitive and affective processes associated with career development. Kuhl's (2000a, 2000b, 2001) PSI theory distinguishes between analytic and holistic information processing (Kazén, Kuhl, & Quirin, 2015) and aims at fostering volitional control (also self-control) and self-growth (also self-regulation) (Alsleben & Kuhl, 2011). Broonen (2015) illustrated the value of the PSI theory for vocational theory and practice: "In the case of difficult intentions in counselling practice, concerned participants could benefit from an approach that considers differential emotional responsiveness as an important parameter of individual functioning of self-control and self-regulation" (p. 83). We want to follow up on these thoughts and – with our Vocational ID – establish a career counselling tool that facilitates working with both the Life Design perspective and the PSI theory. We will explain and illustrate that the two approaches play different roles during different phases of the career counselling process: The Life Design focus on reconceptualising a client's identity narrative comes first, followed by PSI theory methods that foster a deeper understanding of the motivational and volitional processes that clients undergo when making decisions (deciding) and performing actions (doing) based on their reconceptualised identity narrative. Used together, the two approaches are a powerful and creative tool for the career counselling process.

We will first outline the basic theory behind the two approaches and thereby emphasise the underlying processes of self-construction, self-growth, and identity. Then we will introduce the Vocational ID with a special focus on its practical relevance in career counselling. To further demonstrate the practical applications of the Vocational ID, we will present a case study that highlights specific aspects of both the Life Design perspective and the PSI theory.

Life Design perspective and Career Construction Interview (CCI)

The Life Design perspective recognises the challenges of the twenty-first century labour market and offers a new paradigm for career interventions that highlights subjective narrative truths instead of objective scientific facts (Savickas et al., 2009). Life Design sees career as a repeated transition and non-linear progression within an unforeseeable and unpredictable working world that requires great flexibility and adaptability. This results in career development best being described as a unique and individual process. Savickas (2012a, 2015a) depicts *Vocational Guidance* (guiding), *Career Education and Coaching* (developing), and *Life Design* (designing) as three different paradigms for career interventions. Industrialisation and urbanisation introduced a need for Vocational Guidance, whereas specialisation and the rise of hierarchical, multinational organisations saw Career Education and self-actualisation as a complementary method of career intervention. Life Design as a third paradigm answers needs that have newly arisen through the changes of the post-modern world of work. Table 1 contains the theoretical framework of the Life Design perspective including reference to those questions of the CCI that can be attributed to one of the three paradigms.

From a Life Design perspective, Savickas (2011c, 2012a; Savickas et al., 2009) emphasises the individual's own self-making, identity shaping, and career construction as crucial for successful career development. Therefore, he developed the Career Construction Interview (CCI; Savickas, 1989, 2015b), a semi-structured interview technique designed to clarify specific career concerns, to identify idiosyncratic life themes, personality characteristics and manifest interests of clients and, finally, to foster their career construction and work-life management. The CCI is a narrative and constructionist method based on the Life Design paradigm that with its six open questions also attends to Vocational Guidance and Career Education. The Life Design counselling process,

Table 1. Theoretical framework of the Life Design perspective including reference to the CCI questions.

	Paradigm		
	Vocational guidance	Career education and coaching (Career development)	Life design (Career counselling)
Facet of the self / science of the self (Savickas, 2011b, 2011d, 2012a)	Actor, object / objective personality (objective scores)	Agent, subject / subjective personhood (subjective self-estimates)	Author, project / identity (narratives)
Counselling focus (Savickas, 2015a)	Matching, guiding, advising, placing	Self-actualisation, developing, educating, coaching, facilitating, psychological counselling	Self-construction, designing, healing
Perspective (Savickas, 2015a)	Empiricism	Humanism	Constructionism
CCI question (Savickas, 2012b)	Question 2: Early childhood role models	Question 3: Preferred magazines, TV shows, websites	Question 4: Favourite book or movie

according to the Career Construction Theory (Savickas, 2011a, 2013, 2015b) and performed with the CCI, consists of four phases: *construction, deconstruction, reconstruction, and co-construction* (Savickas, 2011a, 2012a).

The process starts with the counsellor asking the client the first, introductory question: How can I be useful to you as you construct your career? After identifying the counselling concern and the problem narrative, the construction phase begins by the counsellor asking the client questions about childhood role models (question 2), preferred magazines, TV shows, or websites (question 3), current favourite story from a book or movie (question 4), favourite motto (question 5), and early childhood recollections (question 6). In the second, deconstruction phase, the counsellor detects in the client's answers patterns of dominance, dissociation, or disorganisation that create expectancies, biases, and feelings that constrain meaning-making options and disrupt the individual's ability to adapt to vocational development tasks, occupational transitions, and work trauma. The counsellor then discusses with the client how a different perspective and adding new meaning to these beliefs might help overcome these self-limitations (Savickas, 2012a). Subsequently, the central meanings from the answers to questions 2 to 6 are extracted. Having gathered these micronarratives, they are then combined and reconstructed into a large, unified *life portrait*, also referred to as identity narrative, or macronarrative. This development of the life portrait represents the third, reconstruction phase. The life portrait comprises the subjective representations of the client's explicit occupational plot, implicit career theme, and character arc. According to Savickas (2012a), the occupational plot adds causality to the client's story, whereas the implicit career theme adds meaning to it, and the character arc shows how a person changes over time. This identity narrative provides orientation and explanation concerning the client's past, present, and future and serves as a compass for the next steps. The fourth, co-construction phase, begins with the presentation, differentiated examination, and modification of the macronarrative together with the client. The results are applied to the client's counselling concern, and future plans (deciding) including concrete next steps (doing) are worked out.

Identity and self-construction from a Life Design perspective

Savickas (2012a) has differentiated between *self* and *identity*. Compared to identity, self is more stable over the lifetime and therefore serves as a compass guiding the individual through upcoming challenges. Identity continuously adapts to a person's social roles and live experiences. Career counselling from a Life Design perspective supports clients to identify their core self and further develop their vocational identity in accordance with the self. The vocational identity is very closely related to other facets of an individual's identity such as family life, leisure time, and spirituality. Savickas contends that self-construction is especially effective for successful career development in a world full of transitions and uncertainties such as the current working world. As stability is oftentimes no longer provided by the labour market, clients seek steadiness at the core of their self by identifying the vital aspects of that self.

Working with the CCI addresses the self in different ways and connects these different facets by constructing the life portrait of the client: self as actor (representing Vocational Guidance), self as agent (representing Career Education and Coaching/Career Development), and self as author (representing Life Design/Career Counselling) (Savickas, 2011b, 2015a). In doing so, Savickas refers to McAdams and Olson (2010), who state that the development of the different selves is connected to different life stages:

> As it develops over the human life course, personality may be viewed as a constellation of dispositional traits (the person as actor), characteristic adaptations (the person as agent), and integrative life stories (the person as author) situated in time and culture. (p. 536)

According to Savickas (2012a) the counsellor takes an active role in the deconstruction process and the reconstruction of the client's life portrait: "Having reconstructed an identity narrative from the client's micronarratives, the counsellor then presents to the client a draft of her or his life portrait, including the occupational plot, career theme, and character arc" (p. 16). In our practical work, we ascribe responsibility to counsellors for guiding the structured process, whereas the client is the ultimate authority for all personal aspects of deconstruction, reconstruction, and co-construction. We consider clients as being the experts of their own lives and therefore invite them to construct their life portrait in collaboration with the counsellor. To facilitate this process and to visualise the life portrait, we developed the Vocational ID presented in this article.

Personality Systems Interaction theory (PSI)

Kuhl's (2000a, 2000b, 2018) Personality Systems Interaction theory (PSI theory) explains differences between persons in behaviour not only by differences in mental content (e.g. beliefs, expectancies, intentions), but first and foremost by the interplay of four cognitive-emotional macrosystems: *Intention Memory* (IM), *Intuitive Behaviour Control* (IBC), *Extension Memory* (EM), and *Object Recognition* (OR). Further, PSI theory postulates that this interplay is influenced by affect-regulation. By definition, each system is associated with a certain affective state and it is assumed that changes in affect enable the activation and deactivation of the systems and the exchange of information between them. In this article, we will illustrate a simplified version of the theory and outline those aspects of PSI theory that are most crucial for working with the Vocational ID. Table 2 summarises these key aspects.

In addition to the distinct functionality of each macrosystem, which will be described further down, the four macrosystems differ in *processing mode* and *processing level*. Not unlike the Jungian typology, PSI theory differentiates between analytic thinking and holistic feeling as processing modes. Two of the systems, EM and IBC, function on a primarily intuitive and holistic level, whereas the other two systems, IM and OR, operate predominantly rationally and analytically. Based on empirical findings and incorporating neurobiological evidence, the PSI theory assumes different functional characteristics of the brain hemispheres and consequently locates the four different macrosystems in their respective hemispheres (Kazén et al., 2015; Kuhl, 2018; Quirin, Gruber, Kuhl, & Düsing, 2013; Quirin, Meyer, et al., 2013): Explicit and analytic, sequential information processing in the left hemisphere (IM and OR) versus mainly implicit and holistic, parallel information processing in the right hemisphere (EM and IBC). This resembles McGilchrist (2009), who supposes that the left hemisphere operates narrowly, sharply, focused, and with attention to detail, whereas the right hemisphere operates with sustained, broad, open, and vigilant attention. Additionally, the four macrosystems operate on two different levels of complexity (Kazén et al., 2015; Kuhl, 2000b): high-level self-representations (IM and EM) and elementary perceptions (IBC and OR). Kuhl

Table 2. Volitional control and self-growth processes according to the PSI theory (simplified).

	Volitional control (Self-control): Concrete behaviour	Self-growth (Self-development, self-regulation): Cognitions and experiences
High-level self-representations	Intention Memory (IM) • making abstract plans • explicit and analytic, sequential information processing (left hemisphere)	Extension Memory (EM) • feeling the integrated self • mainly implicit and holistic, parallel information processing (right hemisphere)
Affect modulation	First modulation assumption: • positive affect (A+) fosters IBC • downregulating positive affect (A+) fosters IM	Second modulation assumption: • negative affect (A-) fosters OR • downregulating negative affect (A-) fosters EM
Elementary perceptions	Intuitive Behaviour Control (IBC) • performing routines, executing activities • implicit and holistic, parallel information processing (right hemisphere)	Object Recognition (OR) • identifying details • explicit and analytic, sequential information processing (left hemisphere)

states that interplay between these four systems is primarily influenced by modulation of *positive and negative affect*. Affect is generated by changes in the discrepancy between actual and desired states on the sub-conscious level of needs and is not always consciously accessible (Kuhl, 2018).

To outline the distinct functionality and the interplay of the four systems, we will focus on two fundamental personality processes that, according to PSI theory, are crucial for the functioning of a person: behaviour-oriented *volitional control* and cognition- and experience-oriented *self-growth* (Alsleben & Kuhl, 2011). Volitional control refers to the process that enables a person to enact difficult (i.e. non-routine) intentions and requires communication between IM and IBC, whereas self-growth (synonymously self-development) refers to the process that enables a person to integrate new experiences into a coherent self-system and requires communication between OR and EM. Taken together, the processes address a central aspect of many career counselling interventions: How can clients successfully implement their career goals (volition control) and thereby undergo a self-congruent career development (self-growth)?

Volition control is primarily affected by the interplay of two macrosystems: IM (analytic, high-level) and IBC (holistic, elementary). Note the contrasting processing mode and level of the systems involved. IM is necessary to formulate abstract plans (e.g. working out a job application strategy), pursue goals (e.g. finding a job in another industry), and retain intentions that cannot or should not be implemented immediately (e.g. implementing a middle-term strategy or searching for the right job to apply for). IBC is essential for implementing intended actions and therefore helps transform plans into concrete action. IM and IBC operate as antagonists: During planning, the act of implementation must be inhibited to prohibit rash actions. On the other hand, planning must be stopped when the moment is opportune for action. Therefore, as one system is activated, the other is simultaneously inhibited. Routine actions, incidentally, are implemented by IBC on its own and do not require the transfer of an explicit intention from IM.

According to the *first modulation assumption* of the PSI theory, it is positive affect that modulates the interplay between the high-level IM and the elementary IBC. Positive affect fosters IBC while inhibiting IM. Downregulation of positive affect, which requires frustration tolerance, fosters IM while inhibiting IBC. Flexible regulation of positive affect is facilitated if an intention is supported by the motives[1] of power and particularly achievement (Alsleben & Kuhl, 2011; Kuhl, 2018): High achievement motivation implicitly ensures that the interplay of IM and IBC works properly. Highly achievement motivated people are well equipped to tackle difficult tasks and face complex challenges. Difficulties along the way implicitly lead to downregulation of positive affect and activation of IM. Once planning is done, the prospect of accomplishing a difficult intention re-induces positive affect and triggers active implementation. For less achievement motivated persons, social support or active imagination of other positive aspects and feelings related to goal-achievement can help to induce the positive affect needed to activate IBC. Additionally, note that according to Kuhl (2000b) "Forming abstract rather than concrete intentions permits greater flexibility and adaptability to future conditions that cannot be fully anticipated" (p. 682). We believe that this can be especially important in the domain of career counselling. Accordingly, we lay a special focus on the crucial step of formulating visions and abstract strategies when working with our clients, before elaborating on concrete plans.

In summary, effective volitional control requires the ability to switch back and forth between IM and IBC. Thus, making coherent plans and implementing them, even if severe challenges arise on the way, is facilitated. Flexible up- and downward modulation of positive affect is of great importance in this process. After having demonstrated the complex cognitive and affective functional processes that underlie volitional control, we will now turn to the processes affecting self-growth.

Self-growth is primarily affected by the interplay of the two other macrosystems: EM (holistic, high-level) and OR (analytic, elementary). Again, the two systems involved are contrasting in processing mode and level. Kuhl (2000b) describes EM as follows: "Extension memory is the repository for extended networks of remote semantic associations such as meaningful experiences, options for action, personal values, and many other aspects of the 'integrated self'" (p. 670). EM is about feeling or having a sense of self within one's social context. In this way, EM offers the best overview of what a person wants (Kuhl, 2000b). In the context of career counselling, EM is related to questions such as: What makes my vocational life meaningful and in line with my personal values, needs, or interests? OR serves as a detector of unexpected or undesired external objects or internal thoughts (e.g. internal thoughts about a dispute with one's supervisor or a lack of meaning at work) and enables contemplation of the object out of context. The terms unexpected and undesired relate to the holistic representations of the rather implicit EM. OR and EM, just like IM and IBC, operate as antagonists.

According to Kuhl's *second modulation assumption*, negative affect modulates the interplay between EM and OR. Negative affect activates OR and inhibits EM, thereby blocking access to the *integrated self* within EM. This can result in career counselling clients limiting all their thoughts to specific undesired objects (e.g. a dispute with a supervisor or their salary) through their OR and losing sight of other relevant aspects of their vocational life. Downregulation of negative affect grants access to EM while inhibiting OR. For self-growth, both OR and EM are indispensable. OR supplies the input required for the integrated self, which is part of the EM. The term *integrated* refers to the ability of the integrated self to reconcile even conflicting information, such as good and bad experiences or conflicting motives. A person can only learn from painful experiences by first tolerating negative affect. Kuhl calls this form of coping *self-confrontation*. It involves looking at the painful experience while negative affect activates OR, followed by downregulation of negative affect and integration of the painful object into EM. This integration makes it possible to avoid repeating the same painful experience in the future.

In summary, effective self-growth derives from the ability to switch back and forth between EM and OR. Thus, details identified by OR, especially distressing experiences, are integrated into EM and the integrated self can grow continuously. Flexible up- and downward modulation of negative affect is of great importance in this process.[2]

Finally, we would like to point to the important impact the two processes have on each other. On one hand, effective self-growth impacts volition control by being a precondition for setting self-congruent goals. On the other hand, effective volition control leads to action and thus to positive and negative experiences that enrich EM. The richer in experiences, the better EM can support self-congruence. To strengthen self-clarity in career counselling, bringing EM to an explicit and vocalised level and thereby integrating important information from OR can be of great importance. Visualising one's EM – as intended with the Vocational ID – can serve as a compass representing key elements of a career counselling client's self. Self-congruent goals facilitate volition because they are supported by the mainly implicit motives and values represented in EM. Lack of access to EM due to persevering negative affect may result in incongruent goals. Kuhl (2000b, 2018) speaks of *extrinsic introjects* or *self-infiltration* when one's own wishes, goals, and choices are confused with those of others (e.g. parental or societal expectations) and therefore are not fully integrated in the EM.

Identity and self-development from a PSI theory perspective

With regard to the great importance of affect modulation for volitional control and self-growth, Kuhl (2018) has stated that "excessive stress and the associated negative affect inhibit high-level holistic processing (self-access), whereas positive affect plays a key role in facilitating behaviour" (p. 558). According to PSI theory, identity and self-development are based upon the complex interplay of the four cognitive systems as well as the affective modulations depicted above. Volitional control and self-growth require activity of both the right and the left hemisphere. Regarding Kuhl's modulation assumptions, we can conclude that career counselling clients need to be able to actively modulate positive and/or negative affect to be successful in setting and implementing self-congruent goals and continuously developing their self and identity. Career counselling clients often state that they more easily operate either in an analytic/left hemispheric (i.e. tend to make plans based on thorough analysis) or in a more holistic/right hemispheric way (i.e. tend to act spontaneously and based on intuition). Furthermore, clients differ in the basic motives (achievement, power, affiliation, or freedom) that shape their perception and behaviour (Alsleben & Kuhl, 2011). By analysing these individual dispositional preferences in combination with the clients' depiction of their central issue, PSI theory can provide counsellors (and clients) with ideas for bespoke interventions for downward or upward regulation of positive or negative affect.

Kuhl (2000b) established eight steps that are crucial for successful self-development: (1) problem perception, (2) realistic goal setting and identification with the goal, (3) persistent goal pursuit, (4) attentive monitoring of available cognitive, emotional, and situational resources, (5) effective self-management of emotional and motivational states, (6) planning and problem-solving, (7) energetic initiative and implementation of plans, and (8) effective use of performance feedback. Implementation of the eight steps requires flexible and adaptive use of all the four macrosystems, supported by effective affect-regulation. Referring to the Vocational ID, we will emphasise the processes of self-growth and volitional control that underlie these eight steps and adapt them to our case study later in this paper.

The Vocational ID – linguistic and visual aspects

We designed the Vocational ID to support effective career counselling and as a facilitator for working with the CCI to form the various aspects of the six questions of the CCI into a consistent and tangible illustration of the life portrait. Furthermore, we use the Vocational ID as a framework to integrate the PSI theory into the Life Design perspective represented by the four phases of the Career Construction Theory (construction, deconstruction, reconstruction, and co-construction). We will now elaborate further on our framework that relates the Vocational ID to the Life Design perspective as well as to the PSI theory and introduce the different areas of the ID depicted in Figure 1. Subsequently, we will discuss our case study Chris.

The Vocational ID includes four areas, which can be attributed, albeit partially overlapping, to the answers to the six questions of the CCI. Consequently, the Vocational ID represents the different facets of the self according to the Life Design perspective (see Table 1) and serves as a structured visualisation of the client's life portrait, comprising occupational plot, career theme, and character arc. In the middle, there is space for a photograph or picture chosen by the client that symbolises either the desired future (e.g. scenery, symbol) or a characterising means of transportation (e.g. airplane, bicycle) that lets the client reach the counselling concern (question 1). Clients can make their own drawing, take a photograph, or search the internet for a fitting image.

As an additional option, we developed a public domain counselling platform containing so-called *resource images*.[3] We instruct clients to select and bundle a set of resource images according to their individual preferences. In a self-directed process, clients select their most appealing resource image and make a reflection thereof. Clients oftentimes choose their resource image as a symbol for their Vocational ID. Taylor and Savickas (2016) showed that the combination of the CCI with *Pictorial Narratives*, a very similar qualitative approach in which clients are asked to draw their current situation as well as their desired future situation, can be very useful.

Table 3 contains the framework that relates the Vocational ID to the Life Design paradigm and the PSI theory. We arrange the framework along the four phases of the Life Design counselling process according to the Career Construction Theory and differentiate between the stages of *establishing the ID*, ranging from construction to reconstruction, and *working with the ID*, primarily consisting of the co-construction phase. In our framework, conducting the CCI and working with concepts of the PSI theory play different roles within different phases of the counselling process: (1) The CCI is crucial to establishing the ID, wherein important aspects of the career client's self are made visible and tangible by means of the Vocational ID. (2) Afterwards, while working with the ID in the co-construction phase, clients make decisions (deciding) and transform their decisions into concrete actions (doing) (Savickas, 2011a). During this stage, the processes of self-growth and volitional control as outlined within the PSI theory are crucial and provide career

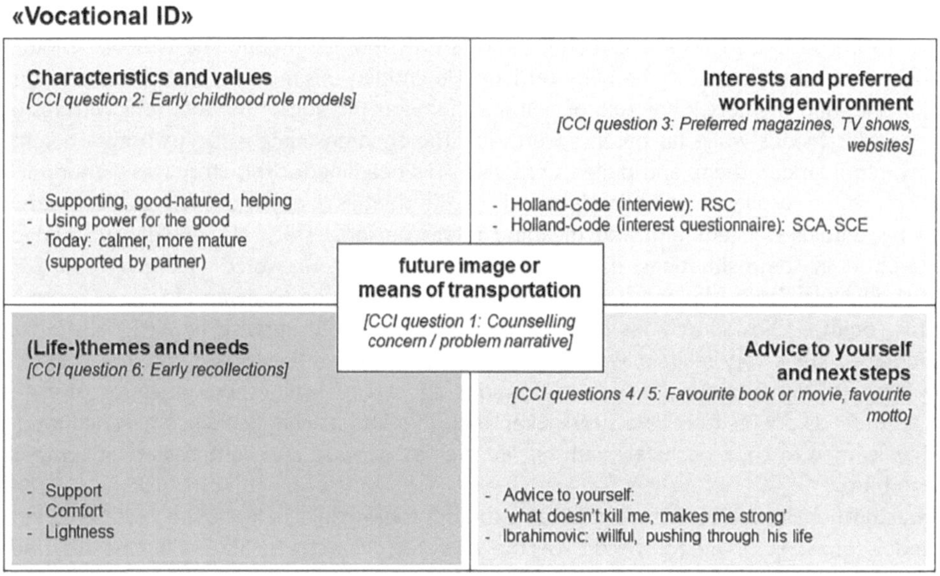

Figure 1. Vocational ID of Chris including attribution to the six questions of the CCI.

counsellors (and clients) with helpful insights. We will now introduce the practical applications of the Vocational ID by illustrating the case of Chris and further explicating the above-mentioned processes and theories. In line with our framework, we have divided the case study into the stages of establishing the ID and working with the ID.

The case of Chris: establishing the Vocational ID

Chris (name changed), a 39-year-old former professional athlete, was on his way to self-employment at the time of his consultation. Together with his partner and a colleague he was in the process of founding a company in the field of sports care (mental training, fitness, nutrition). For financial security, Chris was also looking for part-time employment. His counselling concerns (question 1) were related to taking positive steps in achieving his goal of self-employment as well as to learning more about himself.

The deconstruction of the contents of the CCI was conducted along the four areas in the Vocational ID (see Figure 1). We will subsequently present Chris' answers to the six CCI questions (construction phase). Chris reported the following three childhood memories (question 6), from which his specific life themes and unfulfilled needs could be drawn: In his first memory, Chris is about two years of age. He wakes up thirsty and calls for his father, who brings him water. His title for

Table 3. Vocational ID framework integrating Life Design counselling process, CCI, and PSI theory.

Vocational ID stages	Establishing the ID	Working with the ID
Life Design counselling phases (according to Career Construction Theory)	Construction, deconstruction, and reconstruction	Co-construction
Role of CCI	Information gathering and reconstruction of life portrait. Visualisation in Vocational ID.	Minor role
Role of PSI theory	Minor role	Facilitating deciding and doing by analysing the client's volitional control and self-growth processes.

this recollection was: "Help! I need something". The second situation he could remember was wanting to be pushed in a baby carriage. Although his mother thought he was old enough to walk, he was permitted to sit in the baby carriage. He entitled this memory with "I am too comfortable". In the third memory, Chris told of being at home at the age of three or four with his older cousin and his friends while his parents were out. The children made a ruckus until a neighbour came by, reprimanded them, and pulled Chris's ear. His headline for this story was "Whoop it up". From these three recollections, Chris identified the life themes *support*, *comfort* and *lightness* that hint at his unfulfilled needs and add meaning to his personal story. He would have hoped for more support in some situations, especially from his parents. He noted that giving support to others should play an important role in both his professional and private life. To overcome his need for comfort, Chris sometimes requires time pressure or an impulse by external motivators but, ultimately, he is very reliable, works accurately, and delivers results on time. As a balance to his professional commitment, he sees celebrations and a certain lightness (in terms of an easy-going attitude) as outlets to relieve stress. Even though a lot has changed since his childhood and Chris has learned to cope positively with his life themes, support and lightness are still important topics to him.

Characteristics and values that are applicable to Chris today could be identified from his childhood role models (question 2). One role model was the animated character He-Man, which he described as being tall, blond, muscular and good-natured. United with his sword and tiger, the figure transformed into a hero to fight against evil. Chris also helps and supports others and for him, high-performance sport could be seen as an area that gives him extra powers, similar to what the sword does to He-Man. He said that it was important to him to show his strengths, especially in his company or as a coach. Looking at Chris' second role model, a neighbour and later friend, one can identify an opposing development in the two personalities: Chris described the friend as a quiet person who had gradually opened up and was now a joker. Chris himself had become calmer over the years. His third role model was the Brazilian football player Zico. Chris especially admired Zico's gameplay as a central player and playmaker, and the way he could unfold his strengths in the team. In his own life, Chris could see himself as the central driving force in his company and realised his ability to always see the bigger picture. This is also important to him in his role as a coach.

For the question about favourite journals, TV shows or websites (question 3), which relates to interests and preferred working environment, Chris listed "GQ", "Men's Health", "Facebook", as well as several daily newspapers and sports shows. In the magazines, he is particularly interested in fashion, nutrition, health, trends, and sports. The daily newspaper provides him with short, current information. Sports shows are relevant to him in terms of his own athletic career as well as his occupational future in the field of mental coaching. According to Savickas (2015b), this CCI question also refers to Holland's (1997) RIASEC model. Chris and his career counsellor derived the Code RSC from Chris' answers to this question. Additionally, Chris completed the German version of the Oregon Vocational Interest Scales (ORVIS; Pozzebon, Visser, Ashton, Lee, & Goldberg, 2010).[4] Figure 1 shows that Chris' RIASEC code from the explicit interest inventory (SCA, SCE) differs from the rather implicit RIASEC code worked out with the CCI (RSC). This supports the goal of the ID, which is to portray both implicit and explicit aspects of the self. Discrepancies between these aspects can then be brought up based on the Vocational ID and be discussed with the client.

Finally, the answers to the two questions about favourite book or movie (question 4) and about favourite motto (question 5) relate to advice to oneself and possible next steps. Chris chose the biography of the football player Zlatan Ibrahimovic as his current favourite book. Chris characterised him as a strong-willed person who had to fight his way through, especially during his youth. He grew up in poor conditions but was always supported by his father. This illustrates parallels to Chris' life theme support. He would have wished for more support from his father, but also pushed himself and made his own athletic decisions, including some that went against the wishes of his parents. He was able to overcome difficult phases in life, for example sporting injuries, with the help of his life motto "what does not kill me, makes me strong". This motto underscores perseverance–highly important in performance sport–and an optimistic way of tackling challenges. Chris knows he will end up stronger after difficult situations. He will consistently be confronted with such situations during his self-employment, but he will be able to face them calmly.

To make the different elements of the CCI more real, tangible and visible to Chris, and to mark progression from the reconstruction into the co-construction phase, the results from the CCI process (and from other parts of the counselling process such as the interest inventory) were gathered in the Vocational ID together with Chris. By seeing at a glance his life themes and needs, individual characteristics and values, interests and preferred surroundings, as well as concrete next steps, Chris gained new insights and understanding into his past experiences, current situation, and possible future. In other words, he further developed his inner compass that can support him in making decisions and planning concrete actions. As the ID explicitly relates to both verbalised and visual aspects, it can help him switch more easily from left hemispheric to right hemispheric processes.

The case of Chris: working with the Vocational ID

In terms of the PSI theory, Chris' Vocational ID reflects the aspects of the integrated self (EM) that were made explicit during the CCI process. Additionally, the self-chosen future image or means of transportation itself serves as a holistic and visual representation of the EM. As a pictorial illustration, Chris chose a scooter as his appropriate means of transportation. By choosing a means of transportation instead of a future image he implicitly decided to focus on volition control. The choice of a future image would have focused more on reflecting the characteristics of the desired (vocational) future and therefore on identifying the underlying needs, motives, interests, or (life-) themes related to EM and self-growth. With the scooter, Chris connects and anchors the way of locomotion important and opportune for him in his current situation: flexible, individual, yet fast.

With regard to Chris' situation, we want to point out key elements of the Vocational ID that can contribute to (1) self-growth (second modulation assumption of the PSI theory) and (2) effective volitional control (first modulation assumption) within the co-construction phase.

(1) Self-growth (OR/EM, modulated by negative affect): Chris aims at being self-employed as a consultant within the sports domain. Although he had already established his goal before career counselling, he was able to review it for congruency with his integrated self (EM). It was only after self-confrontation with his life theme support, though, that his integrated self could fully serve in this review for self-congruence. The lack of support from Chris' parents was a painful memory, an undesired object within OR. By contemplating this memory together with his counsellor, Chris realised that despite this difficulty he had become a successful athlete and that he felt forgiveness for his parents. Thus, he could downregulate negative affect, gain access to EM, and complete his integrated self with his life theme support, which was no longer linked to pain. Altogether, his Vocational ID contains many aspects that support his professional goal (e.g. his newly integrated (life-) theme support, his personal characteristics supporting, good-natured, helping, as well as his social interest). To gain access to EM in the future, Chris has two strategies to downregulate negative affect: First, the teamwork with his partner and a colleague relieves him from stress, which is a form of downregulating negative affect. Second, his favourite motto in his Vocational ID (what doesn't kill me, makes me strong) gives him powerful additional orientation.

(2) Volitional control (IM/IBC, modulated by positive affect): In any large undertaking, such as Chris becoming self-employed, frustrations in the form of downregulated positive affect can arise because of severe obstacles hindering goal attainment. Chris reported that he prefers to operate more in a holistic, spontaneous mode than in an analytic mode. His life theme lightness confirms this self-assessment. Therefore, switching to IM and tolerating downregulated positive affect can be difficult for him. With the aid of his counsellor, he became aware of this difficulty. This insight prompted him to regulate his affect more consciously and to sustain IM's planning

mode as long as needed. His chosen picture of the scooter can also help him in this regard: If Chris wants to reach (on his scooter) his abstract "destination" of being a consultant in the sports domain, he needs to stop from time to time to study the map and find the best route. This image helps Chris counteract his tendency toward immediate action and switch to planning mode more easily. Additionally, his strong motto as well as the story of Ibrahimovic support his volition control. Thanks to the Vocational ID, he has picture, motto and the narrative of Ibrahimovic always readily and visually at hand. This helps him tolerate downregulated positive affect and regain positive affect to overcome potential upcoming obstacles.

During his career counselling sessions, Chris was thus able to plan things and set things in motion at the right time, including finishing the administrative work and coordinating the opening of his office rooms. His vision of being self-employed as a consultant within the sports domain is a concretion derived from his life themes, interests and resources summarised on his Vocational ID. This leads him to concrete, meaningful actions to make his vision a reality. After the counselling sessions, Chris stated that with the aid of the Vocational ID, he achieved his counselling concerns of taking concrete steps towards self-employment and of learning more about himself.

Conclusion

We introduced the Vocational ID as a facilitating tool for career counselling based on the Life Design perspective, especially the Career Construction Theory. We emphasised the integration of linguistic and visual aspects of the ID. While linguistic elements embrace the explicit, analytic, and left hemispheric processes accompanying career counselling, visual aspects such as the Vocational ID as a whole or the self-chosen image cover the rather implicit, holistic, and right hemispheric processes. Working with the Vocational ID allows switching from one perspective to the other and – most importantly – allows combining both processes within a single tool to support career counselling matters such as working on vocational identity, goal-setting (deciding), and goal-implementation (doing). The ID provides a framework that integrates cognitive and affective aspects relevant for career development, which always pertains to questions of transition and change. Transition and change can only successfully take place when clients possess or can establish an inner compass indicating in which direction to proceed and how to overcome upcoming obstacles.

The Life Design paradigm (applied through the six open questions of the CCI) represents an effective way to build and strengthen a career counselling client's compass that can then be visualised by compiling the Vocational ID. Savickas (2011a) states that in the co-construction phase, "clients must perform their new meaning" (p. 139) in making a decision based on the key findings of the counselling process (deciding). Furthermore, they should transform their choice into concrete actions for the next days, weeks, and months to come (doing). According to Savickas (2011a), clients' reasons for struggling in doing differ. Some encounter challenges because of negative emotions, such as anxiety, that accompany their phase of transition. For those clients, PSI theory represents a framework that enables interventions focused on client-centred self-growth by targeting the downregulation of negative affect and access to the integrated self (EM). Other clients struggle with "reality that thwarts easy action" (Savickas, 2011a, p. 140). Here, PSI theory rather emphasises interventions that rely on solution-focused volition control that is related to positive affect. The Vocational ID serves as a facilitator to visualise those particular characteristics of a career counselling client that are related to both self-growth and volitional control. This shows that the interplay of the CCI and PSI theory through the Vocational ID can cover a broad range of relevant career counselling topics.

The Vocational ID can also be adopted to other career counselling approaches such as questionnaire-oriented matching (Vocational Guidance), where the ID can be applied as an aggregation of the most important findings of the person-environment fitting process. We therefore also use the Vocational ID to embrace and highlight the findings of psychometric questionnaires. Characteristics of the personality, competencies, interests, values, and motives can be recorded in the corresponding sections of the Vocational ID (see Figure 1). Counsellors that work with their clients on developing (Career Education and Coaching) and defining core competencies can also transfer the relevant findings to the Vocational ID. Whereas the two top sections of the Vocational ID cover general aspects of matching, guiding, and self-actualisation, the bottom sections of the Vocational ID represent important facets of life designing such as crucial (life-) themes and advice to oneself on how to overcome obstacles (see Figure 1).

As process-oriented career counselling has much to do with exploration and concrete action, we also want to point to the uses of the Vocational ID when working with the Cognitive Information Processing (CIP) approach and the CASVE cycle (Communication, Analysis, Synthesis, Valuing, Execution), both proposed by Sampson Jr., Peterson, Lenz, and Reardon (1992), as well as with the Social Cognitive Career Theory (SCCT; Lent & Brown, 2013; Lent, Brown, & Hackett, 1994). Furthermore, we would like to mention the Career Flow approach introduced by Niles, Amundson, and Neault (2011), differentiating between certain stages of the counselling process: self-reflection, self-clarity, envisioning, decision-making, goal-setting, planning, implementing, and adapting. Career counsellors working with these approaches can use the Vocational ID in different stages of the counselling process, to retain the relevant aspects of their clients and their occupational knowledge as well as the crucial metacognitions that are related to decision-making, other forms of information processing, and goal-implementation.

In summary, the Vocational ID is a multifaceted and flexible tool that can be used not only when working with the CCI or the PSI theory, but with a multitude of career counselling approaches. In combining elements of analytic thinking and holistic feeling and making elements of the implicit self visible and tangible, it offers a way of bringing up important aspects during career counselling sessions that can help clients further develop and strengthen their inner compass and their professional goals. In our experience, clients also very much appreciate the fact that with the Vocational ID, they have a tangible and comprehensible tool at hand that they can look at and use anytime, even weeks, months, or years after their counselling sessions. This helps them keep important aspects of their self in mind for difficult professional situations and new challenges, even far in the future.

Notes

1. Very interestingly and congruent with our approach in combining PSI theory with Life Design, Kuhl (2018) suggests that motives should be measured qualitatively: "Motives develop from an extensive web of autobiographical episodes, i.e. from personal 'stories'. The high level of cognitive integration characteristic of motives is best attained by asking respondents to generate stories of their own" (p. 567). Even though the practical implications of the implicit and explicit motives for career counselling are considerable, we will not further elaborate on motives throughout the article because of space restrictions. For an in-depth view of the interplay of motives and affect modulation, see Alsleben and Kuhl (2011).
2. Kuhl emphasises the positive precondition of action-orientation compared to state-orientation as "state-oriented individuals report having uncontrollable ruminations following failure experiences" whereas "action-oriented individuals have no difficulty disengaging from (i.e. 'downregulating') unwanted thoughts and emotions even following aversive experiences" (2000b, p. 672).
3. see www.laufbahndiagnostik.ch/en/tools
4. The German version of the ORVIS has been translated at our institute.

Acknowledgments

We thank the following colleagues for their valuable contributions to this article: Ladina Schmidt of the IAP Institute of Applied Psychology of the ZHAW co-developed the Vocational ID together with the corresponding author. Sonja Schlaepfer, Noemi Blumer, and Ida Marie Mueller edited our case study, being students or interns at that time. We would also like to thank an anonymous reviewer who gave us insightful feedback on the Life Design section.

Disclosure statement

No potential conflict of interest was reported by the authors.

ORCID

Marc Schreiber http://orcid.org/0000-0001-6468-178X

References

Alsleben, P., & Kuhl, J. (2011). Touching a person's essence: Using implicit motives as personal resources in counseling. In W. M. Cox & E. Klinger (Eds.), *Handbook of motivational counseling: Goal-based approaches to assessment and intervention with addiction and other problems* (pp. 109–129). Wiley-Blackwell. doi:10.1002/9780470979952.ch5

Broonen, J.-P. (2015). Motivation and volition in vocational psychology: An action control perspective. In R. A. Young, J. F. Domene, & L. Valach (Eds.), *Counseling and action. Toward life-enhancing work, relationships, and identity* (pp. 69–89). New York, NY: Springer.

Holland, J. L. (1997). *Making vocational choices: A theory of vocational personalities and work environments* (3rd ed.). Odessa, FL: Psychological Assessment Resources.

Kazén, M., Kuhl, J., & Quirin, M. (2015). Personality interacts with implicit affect to predict performance in analytic versus holistic processing. *Journal of Personality, 83*(3), 251–261. doi:10.1111/jopy.12100

Kuhl, J. (2000a). A functional-design approach to motivation and self-regulation: The dynamics of personality systems and interactions. In M. Boekaerts, P. R. Pintrich, & M. Zeidner (Eds.), *Handbook of self-regulation* (pp. 111–169). San Diego: Academic Press. doi:10.1016/B978-012109890-2/50034-2

Kuhl, J. (2000b). The volitional basis of personality systems interaction theory: Applications in learning and treatment contexts. *International Journal of Educational Research, 33*(7–8), 665–703. doi:10.1016/S0883-0355(00)00045-8

Kuhl, J. (2001). *Motivation und Persönlichkeit*. Göttingen: Hogrefe.

Kuhl, J. (2018). Individual differences in self-regulation. In J. Heckhausen & H. Heckhausen (Eds.), *Motivation and action* (3rd ed., pp. 529–577). Cham: Springer. doi:10.1093/oxfordhb/9780199642342.013.034

Lent, R. W., & Brown, S. D. (2013). Social cognitive model of career self-management: Toward a unifying view of adaptive career behavior across the life span. *Journal of Counseling Psychology, 60*(4), 557–568. doi.org/10.1037/a0033446

Lent, R. W., Brown, S. D., & Hackett, G. (1994). Toward a unifying social cognitive theory of career and academic interest, choice, and performance. *Journal of Vocational Behavior, 45*(1), 79–122. doi.org/10.1006/jvbe.1994.1027

McAdams, D. P., & Olson, B. D. (2010). Personality development: Continuity and change over the life course. *Annual Review of Psychology, 61*, 517–542. doi:10.1146/annurev.psych.093008.100507

McGilchrist, I. (2009). *The master and his emissary: The divided brain and the making of the western world*. New Haven and London: Yale University Press.

Niles, S. G., Amundson, N. E., & Neault, R. A. (2011). *Career flow: A hope-centered approach to career development*. Boston, MA: Prentice Hall.

Pozzebon, J. A., Visser, B. A., Ashton, M. C., Lee, K., & Goldberg, L. R. (2010). Psychometric characteristics of a public-domain self-report measure of vocational interests: The oregon vocational interest scales. *Journal of Personality Assessment, 92* (2), 168–174. doi.org/10.1080/00223891.2010.516712

Quirin, M., Gruber, T., Kuhl, J., & Düsing, R. (2013). Is love right? Prefrontal resting brain asymmetry is related to the affiliation motive. *Frontiers in Human Neuroscience, 7*. doi:10.3389/fnhum.2013.00902

Quirin, M., Meyer, F., Heise, N., Kuhl, J., Küstermann, E., Strüber, D., & Cacioppo, J. T. (2013). Neural correlates of social motivation: An fMRI study on power versus affiliation. *International Journal of Psychophysiology, 88*(3), 289–295. doi:10.1016/j.ijpsycho.2012.07.003

Sampson Jr., J. P., Peterson, G. W., Lenz, J. G., & Reardon, R. C. (1992). A cognitive approach to career services: Translating concepts into practice. *The Career Development Quarterly, 41*(1), 67–74. doi.org/10.1002/j.2161-0045.1992.tb00360.x

Savickas, M. L. (1989). Career style assessment and counseling. In T. Sweeney (Ed.), *Adlerian counseling: A practical approach for a new decade* (3rd ed., pp. 289–329). Muncie, IN: Accelerated Development.

Savickas, M. L. (2011a). *Career counseling* (Vol. 74). Washington, DC: American Psychological Association.

Savickas, M. L. (2011b). Constructing careers: Actor, agent, and author. *Journal of Employment Counseling, 48*(4), 179–181.

Savickas, M. L. (2011c). New questions for vocational psychology: Premises, paradigms, and practices. *Journal of Career Assessment, 19*(3), 251–258. doi:10.1177/1069072710395532

Savickas, M. L. (2011d). The self in vocational psychology: Object, subject, and project. In P. J. Hartung & L. M. Subich (Eds.), *Developing self in work and career: Concepts, cases, and contexts* (S. 17–33). Washington, DC: American Psychological Association.

Savickas, M. L. (2012a). Life design: A paradigm for career intervention in the 21st century. *Journal of Counseling and Development, 90*(1), 13–19. doi:10.1111/j.1556-6676.2012.00002.x

Savickas, M. L. (2012b). The 2012 Leona Tyler Award address: Constructing careers - actors, agents, and authors. *The Counseling Psychologist, 41*, 648–662. doi:10.1177/0011000012468339

Savickas, M. L. (2013). Career construction theory and practice. In S. D. Brown & R. W. Lent (Eds.), *Career development and counseling. Putting theory and research to work* (2nd ed., pp. 147–183). Hoboken, NJ: John Wiley & Sons.

Savickas, M. L. (2015a). Career counseling paradigms guiding, developing and designing. In P. J. Hartung, M. L. Savickas, & W. B. Walsh (Eds.), *APA handbook of career intervention: Vol. 1. Foundations* (Vol. 1, pp. 129–143). Washington, DC: American Psychological Association. doi:10.1037/14438-000

Savickas, M. L. (2015b). *Life-design counseling manual*. Rootstown, OH. Retrieved from www.vocopher.com

Savickas, M. L., Nota, L., Rossier, J., Dauwalder, J.-P., Duarte, M. E., Guichard, J., … van Vianen, A. E. M. (2009). Life designing: A paradigm for career construction in the 21st century. *Journal of Vocational Behavior, 75*(3), 239–250. doi:10.1016/j.jvb.2009.04.004

Taylor, J. M., & Savickas, S. (2016). Narrative career counseling: My career story and pictorial narratives. *Journal of Vocational Behavior, 97*, 68–77. doi:10.1016/j.jvb.2016.07.010

Use of narratives and collage in the exploration of the self and the meaning of a career

Anne Chant

ABSTRACT
A methodological challenge during my doctoral research led me to use collage to reflect upon my own life and career. The insights it allowed me into the relationship between who we are and what we do led me to conclude that such methods can also illuminate these connections for clients of career counselling. In this paper I argue that such constructivist approaches allow the examination of that psycho-social space within which career is shaped and understood, allowing access to both the conscious and unconscious meaning made of a career and life story. I further argue that in times of increasing complexity such methods will be an important tool for career counsellors to meet the holistic needs of clients.

Introduction

Over the years that I have practiced as a career counsellor and taught and trained others, I have had a sense that despite numerous developments in career theory which embrace a social constructivist approach to career counselling and guidance, much of this thinking remains the preserve of the academy and is not widely evident in practice, despite research that supports its usefulness (Reid & West, 2018; Reid, Bimrose, & Brown, 2016; Taylor & Savickas, 2016). My own reflections on my life course suggested to me that my career and my need for greater clarity of identity were inextricably linked and had more to do with "who" I wanted to be than a matching of skills or qualities, or indeed my cultural context and expectations. This wondering about such relationships led me to explore the stories and careers of two other participants using loosely structured interviews and this formed the basis of my PhD thesis. The study was entitled, "An exploration of the relationship between personal and career identity in the stories of three women: a counter narrative for career development." However, I soon came upon a problem. The challenge was how to explore my own story with depth and authenticity. The solution was found at a conference (Biffi & Zuccoli, 2014) where I attended a workshop on the use of collage in research.

The epistemological basis of my research was auto/biographical (Bainbridge & West, 2012). My own biography and relationship with my participants connected me to their stories and the interpretation of them, but my story was also separate from theirs. The loosely structured interviews of my two participants were recorded, transcribed and then analysed thematically using the approach by Merrill and West (2009). To examine my own story, as I am not able to interview myself, I set time aside to create a collage in response to thinking reflexively on my life story and my career. The sense I made of this was then explored during an interview with my PhD supervisor; this was recorded, transcribed and analysed using the same thematic approach.

As will be discussed later in the paper, in each of our three stories a resolution of a pre-occupation (Savickas, 2011) was identified, both by my analytical interpretation and by my participants' reflections. In each, notions of identity and the clarification of identity were reflected in the choices made and the facets in each story. This has provided insights into the importance of context and a holistic, constructivist approach to career counselling. As a teacher of career counselling I am aware that, in the UK and possibly elsewhere, there is little time or expectation that such tools and approaches are taught during training (Reid & West, 2011). Part of the aim of this paper is to propose that greater emphasis is given to such approaches, to equip practitioners to respond appropriately in times of rapid change and insecurity. In this paper, I propose that such approaches and tools should include the use of narratives and creative methods such as collage making.

This paper will explore material that examines the relationship between who we are and what we do; that psycho-social space within which I assert career is shaped and understood (Bainbridge & West, 2012; Reid & West, 2016). Embracing a social constructivist perspective, it will examine the use of creative methods including narratives and collage making to access both the conscious and unconscious meaning made of a career and life story, and to reveal that thread that connects the micronarratives of a life and leads to the "active master[y] of what was passively suffered" (Savickas, 2011, p. 11). This search for and interpretation of meaning does not seek a factually truthful account of our stories, accurate in their telling, but a "truth seeking" narrative, that is, what memories and stories mean to the teller (Bruner, 1990).

It is this meaning making that the analysis of narratives and collage making can facilitate, and in so doing provide insights into the conscious or unconscious processes that guide decisions that can shape a life. Such methods offer a critique of the dominant models of professional practice in career counselling such as matching models, following a now well-established paradigm shift in career theory (Savickas, 2011) in response to the changing nature of work and of social structures (Bauman, 2000, 2005: Frosh, 1991), and an increased interest in contextualism in career counselling (Richardson, 2004). Developments in creative narrative methods such as Pictorial Narratives (Taylor & Savickas, 2016) and My Career Story workbooks (Barclay, 2019) suggest that inroads are being made into innovation in practice. However, it is my sense that less of this theoretical advancement and development of social constructivist approaches has been translated into practice than is needed. There remains I believe, work to be done to include such approaches in career counsellor training in the UK.

In this paper, I reflect upon the place of narratives and collage making in the exploration of that most creative process of all, the living of a life. I propose that such creative approaches to understanding of the self and autobiography could, and perhaps should, be added to the toolbox of career practitioners.

Literature review

Before moving to an explanation of the research and its analysis, what follows provides an outline of the literature that underpinned the work. The works of Jung (1938), Adler (1923), Frosh (1991) and, in particular, Savickas (2011) provide theoretical perspectives for understanding the relationship between personal identities and career. Each offered helpful insights into the participants' stories by providing an illumination of the processes at work in this shared psycho-social space between the micro and macro worlds. Adler (1923), congruent with his notions of Individual Psychology, has provided a forward-looking focus, towards an individual's goal and the achievement of the "self-ideal". Savickas (2011) highlighted the perspective this provides for career in the broadest sense. Jungian ideas on individuation and personas (Jung, 1938) also further the understanding of the complexities of identity construction. Frosh (1991) suggested that the nourishing of the self creates an "inner identity" (p. 183) which in a time of social fluctuation can offer some stability in a world of fractured or fluid boundaries, which Bauman has described as liquid modernity (2000). Frosh points out that many of the social and cultural structures within which identities could in the past have been securely constructed, have become less robust, more fractured and in places porous. He notes that the excitement and the possibilities of what, he calls, "the modern world" offers, can be both the motivator and the downfall of the individual. Moreover, he asserts that personal integrity (and therefore perhaps identity) can only survive "the monstrous aggression of the world" by "keep[ing] on keeping on" (p. 21). Such a world, where previously unchallenged structures and establishments are dismantled, can at the same time be liberating and entombing. Critical theory, feminist and secular discourses may provide individuals with alternative narratives, possibilities and identities but also shake the foundations of the selfhood that brought that individual to the point of questioning. Frosh questions how identities are to be established, re-established, constructed and reconstructed in such an unstable world. Savickas (2011) has also written about the process of deconstructing narratives and co-constructing new interpretations of them to examine new possible selves. Within such a context, it would not be surprising if many of us are engaged in a struggle with clarity of identity or selfhood. Whether that identity is one of ambiguity (the selfless daughter or the patriotic child that will be explored in this paper), careers practitioners need to pay attention to such currents of influence.

In this paper I explore why, far from being an odd and even frivolous activity to be asked to engage with, a creative tool such as collage for exploring the meaning of a person's career to them, and its possible trajectory, is an increasingly common tool in this career counsellor's practice. To place such an approach within a broader context of career, it is important to examine the possible meanings of career within an individual's life course. Definitions of career abound, as do the metaphors we use to try to capture its meaning (Inkson, 2004). However the philosopher Arendt (1958) in her exploration of Vita Activa, the psychologist Adler (1923) in his work on "Individual Psychology" and others (Weil, 1978; Wright-Mills, 1959) place career (or work) within the frame of those activities that are necessary to connect us with the rest of society; the shared or meso space between the personal (micro) and the social (macro) spheres wherein we construct our contribution to and identity within our world. For many, work may frame the process of earning a living and offers feedback to the individual as to the value that society, or market forces, give to their contribution by rewarding it accordingly. The focus of career guidance and counselling is often on the maximisation of an individual's achievements and to make informed choices towards a successful career. One definition of career guidance and counselling is an example of such an emphasis on access to and advancement within a labour market; "A range of activities designed to help individuals make educational, vocational or personal decisions and carry them out before and after they enter the labour market" (McClean & Wilson, 2009, p. 59). Notions of what might be meant by "success" are wrapped up with those of earning, status, personal fulfilment and agency, supported by policies that have at their heart principles of national economic benefits and competivity. For reasons of pragmatism and output, matching theories that encourage individuals to make choices based on their skills and aptitudes make fiscal and procedural sense.

However, if we examine this psycho-social space differently we may come to an alternative conclusion about the nature of career and how to support its construction. As a place that is vital to the development of social and cultural identity, it is where our self-confidence, agency and self-ideal (Adler, 1923) are housed. It is also the space in which effective careers work can take place. Meijers and Lengelle (2012) have defined Career Identity as "a dynamic multiplicity of personal (in contrast to social and cultural) positions or voices regarding work" (2012, p. 157). If career, and more particularly career identity, is constructed in a psycho-social space rather than in an objective, individualistic neoliberal one, then I argue that it is a mistake to separate personal constructs of work or career, from social or cultural contexts. That is not to promote deterministic ideas or those that may abandon hope in the face of socially constructed opportunities, or to exclude the impact of social structures on individual agency and decision making (Roberts, 2005), but rather to include in our gaze the socially constructed identities that could perpetuate them.

As Patton and McMahon (2006), Robinson, Moore, and Hooley (2018) and Arulmani (2018) have urged, the process of making career decisions and crafting our pathway in life is not simply a product of one or two theoretical processes such as matching skills and qualities or identifying personality traits. Contextual factors such as socioeconomic position and culturally held beliefs play a crucial role. Objective notions of matching are useful in helping to understand some aspects of this complex process, but relying so heavily if not exclusively upon them, risks ignoring these other aspects of an individual and their identity, alongside aspects such as gender, faith and ethical values. All these, Patton and McMahon (2006) argued, are at work in the construction of a career. It is therefore crucial that all these influences should be appropriate areas to be examined and illuminated and their contribution to the "who" and not only the "what" highlighted.

A client may not be aware of the spheres of influences s/he is subject to and so may present complex career decisions in a reductive and objective form; matching qualifications and interests to jobs and professions. And all the while in the broader context, practitioners notice and policy makers confirm (Social Mobility Commission, 2019) that social mobility is at best stagnant and at worst declining; that gender and social stereotypes are still not only prevalent, but also engrained in even our youngest children (Bobbitt-Zeher, 2011), and that young people from disadvantaged backgrounds still underperform in education and the labour market (Friedman & Laurison, 2019).

So far from being an indulgence, a creative approach to career conversations based on constructivist principles is a way of bringing the full range of influences and voices into the process of career counselling and involving them in the discussion. The systems theory approach (Patton & McMahon, 2006) highlights the wide range of influences that there are on career choices, and how these are "in the room" when guidance or counselling is taking place, and goes a long way to include sociological, psychological and contextual factors in such processes. Others also strive to describe the complex and often chaotic processes at work. Pryor and Bright's (2014) chaos theory, and Krumboltz, Foley, and Cotter's (2013) "planned happenstance", acknowledge the subjective nature of career and its understanding and meaning. Hodkinson and Sparkes's "careership" and "horizons for action" (1997) echo the sociological limitations around opportunities that Roberts (2005) described, but offer thoughts on how movement into new spaces can broaden horizons and provide access to hitherto unknown or "othered" opportunities. Although Hodkinson and Sparkes's approach is, like Roberts, largely sociological, it draws upon notions of cultural capital and/or "habitus" (Bourdieu & Passeron, 2000) and therefore suggests a process of changing or reconstruction of identity at work too. Bimrose et al. (2019) have concluded that within challenging professional contexts the re/construction of career identity for career practitioners is as important as to that of their clients. They also point out that Career Construction Theory (Savickas, 2013), while offering a useful tool in practice, is less well-integrated into practitioners' own professional development and that of their work with clients.

It is the work of Savickas (2011), building on Adlerian Individual Psychology principles (1923), that is most illuminating in the exploration of life narratives in my research, including the contribution of collage. Adler argued (1923) that a prototype adult or "self ideal" is constructed in the mind of a young child as the template of "who I am meant to be", or become. He proposed that choices throughout life are guided by this invisible (and often unknown) hand. He was well known for his analysis of sibling position in the family, claiming that these factors also have an impact upon the shape of the "self-ideal". Whether such prototypes are created by early experience, position in the family or other influences, it is the meaning that is made by the individual of such things that Savickas argues creates the "pre-occupation". This is then the thread that his Career Construction Theory (Savickas, 2011) seeks to illuminate. I suggest that the nature of the "self-ideal" or prototype is the identity that the individual seeks to emulate or become, guided by the thread of the pre-occupation.

Adler (1923) also asserted that all such resolutions are focussed on the regaining of power lost in early life. He was of course well known for his defining of the Inferiority Complex and claimed that this concept led to the need for the amelioration of a felt minus into an active plus. Savickas extended this notion by stating that "in career we actively master what has been passively suffered" (1997, p. 11).

Methodology, method and material gathering

My doctoral thesis began with my own story and evolved to include those of two others; those of my cousin "Sammy" and a friend "Sarah". Our stories are individual but my relationship with each of them meant that my biography was part of theirs and theirs of mine. Although not children or vulnerable adults, the telling of personal histories can and did evoke strong emotions and memories at times from my participants. The research followed my university's ethical procedures for qualitative research. Both participants consented for the transcripts (which they had read and approved) to be used in the research.

This is neither autobiographical nor biographical narrative research, it is an interplay between the two; auto/biographical narrative research. The "/" both connects and separates my story and those of my participants (Merrill & West, 2009). The stories of my participants, gathered through loosely structured interviews are rich in themselves, but their intersection with my own story is also part of the hermeneutic nature of the methodology. This is a methodology that has been used with groups from marginalised communities and embraces rather than trying to minimalise, the subjective relationship between the researcher and the researched (Merrill & West, 2009; West, 2016). It also acknowledges the micro story within a macro setting; the individual's story within the context of society and community. Such a methodology "form[s] part of an interpretive repertoire that, [for present purposes], draws on psychoanalysis, narrative psychology and critical theory" (Reid & West, 2018, p. 228)

Collage

To examine influences or pre-occupations, they must be identified. Loosely structured interviews served to illuminate the stories of my participants. However, including my story posed a problem, because as said previously, I could not interview myself. Furthermore, some of the threads of the story may remain unconscious and non-verbal techniques may be more helpful than verbal questioning and exploration. After experiencing the workshop on the use of collage I decided that this, rather than any other creative method would enable me to reflect on my own story and career. Collage has been defined as:

> an arts-based research approach to meaning-making through the juxtaposition of a variety of pictures, artefacts, natural objects, words, phrases, textiles, sounds, and stories. It is not meant to provide one-to-one transfer of information; rather, it strives to create metaphoric evocative texts through which readers, audiences, and patrons create their own meanings on a given research topic. (Given, 2008, p. 95)

Biffi, Gerber, Biondo, and Zuccoli (2019) have explored the wide range of research contexts where creative approaches can offer new insights, particularly within educational settings. McNiff (2011) concurs that art and creative arts such as fiction can provide windows into understanding where more established methods do not. Along with other creative methods, collage making is a constructivist approach, linking experiential knowing and understanding with the action of choosing and placing of pictures, images or other artefacts. As Butler-Kisber and Poldma explain, collage and other forms of arts-inquiry "are a means of making tacit ideas explicit and makes new insights possible for both the researcher and the research audience" (2010, p. 2)

Frosh (1991) has related the construction of the self to the construction or creation of a work of art. If, as he asserts, this is as much a process of creativity and construction as it is the clarification of preferences, then use of a creative tool or process may indeed be far from odd or indulgent. Thus there was a theoretical and established rationale for my use of collage but also a practical one. Other creative methods such as dance, musical composition and even mind mapping require other skills and qualities that I did not possess. Moreover, it is likely that this will be the case for many clients of career counselling.

As I engaged with the process of reflection on my own career narrative through collage, I was aware that there appeared to be three layers of meaning making at work. The first is the sourcing of the materials, their choosing of what to include and a quiet contemplation whilst doing so. In this case, I chose sources close to hand; magazines, photographs and newspapers, all reflected something of me and my context. The second layer is how and where I chose to place the selected items, on the page and in relation to each other. It is not, however, the physical elements of the work that are important (Biffi & Zuccoli, 2015) but the meaning of their choosing and placing. In order to examine such meaning I then participated in a loosely structured interview with my PhD supervisor, within which we explored the sense I made of the collage. As with the other participants' interviews, this was recorded and transcribed.

Interviews

Two loosely structured interviews with my participants, lasting one to two hours, were recorded and fully transcribed. The transcripts were shared with my participants to ensure that they agreed about what had been transcribed and to offer the opportunity to withdraw any parts that they subsequently wished to not to include. Follow-up interviews that began by reviewing the first transcripts, but then extended the narratives, were also recorded, transcribed and shared. The analysis of the material from my participants and my own collage and discussion is holistic and considers the ethnography, process and Gestalt of our interactions within the research conversation (Merrill & West, 2009). The meaning in these lives and careers is an interpretation and construction from themes derived from each story. The three stories present windows into very different lives and careers, but also into recognisable and shared struggles and resolutions. Although personal agency is at the heart of each story, this is set within and shaped by the family, history and communities in which each of us grew. From the particularities of each individual narrative it is possible to illuminate what might be universal processes (Reid & West, 2011) that can help to understand the stories of others.

Findings and analysis

'Sammy' is a mixed-race woman and the middle child of three girls, and one boy. She is also my cousin. Her arrival in the world was characterised by stories of the difficulty and pain of her birth and the subsequent depression suffered by her mother. She had been told what a hard time her mother had had, but also that she had had:

> ...but what must it have been like for me ... ... and no one's holding yer – no one's comforting yer ... and you're suddenly in this box ... I mean you're a person – you have sensations! ... ... it was a few days before I was actually held!

A conversation between her and her mother had provided some insight: "it sounded like she had post-natal depression'. Sammy takes the blame, repeating her mother's inability to care for her. The use of the word "couldn't" rather than "wouldn't" is notable:

> She couldn't feed me – I was bottle fed – and I don't think she could really – the sense I got was that she couldn't really ... the love I got I think was mostly from me grandma, because she was too traumatised [by me].

This story seems to have been re-told in the family. She had "nearly killed" her mother and the mother of her siblings. Formenti's thoughts (Formenti, 2011) on the impact of the stories about our births on our identity both within the family and beyond are significant in Sammy's story. She appears to have taken upon herself the role of the problem child, who nearly killed her mother and who caused so much disruption in family life in her early days. This role of the problem child is then illustrated throughout her life as she rebels and takes a very different path from that of her family. Nonetheless her narrative suggests that a tendency to consider others' feelings and predicaments continued through her life. She is clear that the empathy illustrated in engaging in the struggles and rights of others is something she has always been aware of having. It may be that the ability to understand the other from the other's perspective was an early skill:

> Maybe it came from being a youngish child and being – you know for a while – for 9 years being aware of stuff going on around me. Maybe it was about being responsible for my mother – my mother's state of mind or

> whatever. I don't know where it came from but ... I was very responsive like 'I'll do the washing up – keep my mum happy ... '

'Sammy's' story has other themes, some relating to her mixed-race identity, but the need to help others, take responsibility for solving others' problems was evident throughout her story. Moreover, the career choices she made also followed what could be described as this invisible camber in her pathway. She had been involved in many areas of work when we spoke: teaching adults, running refuges for ethnic minority victims of domestic violence, and she also trained and practiced as a psycho-therapist.

The second of my participants was "Sarah", a friend of mine with whom I had had many discussions about our shared ambiguities of place and identity. She is the daughter of an Israeli diplomat. She spent much of her childhood and early adulthood living in many different countries; always the outsider and always aware of her responsibility to be a good representative of Israel. However, on returning to Israel she realised that she was an outsider there too; not speaking Hebrew as the other young people did. National Service enabled her to re-establish her Israeli identity but the notion of being the outsider and "different" stayed with her and she was comfortable with that.

'Sarah' explained how this feeling had manifest itself in terms of her relationships with others and how she approached these 'others'. She explained that it was an approach based upon caution:

> i [I] waited for people to come to me, waited for to know where I was, I understood the layout, you know, understood the dynamics so that I could .... that were in front of me ... and I think I still do it to this very day ...

However, it was not because she blamed others for making her feel this way, on the contrary she rationalises this expected rejection:

> I suppose it's just rejection .... afraid that you're not going to be accepted, that people will think you're strange or different – but you are [smiles] ...

Her identity, although strong in its essence, was that of the "different" one, even within her own country and culture. Her goal was perhaps to embrace difference rather than eliminate it as others may have done. Something in her character, upbringing or experience led her to be determined to embed difference into what she did and who she is. Although interested in Law, Education and International relations, and perhaps expected to follow one of these paths, she had, at the time of the research, amalgamated these areas of skill and interest into a different presentation of them all. She was a quality officer in a Jewish college; teaching adults (not children), maintaining the rules of awarding bodies (not Laws) and working with students from all over the world who, like her, knew feelings of being the "outsider". She had her own explanation:

> ... we are made up of these sort of mosaics where you overlap one thing with someone and overlap something else with someone else.
>
> ... and I think ... I think that's how one's life is ... how one's identity is constructed ... so it's infinite ... there are infinite patterns er living now in a Surrey village will be again er of those encounters where, on the face of it, I don't have too much in common with, in terms of my biography here, although with time I suppose there is a kind of Surrey identity that builds up and it becomes part of me and I become part of this ... world here.

The themes from my collage and subsequent discussion were identified as identity, recognition, family background and damage. Speaking about the choice of some pictures of flowers; a bunch of mixed blooms and a single floret I suggested:

> ... there's also a self-justification that mixture's OK, mixture can be wonderful and um people might say things like 'it's much healthier to be mixed' and that sort of thing. So maybe it's a bit of self-justification but also that colours in this case and people in other cases, do quite well when they're with others of the same. Because it enhances you ... I mean one of these little flowers on its own would be ignored but there's a whole load together they look stunning and have an impact.

The theme of recognition of myself as a mixed-race woman in England was illustrated in my explanation of the significance of the picture of the "Blue-footed Booby" I had chosen in terms of discomfort but also recognition.

> It is about what I looked like and what that might mean to others and about acceptance … a creature put together [laughing] by two completely different species. And – er – that's how I've felt for a lot of my life - a bit um – um – rather than the beautiful bouquet – more the blue footed booby! [laughing] and although I wouldn't say it's a painful memory it's not a comfortable feeling. You're neither one thing nor another and … look a bit odd let's be honest … look like you don't really fit in.

I also talked about my family and background, and my awareness of the damage done when I embraced or turned away from the two ethnicities I recognised in my own identity. Explaining the inclusion of a photograph of my parents when they first met I said:

> … what really stood out was this sign behind my parents' head saying 'this footpath is dangerous'. And there's this coloured man with a white woman looking very confident, but I don't know if they realised how different that relationship was from others and what that might mean for them and for the rest of their family.

And of the inclusion of a picture of an eraser:

> … I think what I often do is when I'm with people from one part of my world to another, I erase the other side. … That can be damaging – like the blue end of the rubber because it can tear bits off. ..and that leaves you with various holes which um – which you have to fill in when you return to that world … so um … talking to family you … there are bits of life that aren't understood and then you fill them with other bits so um … It's the notion of not only building but having to get rid of things as well. A constant process of editing and self-editing of identity as you engage with relationships …

The discussion was then able to develop into one about the possible relationship between my perceived ambiguous identity, and my determination to find clarity within my career. The pre-occupation in life, revealed in the Gestalt of the collage seemed to be "a search for clarity of identity and purpose".

> Now in my story … that's been very clear in so many ways but in particular in terms of having two very different sorts of career.

> … so the mixtures and the conflicts and the searches for identity are all quite different types I think and um – I think this one [pointing to collage] just shows the influence on career a little more starkly

I noted in all these research stories what Savickas (2011) calls a "pre-occupation". This thread or common theme appeared to guide or influence decision making either consciously or unconsciously throughout each of our lives. A "preoccupation" in day-to-day language is that thought or idea that is hard to remove from our thinking. We become "preoccupied" with that idea or thought such that other activities or thoughts become difficult to engage with. A "pre-occupation" in the context of career is a "precursor" to notions of career and working life. Savickas (2011) brings these two meanings together when he refers to the Adlerian notion of the "self-ideal". In each of our stories the pre-occupation of "who" we are connected clearly with "what" we did and the choices that were made.

Discussion

Career in each of these three research narratives has been interpreted as a means of resolution and an integral part of their lives and stories. This is both my interpretation of the material and recognised, on reflection, by the other participants. Goffman's (1959) notion of the masks we wear in society could include those we "wear" in career; relating the "what" we do with the "who" we are and extending this sociological concept to a psychological one. Taking such a psycho-social perspective on career presents the careers profession with an opportunity to adapt to the broader needs of clients; placing career decisions within the broader landscape of a life course.

This context for careers work is not only very different to that of the early pioneers but it also continues to change rapidly. The post-modern world with few and porous boundaries and structures with which to frame our lives, provides little stability in which to understand ourselves in its context (Bauman, 2000; Frosh, 1991). As opportunities change and, we anticipate broaden, liberation is accompanied by insecurity, flexibility allows for diversity but also allows for less delineation between work and the rest of life. As work sustains us financially and also with regard to our identity (Noon & Blyton, 1997) then a flexible, fractured and less predictable world of work has an impact on both of these aspects of our lives. Work may be less of a point of reference and source of community and identity (Garsten, 2008), so where else might that sense of "who" come from?

In my research, I explored the notion of "mixture", of ethnicity, place and identity in my story and those of my participants. As the world of work and the world itself is more connected by migration and technology, this leads potentially to more "mixture" of race, culture, religion, identity and family shape. With an increase in mixture, complexity of identity and lives, an accompanying reduction in the stability of the homogeneous factors in a person's life may have an impact on clarity of identity and sense of selfhood or rootedness in the past. If careers practitioners are to support people in this context we need to be cognisant of these changes and understand the implications for the development of an individual's personal and career identity. Although there will always be a place for established and traditional activities and services in careers work, at relevant points of need, as a profession we need to be ready to respond to clients' needs as they evolve in response to changes in the world of work and in society more broadly. Developments in practice must, therefore, keep pace with theoretical paradigm shifts illustrated by developments in narrative career counselling and the Life Design approach (Nota & Rossier, 2015).

The use of narratives including non-verbal creative narrative such as collage were used in my research to explore lives and the meaning made of our careers. These methods helped me to understand the links between personal and career identity and their meaning. Thus, as Reid (2016) proposed, if such creative approaches as collage making can illuminate meaning in research, then they can also be used in practice. My own experience of using collage in my own practice bears this out.

But there is a place here for a critique of the movement toward social constructivist approaches. The first is a recognition that not all clients will feel comfortable with techniques that require them to reflect on their lives and their family and community in a personal way. Some may find such storytelling stressful and prefer a more objective approach. Practitioners must retain the full range of tools and approaches to meet the needs of individual clients.

Concerns expressed over neoliberal agendas (Hooley & Sultana, 2016; Irving, 2009) and their impact on careers work, include the focus on the subjective individual (and in this case a highly subjective process) and their construction of career. Some (Hooley & Sultana, 2016) argue that subjective approaches move careers work increasingly away from its responsibility for social justice and equality. A view that a subjective, narrative approach can pander to the individualistic "each person for themselves" resilience agenda has some justification. However, society is made of individuals, some are privileged and others marginalised and disadvantaged. Many are somewhere in-between or unaware of their position on such a continuum. Some may be privileged in some regards (a good education and supportive families for example) and marginalised and disadvantaged in others (racism or sexism). The counter narrative to individualisation I would argue is not in denying it, but embracing it as the construction of identity through a connection or re-connection with the biography of the person and their community, their family and their roots. This is not about restriction or "knowing your place". It does not ignore the realism of Roberts (2005) spotlight on how the structures of the labour market can restrict access to some opportunities, but rather it is about reconnecting who people are with what they do. This can be liberating rather than restricting as it allows people to regain some agency as they have increased awareness of the whole picture rather than an expectation to make career decisions in a cultural vacuum, ignoring subliminal but very significant drivers and motivations that creative methods such as collage and narratives can reveal. The very notion of choice is contestable as cultural and other stereotypes and expectations persist in the decision-making process. Therefore, a reconnection with the social and cultural contexts of individuals, identifying pre-occupations and threads of meaning in their stories may help careers work to re-inhabit its social justice responsibility. Making restrictions, challenges and structures of opportunity more transparent to the client themselves can provide valuable insights for the practitioner to ask different questions.

In essence, as many practitioners know, it is not the answers that matter, but the questions that are asked. Creative methods such as collage can ask different questions and in more insightful ways. My own reflections on the relationship between my career and identity were illuminated by the use of collage because, I suggest, it was a method that allowed a range of contextual aspects of a lived life to be seen in relation to each other and to life events and identity construction. The pre-occupation (Savickas, 2011) of the narrative was visible, not only verbalised so that its resolution through career could be brought into the centre of subsequent discussions. The use of collage in my own practice as well as in this research has reinforced my view that this can be a powerful tool for career counselling, where established approaches are limited in their effectivity and inadequate in their ability to meet the needs of the client. But in order for such approaches to be a regular feature of careers practice in the UK it must move from the fringes into the mainstream. This requires the inclusion of this and other constructivist approaches in the professional education and training of practitioners in my own and other centres and HEIs.

Acknowledgement

I would like to acknowledge the help and support of Emeritus Professor Hazel Reid in the preparation of this article. Discussions about its content and structure were invaluable and I would like to offer her my sincere thanks.

Disclosure statement

No potential conflict of interest was reported by the author.

References

Adler, A. (1923). *Individual psychology*. London: Routledge and Kegan Paul.

Arendt, H. (1958). *The human condition*. Chicago: University of Chicago Press.

Arulmani, G. (2018). The cultural preparedness model of aspiration and engagement: Understanding the dynamics of integration. *British Journal of Guidance & Counselling*. doi:10.1080/03069885.2018.1513284

Bainbridge, A., & West, L. (2012). *Psychoanalysis and education: Minding a gap*. London: Karnac Books.

Barclay, S. R. (2019). Creative use of career construction interview. *The Career Development Quarterly*, *67*(2), doi:10.1002/cdq.12176

Bauman, Z. (2000). *Liquid modernity*. Cambridge: Polity Press.

Bauman, Z. (2005). 'Education in liquid modernity. *Review of Education, Pedagogy, and Cultural Studies*, *27*(4), 303–317. doi:10.1080/10714410500338873

Biffi, E., Gerber, N., Biondo, J., & Zuccoli, F. (2019). 'Art-based methods. An approach to educational research'. In A. Luigini (Ed.), *Proceedings of the 1st international and interdisciplinary conference on digital environments for education, arts and heritage* (pp. 249–252). Joensuu: Springer Verlag.

Biffi, E., & Zuccoli, F. (2014). *'Using collage as a research method'. Workshop at doctoral studies in research methodologies: Erasmus intensive programme*. Joensuu: University of Eastern Finland.

Biffi, E., & Zuccoli, F. (2015). *"It is not the glue that makes the collage" (Max Ernst): Training in educational research as an artistic process* Joensuu: (Unpublished).

Bimrose, J., Brown, A., Mulvey, R., Kieslinger, B., Fabian, C. M., Schaefer, T., ... Dewanti, T. (2019). Transforming identities and co-constructing careers of career counselors. *Journal of Vocational Behavior, 111*, 7–23.
Bobbitt-Zeher, D. (2011). Gender discrimination at work: Connecting gender stereotypes, institutional policies, and gender composition of workplace. *Gender & Society, 25*(6), 764–786.
Bourdieu, P., & Passeron, J. (2000). *Reproduction in education, society and culture*. London: Sage.
Bruner, J. (1990). *Acts of meaning*. Cambridge, MA: Harvard University Press.
Formenti, L. (2011). *How do we honor the systemic nature of the subject? Ethical, aesthetic and epistemological presuppositions in the making of auto/biography*. Paper given at ESREA – European Society for Research on the Education of Adults, 'Life History and Biographical Research Network' conference entitled 'Human agency and biographical transformations: adult education and life paths', March 3–6.
Friedman, S., & Laurison, D. (2019). *The class ceiling: Why it pays to be privileged*. Bristol: Policy Press.
Frosh, S. (1991). *Identity crisis: Modernity, psychoanalysis and the self*. London: Palgrave MacMillan Press.
Garsten, C. (2008). *Workplace Vagabonds*. London: Palgrave Macmillan.
Given, L. M. (ed.). (2008). *The Sage encyclopedia of qualitative research methods*. London: Sage.
Goffman, E. (1959). *The presentation of self in everyday life*. London: Penguin.
Hodkinson, P., & Sparkes, A. C. (1997). Careership: A sociological theory of career decision making. *British Journal of Sociology of Education, 18*(1), 29–44.
Hooley, T., & Sultana, R. (2016). Career guidance for social justice. *Journal of the National Institute for Career Education and Counselling, 36*, 2–11.
Inkson, K. (2004). Images of career: Nine key metaphors. *Journal of Vocational Behavior, 65*, 96–111.
Irving, B. (2009). *Careering down the wrong path: (Re)positioning career education as a socially just practice*. Paper presented at CDANZ Career Research Symposium, Otago.
Jung, C. G. (1938). *Psychology and religion*. New Haven: Yale University Press.
Krumboltz, J. D., Foley, P. F., & Cotter, E. W. (2013). Applying the happenstance learning theory to involuntary career transitions. *The Career Development Quarterly, 61*(1), 15–26.
McClean, R., & Wilson, D. (2009). *International handbook of education for the changing world of work: Bridging academic and vocational learning*. Dordrecht: Springer.
McNiff, S. (2011). Artistic expressions as primary modes of inquiry. *British Journal of Guidance & Counselling*, l(5), 385–396.
Meijers, F., & Lengelle, R. (2012). Narratives at work: The development of career identity. *British Journal of Guidance & Counselling, 40*(2), 157–176.
Merrill, B., & West, L. (2009). *Using biographical methods in social research*. London: Sage.
Noon, M., & Blyton, P. (1997). *The realities of work*. Basingstoke: Macmillan.
Nota, L., & Rossier, J. (eds.). (2015). *Handbook of life design; from practice to theory and from theory to practice*. Gottingen: Hogrefe Publishing.
Patton, W., & McMahon, M. (2006). The systems theory framework of career development and counseling: Connecting theory and practice. *International Journal for the Advancement of Counselling, 28*(2), 153–116.
Pryor, R. G. L., & Bright, J. E. H. (2014). The chaos theory of careers (CTC): Ten years on and only just begun. *Australian Journal of Career Development, 23*(1), 4–12.
Reid, H. (2016). *Introduction to career counselling and coaching*. London: Sage.
Reid, H., Bimrose, J., & Brown, A. (2016). Prompting reflection and learning in career construction counseling. *Journal of Vocational Behavior, 97*(1), 51–59. Retrieved from: http://search.ebscohost.com/login.aspx?direct=true&db=eoah&AN=40502405&site=pfi-live
Reid, H., & West, L. (2011). "Telling tales": Using narrative in career guidance. *Journal of Vocational Behavior, 78*, 174–183.
Reid, H., & West, L. (2016). Negotiating professional and personal biographies in a liquid world: Creating space for reflexive innovation in career counselling. *British Journal of Guidance & Counselling*. doi:10.1080/03069885.2016.1145014
Reid, H., & West, L. (2018). Connecting big and intimate worlds: Using an auto/biographical research imagination in career guidance. In T. Hooley, R. G. Sultana, & R. Thomsen (Eds.), *Career guidance for social justice; contesting neoliberalism. 1. Context, theory and research*. Abingdon: Routledge.
Richardson, M. S. (2004). The emergence of new intentions in subjective experience: A social/personal construction and relational understanding. *Journal of Vocational Behaviour, 64*(3), 285–498.
Roberts, K. (2005). 'Social Class, opportunity structures and career guidance. In B. Irving & B. Malik (Eds.), *Critical reflections of career education and guidance: Promoting social justice within a global economy* (pp. 130–142). London: Routledge Falmer.
Robinson, D., Moore, N. and Hooley, T. (2018) Ensuring an independent future for young people with special educational needs and disabilities (SEND): A critical examination of the impact of education, health and care plans in England. *British Journal of Guidance & Counselling, 46*(4), 479–491. doi:10.1080/03069885.2017.1413706
Savickas, M. L. (1997). Career adaptability: An integrative construct for life-span, life-space theory. *Career Development Quarterly, 45*, 247–259. doi:10.1002/j.2161-0045.1997.tb00469.x
Savickas, M. L. (2011). *Career counselling*. Washington, DC: American Psychological Association.

Savickas, M. L. (2013). Career construction theory and practice. In R. W. Lent & S. D. Brown (Eds.), *Career development and counseling: Putting theory and research to work* (2nd ed.), 147–183. Hoboken: John Wiley & Sons.

Social Mobility Commission. (2019). *State of the Nation 2018-19: Social mobility in Great Britain*. London: Her Majesty's Stationary Office.

Taylor, J. M., & Savickas, S. (2016). Narrative career counseling: My career story and pictorial narratives. *Journal of Vocational Behavior, 97*(1), 68–77. Retrieved from http://search.ebscohost.com/login.aspx?direct=true&db=eoah&AN=40502402&site=pfi-live

Weil, S. (1978) *Lectures on Philosophy*. Cambridge: Cambridge University.

West, L. (2016). *Distress in the city; racism, fundamentalism and a democratic education*. London: UCL Press.

Wright-Mills, C. (1959) *Sociological imagination*. Hardmondsworth: Penguin.

Bridging cultural divides with the power of poetry: an educator's reflection

Caylee Kreller

ABSTRACT
In this article I discuss the ways in which writing poetry and reflecting on its meanings may be a valuable tool for promoting an educator's reflexivity surrounding issues of reconciliation. As Canada embarks on the work of healing the difficulties its colonial past has caused its original inhabitants (i.e. Indigenous peoples), educators must explore ways in which they can contribute to a more socially just, democratic, and healthy society. By utilising the theoretical framework of Dialogical Self Theory (DST) to describe and explore identity and the writing of poetry as an exploration of self, it becomes possible for myself, as an educator, to unearth my own biases and begin to create safe spaces for identity exploration, learning, and healing.

Introduction

Poems suggest; they move us towards a sense of completion. They also leave room for open-ended exploration and the reader's own interpretation.
—Reinekke Lengelle, Blossom & Balsam

As our schools become more diverse, creating safe spaces where students can explore cultural identities and relationships to one another is essential. According to Rehm and Alison (2006), educators find themselves having to navigate the dynamics of an increasingly culturally diverse student body (pp. 260–275). However, the subjective experience of educators around their own cultural identities may limit their ability to create inclusive classrooms where conversations about histories, identities, and diversity can occur. Therefore, pedagogical tools that enable relationships that foster a space where students and educators alike can gain an awareness of their own prejudices and share in dialogue is critical to creating welcoming, open and equitable classrooms. In this article, I propose that poetic forms of creative writing can serve as a way to make professional reflexivity possible (Bolton, 2010); other authors have suggested that such creative reflection through writing can contribute to cultural healing in educational contexts (see, for instance, Lengelle, Jardine, & Bonnar, 2018).

I contend that writing poetry in particular can initiate and support the development of self-awareness and professionalism. By exploring *Dialogical Self Theory* (DST)[1] as a foundation for reflection on my own personal poetry, I seek to move myself towards openness and understanding. Poetry can stimulate profound self-understanding and invite us to re-examine our unquestioned prejudices, which can improve our relationships with others (Lengelle, 2008). This, along with self-care and the ability to see the self as "other", helps one to develop empathy that can create a cultural *Umwending* (Meijers & Hermans, 2018, p. 66).[2] According to Furman (2005), writing poetry helps students develop empathy, which "is a requisite feature in the possession of social consciousness" (p. 103).

Building a social consciousness based on individual self-awareness and relationship to the "other" is what this process of writing and reflecting upon my poetry hopes to achieve. Moreover, this article aims to show how writing poetry may therefore be an effective medium for change within myself, and in future, the classroom.

In order to demonstrate how writing poetry can be a key to unlock the self, I will speak of my own experiences as a female of white European ancestry working with Indigenous students in Canada. In the current Canadian context, Indigenous cultural groups are raising their voices to question and oppose assimilation, and the process of decolonisation is necessary to move towards healing and reconciliation. Their activities raise awareness of the effects and the reality of colonisation. Being a part of the Canadian community means I need to support the reclaiming of cultural identities in order to break down barriers caused by Eurocentric hegemony. To contribute to this process, the Indigenisation of my work of self-exploration by embracing the traditional practices of orality is useful. Stories must be told in order to promote healing, and writing/saying poetry is one way I can face my own internalised story in relationship to the "other".

Canada is in the midst of a Truth and Reconciliation movement,[3] where there is hope for a future founded on the principles and practices of equality. To move towards actual equality, seeking out and identifying biases, judgements, and misconceptions as an educator is integral to designing and implementing fair and just teaching practices. In order to do this, I am looking to investigate the following two questions: (1) "How do I create a space of respect for various Indigenous cultures when my internalised belief system has been largely inherited from Eurocentric and colonial foundations?" and (2) "How might the practice of writing poetry for personal development act as a bridge to help me examine and undo the effects of those foundations and make me a better educator?" My approach to these questions is inspired by current research that examines the use of writing for personal development to unearth internalised beliefs that might stand in the way of cultural healing and connection (e.g. Lengelle et al., 2018).

Exploring how poetry can cultivate an internal dialogue regarding misconceptions of Indigenous cultures, and simultaneously become the catalyst for overcoming prejudices and developing meaningful relationships, will hopefully contribute to an in-depth reflection that may be of use to other educators and students. Poetry as an exploratory medium may instil and enhance a sense of recognition of identity in its various forms; as Jardine explains in Lengelle et al. (2018),

> Writing can provide the means through which we detach ourselves from outmoded identities; we write, we read it over, and we also become an observer (i.e. in DST terms, we develop meta-positions) with the ability to see the bigger picture. (p. 87)

Emotion, feelings, and phenomena that are a source of inner conflict or confusion can be explored, and in some cases resolved, by reflecting on what is revealed when one writes poetry. By becoming an observer of how we shape our own identities and those of others, we can move towards greater awareness, understanding, and empathy.

Poetry, self-reflection, and the dialogical self

As Giuseppina Marsico has explained, "education is the way to free one's self from the oppression of rigid forms of thinking and narrow-minded definitions of the self and other" (as cited in Meijers & Hermans, 2018, p. viii). Meijers and Hermans (2018) confirm this idea by explaining that learning for personal development should be the basis upon which students are taught, rather than focusing on rote memory practices (p. 3). These scholars argue that there should be "a dialogue between teachers, between students and between teachers and students" (p. 6). The dialogue they espouse focuses not only on seeking consensus, but also on welcoming conflict. Creating "practice-relevant learning environments" fosters innovation, collaboration, and understanding – and, as Meijers and Hermans go on to explain, "recent research shows that educational innovation is only possible on the basis of collective learning where teachers gradually develop new practices and a new sense of identity" (p. 6). In order to create a new identity, the individual needs not only to converse with the 'other', but also with the self (p. 6). Moreover, social and emotional learning, as Dymnicki, Sambolt, and Kidron (2013) state, "is the process through which [individuals] effectively apply the knowledge, attitudes, and skills necessary to understand and manage emotions, set and achieve positive goals, feel and show empathy for others, establish and maintain relationships and make responsible choices" (p. 2). Poetry is therefore a suitable pedagogical tool for the development of such qualities in relation to professional identities; poetry makes use of metaphor, which helps an individual make new meanings, and it explicitly makes room for exploration of emotion in a positive and meaningful way. It is an artistic medium that enables individuals to explore facets of the self that they might not otherwise be interested in sharing or that they are not aware of.

Dialogical Self Theory (DST) helps us make sense of how poetry leads to self-awareness and reflection, and promotes cultural healing and connection. Meijers and Hermans (2018) state that DST "weaves two notions, self and dialogue, together in order to create a bridge between the individual and society" (p. 7). Instead of looking at "you" and "I" as separate entities, there is a shift towards focusing on how "I" as an individual can enact change on society by having an awareness and understanding of the relationships and dialogue within myself (p. 7) and create a place were the focus is on *we*. DST is based in part on Mikhail Bakhtin's analysis of the works of Feodor Dostoevsky, which often feature multiple narrators; the self is a "dialogical narrator" that expresses thoughts in a form of internal language and "dialogical relations spontaneously occur between this utterance and the utterance of imaginal others" (as cited in Hermans, Kempen, & van Loon, 1992, p. 27). Meijers and Hermans (2018) add to this explanation: "In the most succinct form, the dialogical self can be defined as a dynamic multiplicity of I-positions in the society of the mind" (p. 7). What is meant by this statement is that within my mind, there are various "I-positions" from which I can reflect on my understanding of the world and my experiences; each I-position within this multiplicity can converse with other I-positions to build relationships between them (p. 8). This multiplicity of voices or "society of mind" becomes one voice in the arena of reality (p. 8): for example, "if I am having an imagined conversation with another, they are in my mind, but still external to the self, or in other words, the I-position of the self" (p. 7). Meijers and Hermans go on to explain, "An *I*-position as a spatial-relational act exists in the context of the positions of other people. … [P]ositioning is *placing* oneself vis-à-vis with somebody else and, at the same time, toward oneself in the metaphorical space of the self" (p. 8). Through this relational act I am opening myself not only to the other, but also to myself, and to the other in myself.

What this plurality of I-positions creates is a different conceptual understanding of the self and how it interacts: rather than seeing one's self as a singular, unified entity, we can imagine the self as though in a house of dissimilar mirrors, with each I-position of the self reflected differently and individually, while also being able to form coalitions. Poetry allows me to enter this house and dialogue with parts of the self that may not have a voice otherwise. This unearthing of the myriad voices or I-positions of the self allows the self to reflect on what is, not just on what might be, and vice versa. My multiplicity of selves can dialogue with each other and work to create a better understanding of each perspective of self that creates a sense of a narrated whole (i.e. the story of identity). In this way, poetry can become a catalyst for a greater awareness of judgements, biases, and beliefs that may be held so deeply that they rarely see the light of day. Only by shedding light on these deeply buried parts of self can we truly see what is operating behind the scenes – what may be causing behaviour we might not otherwise be able to understand.

In addition, Meijers and Hermans (2018) have explained that there are various levels of consciousness from which I can view my place in the world; I can act upon the world with my consciousness fully engaged in the present moment, or I can view it from a meta-position that allows me to reflect on my practice (p. 9). I can even go one level higher to think about how I want to change my practice in the future (p. 9). By writing poetry, I am engaged in a conscious act, but I can begin to view that poetry from a meta-perspective in order to unearth hidden biases and judgements. From this awareness, I can create open spaces where honest and reflective dialogue may take place. My beliefs require self-reflective inquiry in order for me to begin addressing any internal confusion or lack of knowledge.

Writing the self

As explored in Lengelle et al. (2018), the process of "writing the self" uses creative, expressive and reflective forms of writing to take individuals through the "process of going from a first (i.e. destructive, distressing, victim–laden) to second (i.e. life-giving) story" (p. 85). This process uses creative writing exercises; those participating in the process "progress … through the cognitive steps of sensing, shifting, focusing, and understanding" (Lengelle et al., 2018, p. 85). In order to move from a first story into a second story, people must embark on the work of sensing and shifting their first story in order to transform this first narrative and create a new second story (Lengelle, 2014, p. 26). This "re-storying" of identity in this way can free individuals from, as DST terms it, an "I-prison" to new "I-positions" (Lengelle et al., 2018, p. 82). These meta-narratives are observed and deconstructed first and second stories, and bring about space where holistic and interrogative "third position" narratives can be created and revealed (Lengelle et al., 2018). Poetry can be used to create a safe space where I as an educator, and perhaps also my students, can explore the multiplicity of I-positions through writing and dialogue, moving towards reflexivity and an increased awareness of self. Working through the exercise of creating a series of poems with a specific focus and then reflecting and identifying relationships within the poems might also culminate in coming to recognise a "second story" – an uplifting revisionist story of who I am – that is felt; it is the result of both cognitive and affective reflection through writing, which can lead to the further development of my own identity (Lengelle, 2014, p. 26).

Lengelle's scholarly articles (2003, 2008, 2014) and Lengelle et al. (2018) on the subject of "writing the self" serve as both the foundation and inspiration for the processes documented throughout this paper; therefore, I would like to begin this personal inquiry with a passage from her work:

> [Reflective] writing is in principle non-fiction and requires the questioning and de-construction of existing identifications that might stand in the way of one's own agency.
>
> … [R]eflexive writing, an extension of reflective writing[,] involves 'doubling the self'
>
> … and working directly with the self as multi-voiced, so that we are both 'inside' and 'outside' ourselves simultaneously while also 'retaining a grounding in our familiar sense of self. … In short, reflective writing allows us to watch the many (inner and outer) characters on the stage of our lives, while reflexive writing lets us get on the stage and try on the various selves'. (Lengelle, Meijers, Poell, & Post, 2014, p. 76)

Writing the self in both reflective and reflexive ways allows me to explore my identity in relation to others and the world. Writing "proprioceptively", for instance, can, as its creators Metcalf and Simon (2002) explain, enable the writer to explore the thoughts that arise and to ask the deepening and broadening proprioceptive question, "What do I mean by _____?" and later also additional questions, one of which is, "What thoughts were heard but not written?" (pp. 34–39). By reflecting on assumptions that are often only half conscious, I can begin to see what may be driving my teaching behaviours and attitudes. In this way I can use my poetry as an outlet to bring about real-world positive change in myself and then in my actions in the world. This exploration and self-awareness will help me move beyond misconceptions or preconceived notions of the world that may inhibit me as a professional. I have an obligation to unearth parts of myself that are limiting, but also to celebrate when openness and dialogue are achieved.

Poetry as self-reflection: a personal exploration

Bridging the gap between differences in cultural ways of knowing is a lofty goal, but one that educators should strive for in order to create cohesive and respectful classrooms. As Lengelle et al. (2018) have contended, being able to unearth the hidden stories and identifications we have about race and "the other" is essential to making an impact in the context of reconciliation: the stories we are able to reconcile within ourselves make reconciliation with others more likely (Lengelle et al., 2018, p. 88). When I started developing this project of writing self-reflective poetry, I imagined using it with my students, but realised I needed to do the work myself; the process of "writing the self" is not something one can teach without personal experience. So, I first sought to explore and undo some of my own Eurocentric, colonial-influenced thinking. My trepidation about this project is something I cannot fully convey in words. And, as Bolton (2010) posited,

> Self-protectiveness against exploring unknown aspects of oneself arises from fear of unpalatable selves. . . . [A]n examination of our taken for granted psychological and social structures does not, however, let [one's] ungovernable demons [out], though the uncertainty it occasions can be uncomfortable. (p. 73)

In other words, Bolton recognises that it can be unnerving to cast a light on one's thinking and to note that one is expressing ideas or biases that may disadvantage and discriminate against others. However, it is only in exploring the uncomfortable parts of my psychological and social constructs that I can begin to understand the multiplicity of selves that is a part of my psyche, and the motivations, fears, and desires that guide my actions. As Lengelle et al. (2018) have explained, "it is naïve to think that cultural competencies can be learned in [a] reproductive learning process where information is provided about difference and diversity and discussions do not unearth unconscious identifications" (p. 82). I will illustrate now how poetry is a place where these unconscious or conscious identifications can be brought to the forefront of awareness in order to inspire reflective and reflexive personal work. The first poem is an invitation to dare to open the door to this potentially uncomfortable realm.

–Haiku

> Fearing what is here
> Previously unwritten
> Words now on the page

The first poem is a Haiku, a short yet structured form of three-line poetry developed in Japan. The form of Haiku is meant to express mood; the simplicity of the words and structure convey tone or feeling to the reader rather than focusing on devices such as simile and metaphor (Higginson, 1985, pp. 2–3). Although I wrote many of the poems for this project in free verse, I specifically included Haiku – a poetic form that may easily be practiced orally – since this work focuses broadly on students from cultures where oral traditions play a prominent role. When using Haiku to muster the creative spirit, I wanted to make my lines short and simple, while embedding imagery into my poems. As Bolton, Field, and Thompson (2006) contended, "Haiku encourages a dwelling in the now" (p. 127). Although Haiku is best known for a focus on nature, I bent this rule to focus on the *nature of the self* in order to express how I feel here and now, in this moment.

Beginning the process of introspective creative writing, by writing this Haiku, I can see that right now, in this place, there is fear of what others think of me. I have come to the knowledge that fear is the biggest barrier to overcoming biases, judgement and misconceptions; it is not fear of the other, rather, it is the fear of how I will be perceived by the other in my attempts to bridge cultural divides; to be seen as a fake and fraud, or even more so, seen as a perpetrator of institutionalised power structures. This inner conflict is not easily encountered in a society where soundbites and ideas of what is or is not politically correct can derail one's own professional track and future by simply saying something the wrong way. As a Caucasian female in a position of power within the classroom – how could I possibly understand the hurt others have faced – there is fear of being inept, culturally insensitive, and even so far as being perceived a racist. By delving into an issue that is generally uncomfortable for most, silencing the ego that detests embarrassment or shame and wants to consider self as most important, and calming the inner child that wants to run and hide, the apparent conflict inherent in my psyche is enough to walk away. But by saying "I fear", in verse, I have given these words the opportunity to be observed, contemplated, and re-worked.

I could easily have given in to the powerful voice of my fear and stayed locked in a prison of my own making. However, confronting my fear of expressing my personal biases or judgements is what "writing the self" sets out to achieve (Lengelle, 2003). I see now that I desire to be knowledgeable in my role. I want to be able to answer difficult questions and, the selfish part of me would like to be seen as someone who has it all together. But I also see that it is this fear of unbecoming that motivates me to learn and grow. I am also motivated by giving others the tools to foster success as I have, but on their own terms. And, I desire to make a positive and lasting impact by creating spaces that are culturally diverse and inclusive. I can only bridge the cultural divide by moving forward into the unknown and facing fears with the knowledge that my heart and intentions are good. And as educators, don't we have an obligation to confront these issues – to not be afraid of failure – and foster dialogue in order to move forward? By creating a space for what was unsaid to now be "left on the page", I can see that fear is a barrier to growing as a professional.

To turn now to the second poem written, for educators, it can be a daunting task to navigate through the raging waters of cultural diversity especially in light of effects of colonisation. There is a path forward, but not knowing how to access the path to reconciliation is difficult. This is how I felt when I wrote this second poem, but as I was writing I noticed that this poem follows no structure and is written in free verse. I began to feel a sense of freedom. As Bolton et al. (2006) stated, "The tension between freedom and control, spontaneity and measured reflection is inherent in all writing practice. Usually, in a therapeutic setting, spontaneity is prioritised" (p. 125). I encouraged myself to freely explore these contentious issues. I wanted to write a free verse poem about my ideal version of reality juxtaposed against what I have learned about the cultural realities of others. Although, I am afraid of judgement and especially afraid of pursuing this work despite having no direct relationship to communities of which my Indigenous students are a part, I have a responsibility to move through the fear toward the uncomfortable and look for commonalities from which a dialogue with myself and others can begin.

–Leaf

Two sides of leaf
One under the sun beautifully brown in colour
The other side, white as snow
They would not be without the other.
Yet both of the same leaf,
Parts intertwined

A force as strong as the wind could not break them apart.

Why the adamant focus on differences then? I ask
To be told, "You have been sutured in"
To an inescapable bond we share
Both not understanding
Not having lived the reality that once was
We have been handed down our places
Like statues made from moulds
Tales told of hate, war and dissent

But you and me, we are the same
So I thought
But I can never be you
And you can never be me
But together, maybe both sides of the leaf
Can we be nurtured at once?
To move beyond the mortar and stone
Into a place of reconciliation and love

To never forget what was done
Where we can be free to dance in the wind as one.

Graham Hartill wrote: "When we make a poem, we make something of ourselves, and the world, anew" (as cited in Hunt & Sampson, 2002, p. 53). This statement aligns with this second poem of self-exploration. Becoming aware of how I value people, diversity and community is integral to this project and I wanted to write a poem that captured the idealist self who I know (or hope) guides most of my actions. Through exploring these issues, I have come to realise that I value the history, culture and ways of knowing Indigenous peoples have shared with settler populations. I value the steadfastness of being able to survive through, as the Indigenous author, Waubgeshig Rice, calls the "apocalypse"[4] in his recent novel, *Moon of the Crusted Snow* (CBC, 2014). I can empathise with the suffering that was faced and support healing and reconciliation by nurturing the process of decolonisation. I also value the steps the Canadian government is taking to right historical wrongdoings through apologies and settlements. However, I also recognise that we have a long way to go yet. By examining my own ways of being, integrating Indigenisation strategies within the classroom and making space for students to just be, will, as my poem states, create room for us to "be free to dance in the wind as one". Writing this poem helped me to understand that equity, social justice and change for a better future are all very important ideas to me and that they have an important place in the classroom. The identification of these values will help me become a better educator.

This poem illustrates that a starting point for understanding the other can be the overarching theme of what it is to be human; focusing on the qualities individuals share can lead to understanding. The imagery of a leaf with contrasting colours on each side, but still representative of a whole structure, is my foundation. Without the baseline of human experience as the bridge between differing cultural identities, I argue we are left in a place of continual cognitive dissonance or an "I-Prison" where a new, second, revisionist story cannot be told.

Creating a contrast between the two sides of a leaf and using colour to do so, I wanted to highlight the beauty of diverse cultural identities, but I must be cognisant that the colour of one's skin has lead to the very colonial power differentials we are trying to dismantle though healing and reconciliation. Writing of his journey to confront the prejudices he had unwittingly internalised, American psychologist Kiselica (1999) explained that he initially failed to recognise his own ethnocentrism and was once blind to racial injustice: "understanding the implications of my physical appearance has helped me to appreciate that the degree of comfort and opportunity provided to people in this nation is partially determined by skin colour" (p. 15). Given my own limited knowledge of Indigenous cultures, seeking out racialized stereotypes that appear in my poetry is a way to shed light on conscious or unconscious narratives of race that I need to explore. I felt an internal tension when I highlighted skin colour in my poem. The internal dialogue left unsaid was,

> As a "polite Canadian" how can I talk about issues of colour? I need to play it safe and not write about how social norms have created internalized biases such as judging quickly based on culturally damaging stereotypes, quickly dismissing the thoughts and ideas of the other as not as important or valid, or not taking into consideration the things I take for granted because of my skin colour.

The inner conflict between who I want to be and who I actually am, coupled with the influence of this time, place and influence of power, privilege and cultural norms causes inherent confusion. However, by being open to this tension and personally acknowledging the trap of ethnocentric views, I have created a space where self-reflexive dialogue can begin.

The second stanza of this poem was inspired by Lengelle et al. (2018); they use the idea of being "sutured in" to a cultural context that is not of one's own making, and this idea resonates with me. Trauma and guilt have been passed down through generations of Canadians because of the history of residential schools and the treatment of Indigenous communities across the country. According to CBC's (2014) timeline of residential schools, the Gordon Residential School in Saskatchewan – the last federally-run residential school – was closed in 1996 (para. 35). This painful history is one I have been "sutured in" to – in this context, being "sutured in" refers to being captured in a narrative I did not choose, while still having to carry a certain responsibility for being implicated by my background and internalised identifications. I live with the feeling of being "guilty by association" but by writing this poem, the questions left are worth exploring. I ask myself,

> Has this guilt stopped me from confronting my own beliefs about power, privilege and authority? How has the colonial subjugation of Indigenous peoples benefitted me personally in my career, positionality within society, and the mitigation of challenges faced as a person of privilege? How has the misuse of trust caused immense pain and suffering for numerous Indigenous nations across Canada

and finally "how can I even pretend to understand the effects of this trauma?" By facing this guilt, I have come to realise that I am in this narrative and regardless of being "sutured in", I have an obligation, as a citizen of this community, to learn about the past in order to use my personal agency to create change.

Intergenerational trauma is a major contributor to many issues haunting Indigenous communities.[5] As Lengelle et al. (2018) have contended: "Because of the colonial foundation on which we tread, the divide persists. … The fallout of the experiences of their parents and grandparents is passed on to [Indigenous peoples] in the form of intergenerational trauma" (p. 90). Santner (1990) too talked about how intergenerational trauma can affect subsequent generations and points to the legacy of trauma; he argued that if trauma is not dealt with, the second and third generations are left to deal with the aftermath. Santner explains that trauma can induce a state of forlornness where the trauma victim is not fully present; when this absence of being is experienced by a parent, it can have dire consequences for children, as future generations are left to function on their own (p. 37). The loss or fragmentation of identity plays a significant role in the disconnection trauma victims suffer, and the focus on reclaiming what once was can leave victims in a state of continual looping, where they are never really able to accept the loss and move forward. Understanding that many of the struggles Indigenous communities face are intergenerational in nature creates the context from which I can face the atrocities of the past brought about by Euro-Canadian settlers, such as those from whom I am descended; it is the place of recognition where I can ask for forgiveness for past sins and reconcile my own feelings of guilt in order to move forward. It is one thing to learn about the past through history, but it is another to personally feel and acknowledge one's part in the meta-narrative of Canadian culture. It is not that I am personally "at fault" for past injustices, but the unquestioned narratives I carry as part of my inheritance can put me at risk of perpetuating injustices without my conscious will.

In current Canadian culture, many Indigenous communities are embracing the healing process by talking about residential schools, colonisation, and the history of Indigenous peoples more broadly. In Manitoba, the Canadian Broadcasting Corporation (CBC) covers events where these dialogues are taking place; as the CBC's Carreiro (2017) reported, "Fontaine, an Ojibway NDP MLA[6], said while these stories are hard to hear, they're important to hear. Without, she added, 'dismissing or minimising' them" (para. 8). Fontaine continues: "As Indigenous people, we hear all the time, 'Why don't you just get over it?' Instead, why don't we just be honest – even though it's an uncomfortable truth, embrace and learn from it?" (as cited in Carreiro, 2017, para. 9). Such dialogue, frankness, and openness about the atrocities of the past appear to allow each generation the opportunity to acknowledge and accept the past and move towards a more hopeful future. And, as Carreiro reported: "Fontaine said there are signs of hope in the fight against racism; the very fact that people stood up and shared their stories at the CBC Town Hall forum – and that others listened – is progress" (para. 10). This is a conversation that must take place in order for us all to move forward as equal citizens of Canada.

The last stanza of the poem *Leaf* reflects my awareness of difference but alludes to a moving forward into a place of, as Meijers and Lengelle (2012) described it, "re-storying" identity, without dismissing the past (p. 158). This is an important part of healing and reconciliation. When she relaunched the Indian Residential Schools Truth and Reconciliation Commission on 15 October 2009, former Canadian Governor General Michaëlle Jean said: "When the present does not recognise the wrongs of the past, the future takes its revenge. … [F]or that reason, we must never, never turn away from the opportunity of confronting history together – the opportunity to right a historical wrong" (as cited in CBC, 2014, para. 9). Using poetry to "re-story" identity allows me the opportunity both to confront the past and to identify my desire to create hope for the future. This poem helped me to look at the relational dynamics between Indigenous peoples and myself, but showed me that I am part of a larger story that I can, in some small way, influence. I can be a vessel of hope for the future by grappling with tough issues and working to create space to hear each voice.

However, it must be mentioned that as Bolton (2010) has argued, ethnographic writing can never be fully truthful, as an individual's subjective experience cannot capture the entirety of an event; rather, such writing is based on the experience of the individual writer (p. 214). She explains that, "Told from the narrator's point of view, [their writing] contains the details they noticed and remembered, interwoven and shot through reflexively with their memories, dreams, prejudices, personal and cultural values, and so on" (p. 214). If I am to "undo" these prejudices in my own thinking, I must be willing to tackle the assumptions I have held about the "Other" and deconstruct them to make new meanings by comparing them to the voices and stories of the other. Deconstructing these biases and assumptions cannot happen in one individual moment; rather, it will take time for me to grapple with all the issues that are entwined in the development of personal and cultural freedom. It must become a reflexive practice and I will continue to write as I uncover further layers of my thinking and its associated limitations and possibilities.

Using DST, I am able to "study the self as a society of 'I-positions'" (Meijers & Hermans, 2018, p. 7). Exploring this poem has identified where more learning, association, and dialogue can help me move forward and let go of fear and guilt in order to "re-story" my own cultural awareness in order to tell a new story. As Bonnar explains in Lengelle et al. (2018),

> The research method of autoethnography and 're-storying' is culturally appropriate because storytelling is an essential part of learning and teaching in Aboriginal cultures, and as one of my mentors reminds me, in the oral tradition, we learn indirectly through the telling and re-telling of stories. As a member of the dominant culture, I have the opportunity to give voice to the assumptions of the colonizers and try to undo them in myself, thereby creating possible solutions based on new conceptions. (p. 90)

By addressing the assumptions of current I-positions, I can see that the emotions I was holding on to can be worked through in order to move forward into a place where "new conceptions" occur. Consistent with DST, the Haiku and the poem *Leaf* demonstrate the position that the dialogical self is able to transcend the self/dialogue dichotomy by "bringing the external to the internal and, in reverse transporting the internal to the external" (Meijers & Hermans, 2018, p. 7). I have unearthed internal subject matter that is difficult, but confronting these issues and having dialogue around them clarifies the internal thought process and identifies the motivations behind subsequent behaviour. Future metaphors and free verse writing are a way for me to pay homage to a diverse array of cultures and environments from a different perspective and to be able to express what is internal in an external place that others can understand.

Transformational learning, in this sense, has occurred when I reflect on the poetry I have written based on my own personal experiences – both internal and external. Breaking down barriers is what this "writing the self" process is all about – initiating a transformational experience where knowledge, understanding, and self-reflectiveness can bridge cultural divides. The self-reflexivity possible through DST has enabled me to better relate to students, parents, colleagues, and others, and those experiences of relating, in turn, create new inspiration for reflective writing. And by creating space to listen to the stories being told, we can each individually "re-story" our identities and co-construct a new reality.

Notes

1. For an in-depth look at Dialogical Self Theory, please refer to Hermans and Konopka (2010).
2. "Umwending" is a German term Barbara Schellhammer (2018) uses to describe an individual's consciousness turning away from the discomfort that arises through the recognition of the "strangeness" of other, towards a "caring for self" (Meijers & Hermans, 2018, p. 66).
3. For more information on Canada's Truth and Reconciliation movement, please refer to www.trc.ca.

4. Waubgeshig Rice's novel, *Moon of the Crusted Snow*, is a dystopian drama where outside forces are causing impending peril to a reserve. In a recent interview with CBC Waubgeshig states,

   > A lot of Indigenous communities, like the one in this story, are overcoming the negative, brutal effects of being colonized. This includes being displaced from their homelands, having children taken away, being shamed out of their culture and being legislated out of their culture in many ways ... It's a world that I'm familiar with. It's set in an Anishinaabe community that's dealing with the impact of being displaced and the effects of colonialism. It's a dystopia that's already here. (Patrick, 2018)

5. To see the TRC final report, please refer to www.trc.ca.
6. NDP refers to the New Democratic Party of Canada and MLA refers to a Member of the Legislative Assembly.

Disclosure statement

No potential conflict of interest was reported by the author.

References

Bolton, G. (2010). *Reflective practice: Writing & professional development*. London: Sage Publications.

Bolton, G., Field, V., & Thompson, K. (2006). *Writing works: A resource for therapeutic writing workshops and activities*. Philadelphia, PA: Jessica Kingsley Publishers.

Carreiro, D. (2017, March 13). Healing the powerful pain of racism through frank talk. *CBC News*. Retrieved from https://www.cbc.ca/news/canada/manitoba/town-hall-racism-frank-talk-1.4022638

CBC News. (2014, March 25). A timeline of residential schools, the Truth and Reconciliation Commission. Retrieved from https://www.cbc.ca/news/canada/a-timeline-of-residential-schools-the-truth-and-reconciliation-commission-1.724434

Dymnicki, A., Sambolt, M., & Kidron, Y. (2013). *Improving college and career readiness by incorporating social and emotional learning*. American Institutes for Research Issue Brief. Retrieved from https://files.eric.ed.gov/fulltext/ED555695.pdf

Furman, R. (2005). Using poetry and written exercises to teach empathy. *Journal of Poetry Therapy, 18*(2), 103–110.

Hermans, H. J. M., Kempen, H. J. G., & van Loon, R. J. P. (1992). The dialogical self: Beyond individualism and rationalism. *The American Psychologist, 47*(1), 23–33. doi:10.1037/0003-066X.47.1.23.

Hermans, H. J. M., & Konopka, A. (2010). *Dialogical self Theory: Positioning and counter-positioning in a globalizing society*. Cambridge, UK: Cambridge University Press.

Higginson, W. J. (1985). Guidelines for writing haiku in English. *The Haiku Foundation*. Retrieved from https://www.thehaikufoundation.org/edwall/higginson_guidelines_for_writing_haiku.pdf

Hunt, C., & Sampson, F. (2002). *The self on the page: Theory and practice of creative writing in personal development*. London: Jessica Kingsley Publishers.

Kiselica, M. S. (1999). Confronting my own ethnocentrism and racism: A process of pain and growth. *Journal of Counselling and Development, 77*(1), 14–17.

Lengelle, R. (2003). *MAIS 616: Writing the self: The experience and potential of writing for personal development [Course guide]*. Athabasca, AB: Athabasca University.

Lengelle, R. (2008). *Blossom & balsam: Poems that reveal and heal*. Edmonton, AB: Black Tulip Press.

Lengelle, R. (2014). *Career writing: Creative, expressive, and reflective approaches to narrative and dialogical career guidance* (Published doctoral dissertation). the Netherlands: Tilburg University.

Lengelle, R., Jardine, C., & Bonnar, C. (2018). Writing the self for reconciliation and global citizenship: The inner dialogue and creative voices for cultural healing. In F. Meijers & H. J. M. Hermans (Eds.), *The dialogical self in education: A multicultural perspective* (pp. 81–96). New York, NY: Springer.

Lengelle, R., Meijers, F., Poell, R., & Post, M. (2014). Career writing: Creative, expressive and reflective approaches to narrative identity formation in students in higher education. *Journal of Vocational Behavior, 85*(1), 75–84.

Meijers, F., & Hermans, H. (eds.). (2018). *The dialogical self theory in education: A multicultural perspective*. Cultural Psychology of Education Series, Vol. 5. New York, NY: Springer.

Meijers, F., & Lengelle, R. (2012). Narratives at work: The development of a career identity. *British Journal of Guidance and Counselling, 40*, 157–176.

Metcalf, L. T., & Simon, T. (2002). *Writing the mind alive: A proprioceptive method for finding your authentic voice*. New York, NY: Random House.

Patrick, R. (2018, October 09). Why Waubgeshig Rice wrote a dystopian novel about the collapse of society from an Indigenous perspective. Retrieved from https://www.cbc.ca/books

Rehm, M. L., & Allison, B. (2006). Positionality in teaching culturally diverse students: Implications for family and consumer sciences teacher education programs. *Family and Consumer Sciences Research Journal, 34*(3), 260–275.

Santner, E. L. (1990). *Stranded objects: Mourning, memory, and film in postwar Germany*. New York, NY: Cornell University Press.

Schellhammer, B. (2018). The experience of the other and the premise of the care for self. Intercultural education as *Umwending*. In F. Meijers & H. J. M. Hermans (Eds.), *The dialogical self theory in education: A multicultural perspective* (pp. 81–96). New York, NY: Springer.

Dialogical Temporal Chair Technique

Małgorzata Łysiak

ABSTRACT
The Dialogical Temporal Chair Technique (DTCT) is a method based on Hermans's dialogical self theory combined with Gestalt and cognitive–behavioural therapeutic techniques. The Dialogical Temporal Chair Technique is a method of activating temporal voices. Three chairs symbolising the past, present and future are used to help subjects create a temporal dialogue. Participants are asked to take a specific I-position and to construct a temporal self-dialogue by changing chair (and hence I-position). The DTCT can be used to solve undefined problems or to explore new ways of thinking, but it may also be used to review important life decisions or enable integration of, or detachment from, ambivalent feelings and attitudes.

The ability to dialogue is a specific human capability. Observations indicate that from early childhood humans have the capacity to take part in dialogues with others and to conduct internal dialogue. Hermans's dialogical self theory (1996, 2001a, 2001b) proposes the existence of a polyphonic self, such that 'I' consists of many relatively independent positions representing a range of perspectives. Internally the 'I' has the capacity to move freely within time and space and 'without time there is no story' (Hermans, 1996, p. 33). Spatial and temporal variables are essential to the creation of narratives and stories based on personal experiences. In imaginative space an individual can move backwards and forwards in time, between past, present and future; such movements lead to change through a dialogical process. Hermans (1996, p. 33) explained:

> For example, I can imaginatively move to a future point in time and then speak to myself about the sense of what I am doing now in my present situation. This position, at some point in the future, may be very helpful to evaluate my present activities from a long-term perspective. The result may be that I disagree with my present self as blinding itself from more essential things.

The voice associated with each position can communicate desires, expectations, fears or needs and contribute to a conversation between the various voices. This form of communication is called internal dialogue. There are I-positions that are grounded in the past or future as well as in the present.

The internal dialogue between the 'I's associated with the different temporal positions is called a temporal dialogue. The exchange of perspectives, opinions and arguments between the different temporal positions can initiate a process of change. For example, a young woman who is bored with her job in a shop might contemplate the future, picturing herself as a stockbroker, feeling the adrenaline rush of trading and risk-taking every day. This kind of dialogue between *present-I* (salesperson) and *future-I* (stockbroker) leads to some sort of internal debate about whether to change job or career path and may prompt behavioural change (e.g. change of job). Similarly, a person might look back at the past and remember who his or her past self was, what decisions he or she took, and whether they turned out well. The dialogical self can revisit the past as well as project forwards into the future. Despite the autonomy and varied desires of the different temporal selves, they can be integrated into a single 'I'. Of course, during the temporal dialogue some of I-positions are easy to integrate, (e.g. me as beloved child and me as a beloved wife) and some of them are not (e.g. me as a beloved wife and me as an aggressive, old widow) (Oleś, Brygoła, & Sibińska, 2010; Sibińska, 2012). Dialogical activity may reveal a variety of relationships between I-positions: agreement or disagreement, dominance or dependency, partnership or separation.

When viewing these various temporal perspectives, the individual looks for ways to create bridges between them and synthesise the various experiences they represent. This bird's-eye perspective which enables one to integrate the different internal voices is referred to as the 'metaposition'. Hermans (2001a) described meta-reflection as a very adaptive process involving an overview of the various dialogues. The main functions of the metaposition are: 1) to achieve detachment from other positions; 2) to provide an overarching view of their relationships; 3) to build bridges between contradictory points of view; 4) to provide a broader view of the issues in order to facilitate decision-making. In the terminology of counselling or psychotherapy the dialogical metaposition is a way of achieving deeper self-reflection and greater insight.

Dialogical self-theory recognises the plurality of human experience: unity and multiplicity, continuity and discontinuity (see also Hermans, 2003). The personal ability to establish imagined inner dialogues between temporal I-positions is the main framework for constructing the Dialogical Temporal Chair Technique. Confronting the past, future and present I-positions allows people to express their life experience and explore different emotional states. In order to explore these experiences by internal temporal dialogues, the main research focus was whether the confrontation of the past, future and present I-positions relates to affective states and/or the meaning of life. Moving along a time line can activate analysis, organisation and exploration of new perspectives and may generate differences in the experience of the meaning of life. Reminding oneself of the past has more to do with life review and is based on a realisation of choices and values therefore it should enhance the meaning of life. Constructing a possible future perspective will promote a choice of life goals which are in harmony with personal needs and aspirations. This should influence the meaning of life in broadening the temporal perspective, which allows one to find basic values and other anchors for a personal meaning of life. Taking a starting point in temporal dialogical relationships, activating all three time-related I-positions and using spatial relationships the DTCT was constructed.

The next research aim of constructing the method was reviewing the process of activating the voices (past, future and present) and analysing the possibilities for integrating the voices representing different temporal perspectives.

The method of activating the voices of the self was used to facilitate clients' integration of different temporal aspects of the self. The rationale behind constructing the DTC technique is to help people move from talking about something from their past/future experience – using sensation, affect, cognition and movement, towards the present voice in order to gain further insight. The emphasis is on what is being done, thought, and felt at the moment, or occurring in the past or what might happen in the future. Moreover, activating temporal positions at the same time is an experience of taking a brief look at the problems, decisions, goals or aims you want to achieve. Using people's natural ability to conduct an internal dialogue using the constructed method may help to integrate experiences from the past with the present situation and aid the formulation of a positive future.

DTCT – instruction

The Dialogical Temporal Chair Technique (DTCT) is a procedure for activating the temporal voices of the self. It was inspired by several communication and psychotherapeutic techniques. Firstly Linell and Markova's (1993) three-step model of communication, step 1: A to B; step 2: B to A; step 3: A

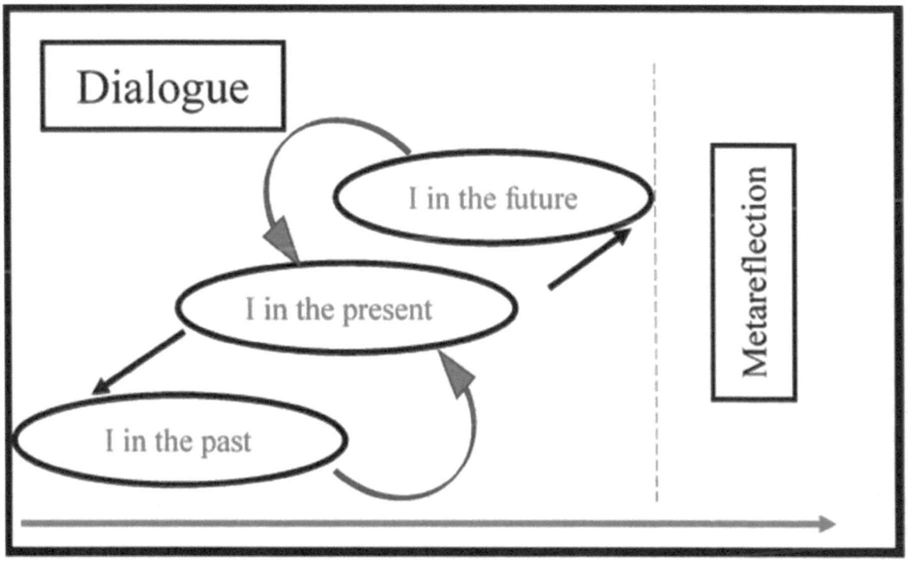

Figure 1. Schematic procedure for activating temporal dialogue based on Dialogical Temporal Chair Instruction.

to B. The essence of this cycle is that A is not the same person as in the first step. The dialogue with B has an influence on A. Hermans (2006) concluded that this model implies that an initial utterance is changed to some extent by the dialogical process itself. This kind of transaction can be observed in everyday conversations, as people permit themselves to be influenced by other people's points of view.

Another inspiration was the Gestalt therapy 'empty chair' technique in which the client engages in an imagined dialogue with his or her self. The client sits in front of the empty chair, which symbolises another person or a part of the self that is unacceptable in the process of therapy and tries to verbalise thoughts and feelings which are difficult to say in real life. During the procedure the client switches between the chairs representing the different parties in the dialogue; the chairs are a way of increasing the immediacy of the experience.

The final inspiration for DTCT was a double-column technique used in cognitive–behavioural therapy. The patient writes his or her unreasonable, automatic thoughts in one column and the counterarguments in the opposite side. It is a method of controlling negative thoughts and replacing them with a more adaptive perspective.

Dialogical Temporal Chair Instruction provides four elements of the procedure concerning temporal 'I' positions: past, future and present. The participant is instructed to imagine him or herself at a well-defined point in time and formulate messages to *past-I* and *future-I* and to respond to their messages as *present-I*. The procedure ends with holistic reflection on the temporal positions, finding new qualities or connections. The instruction of activating voices called Dialogical Temporal Chair Instruction assumed four steps (see Figure 1):

Step I: introduction

There are three chairs in front of you. Each of them represents a certain time in your life. The chair in the middle represents you in your current self or life situation, and we will refer to it as *present-I*. The chair on your left represents you at time of your choosing in your past and we will refer to it as *past-I*. The chair on your right represents you at a time of your choosing in your future and we will call it *future-I*. As you construct the dialogue I will ask you to switch between the chairs. Is everything clear to you?

Step II: dialogue with the past

Please sit in the left-hand chair. Imagine yourself at any important moment from your past. It might be a situation, experience or any period of your life which was different from your current situation and important to you. Please describe it giving all the details you can remember – emotions, behaviours, thoughts. [*The description is audio-recorded or the researcher administering the procedure takes notes*]

(A) What do you think your *present-I* would say to your *past-I* on hearing this story? Please sit in the middle chair to respond.
(B) Now imagine yourself as your *past-I* again. How would your *past I* respond to your *present-I*? Please move to the left-hand chair to respond.
(A) And how would your *present-I* reply? Once again, please change chairs and sit in the middle chair to respond.
(B) (carry on the discussion as above)

Now that you've constructed this dialogue and heard this internal conversation, can you find a way of combining what the various voices have said into a single reflection or message? What would that be?

Step III: dialogue with the future

Now please sit in the right-hand chair. Imagine yourself at any moment in your future. Please describe yourself in your imaginative future giving any details you want – emotions, behaviours, thoughts. [*The description is audio-recorded or the researcher administering the procedure takes notes*]

(A) What do you think your *present-I* would say to your *future-I* on hearing this story? Please sit in the middle chair to respond.
(B) Now please go back to your *future-I*. How would it respond to your *present-I*? Please switch chairs and sit in the right-hand chair to respond.
(A) And how would your *present-I* reply? (Once again, please change chairs and sit in the middle chair to respond.
(B) (carry on the discussion as above)

Now that you've constructed this dialogue, heard this internal conversation, can you find a way of combining what the various voices have said into a single reflection or message? What would that be?

Step IV: meta-reflection

Now please sit in the middle chair, which symbolises you in your present situation and consider your reflections on the two dialogues, with your past self and with your future self. Is there any way of combining them into a single message, or insight or piece of information? Does reflecting on the combination of voices give you any new insight? [*The description is audio-recorded or the researcher administering the procedure takes notes*]

Is there is anything you would like to add?

The procedure concerns two processes: activating and integrating temporal positions. Activating the dialogue starts with a process of remembering a situation from the past or creating a situation from the future aloud and constructing the conversation between temporal (past/future and present) positions and changing the chairs at the same time. Characteristic questions for activating dialogue are *what would your present -I say to* or *how would you respond*? At the end of the procedure one element appears (step IV) called meta-reflection. The participant answers a question concerning meta-reflection on the effects of what has taken place just before: *What is the result of confronting those voices? Does reflecting on the combination of voices give you any new insight?* By this new combination (question, answer) of temporal positions it is hoped to test whether integration of the voices emerging from different temporal I-positions is possible.

The DTCT is a method which can be used by counsellors, psychologists or advisors working with people who are seeking to change something in their life, dealing with difficult situations from their past, overcoming fears about the future or in the process of making a decision. It can also be used to help an individual gain perspective on his or her current situation. The therapist, counsellor or advisor acts as a Rogerian partner, listening carefully and showing empathy, helping the client or patient to explore dialogues as he or she wishes. After the procedure, within the counsellor – patient/client relationship, it is good to discuss the feelings and thoughts which arose and the willingness to practise the method in real life or real situations.

In this study the DTCT was used with adolescents and young adults and the methodology is presented below.

Method

To explore the method of understanding the temporal dialogical activity of the self the experimental procedure was done. The main aim of the research was to explore how well people construct temporal dialogues and to what extent they are able to integrate the temporal positions and what factors influence this integration. We hypothesised that activating inner temporal dialogue causes a positive increase in one's perception of the meaning of life measured as a state and influences emotional states (H1) and that integration of temporal I-positions has a positive impact on one's perception of the meaning of life and emotions, both measured as states, whereas lack of integration of temporal I-positions causes negative changes (H2).

The participants were students ($n = 100$, M age = 17.92 years; $SD = 1.01$) and young adults ($n = 100$, M age = 22.96 years, $SD = 2.38$) who were asked to define personally important I-positions, one in the past and one in the future, and then to construct a dialogue between these past and future selves and their current self. Participants were recruited through advertisements at universities and by school counsellors who invited younger people to participate in the dialogical study. Qualitative data, in the form of dialogues, were gathered using the DTCT and quantitative data was collected using paper-and-pencil questionnaires. Before and after the DTCT participants completed two scales: a 30-item scale measuring perception of the meaning of life (MLS-S; Oleś et al., 2010) and the State Personality Inventory (SPI; Spielberger & Reheiser, 2003, 2009).

The MLS-S (Oleś et al., 2010) was based on the Purpose in Life Test (PLT) developed by Crumbaugh and Maholick (1981). The difference between them is that the PLT measures stable beliefs and a general attitude towards one's own life whereas the 30-item MLS-S measures meaning of life as a state i.e. current perception of the meaning of one's life. Participants respond to items using a five-point Likert scale (1: *I definitely do not agree* to 5: *I definitely agree*) and the total score (range: 30150) is used. The scale has high internal consistency (Cronbach's $\alpha = .95$).

The SPI (Spielberger & Reheiser, 2003) is a 40 item questionnaire measuring four emotional states: anxiety, anger, depression and curiosity (10 items per state). Responses are given on a four-point scale and refers to the intensity of the current emotions. The Polish version was developed by Wrześniewski and Oleś. The internal consistency (Cronbach's α) for the various subscales is as follows, anxiety: .75; anger: .68; depression: .85; curiosity: .75.

Participants' ability to adopt a metaposition was assessed. Participants were considered to have demonstrated the ability to adopt a metaposition when, in the fourth stage of the procedure, they were able to create a single message from the various dialogues and confrontation, when the dialogue was not conclusive. Participants created meta-reflection formulated from the present position (step IV) which was an indicator of temporal integration – a new message was formulated as the combination of voices at the end of the procedure.

Results

Analysis of data from the whole sample ($N = 200$) confirmed the first hypothesis: the process of constructing temporal dialogues between past, present and future selves resulted in a positive increase in one's perception of the meaning of life measured as a state ($F_{[1,194]} = 212.35, p < .001, \eta^2 = 0.52$) and increase in curiosity ($F_{[1]} = 7.48, p < .01$).

As stated in dialogical self-theory where autonomic temporal I positions communicate with each other to find a common new quality, new solutions for diverse points of view, this result improves the impact of internal dialogicality on individual's self-reflection. Self-reflection is conducive to personal development and to broadening one's life-wisdom (Baltes & Staudinger, 1996). The process of constructing a temporal dialogue involving exchanges between different perspectives gave participants the chance to take a look at their life in a different way. Changing perspective verbally and physically enabled participants to identify more closely with the different temporal I-positions. In agreement with Hermans that story is built in time frame, the person has the potential of becoming someone better in certain conditions of time and space. The process of voicing the different temporal perspectives seems to produce an increase in the quality of perceptions about the meaning of life.

The second hypothesis was that integration of temporal I-positions causes positive change in feelings about meaning of life and emotions, both measured as states, whereas non-integration of temporal I-positions causes negative changes. A qualitative analysis was based on the indicator for temporal integration, that is, a new message formulated as the combination of voices at the end of the procedure. Meta-reflection was formulated from the present position showing a new quality derived from confrontation of the past, present and future self. Meta-reflection was evaluated by five independent judges with a thorough knowledge of the procedure using a four-point scale. Based on these evaluations participants were assigned to the 'integration' group (51%) or 'non-integration' group (49%). There was no group difference in gender distribution ($\chi^2_{[1]} = 1.21, p < .27$).

It is notable that although both groups showed an increase in perception of the meaning of life ($F_{[1,194]} = 212.35, p < .001, \eta^2 = 0.52$); see Tables 1 and 2) there were group differences in affective states. Participants who were able to integrate the voices better differ in affective states and showed an increase in curiosity and decrease in anger. There are no significant differences in anxiety and depression.

Significant differences were also found for the non-integration group where the results were quite unexpected. An increase in perception of the meaning of life, curiosity and anxiety and no differences in anger and depression were revealed after the DTCT procedure (see Table 2).

The main interesting result in the non-integration group was the increase in anxiety. We assume that this is because reimagining one's past may involve recall of negative as well as positive experiences, perhaps eliciting frustration at the difficulty of the problems to be solved. The nature of the procedure makes it likely that participants had to confront existential dilemmas. Some people may find looking into the future terrifying, particularly when they compare possible futures with their present situation. It is also an interesting element of work for counsellors and advisors.

Table 1. Descriptive statistics for perception of meaning of life and affective state scores before and after inner temporal dialogue in the integration group.

	Integration group					
	Before Dialogue		After Dialogue		Differences	
Variable	*M*	*SD*	*M*	*SD*	*t*	*p*<
Meaning of life	78.1	11.75	104.59	10.81	−27.46	0.001
Anxiety	14.43	3.37	15.05	3.33	−1.60	–
Curiosity	29.08	6.19	30.48	5.38	−3.28	0.001
Anger	15.60	3.62	13.81	2.92	−1.78	0.001
Depression	13.98	3.66	13.44	3.00	1.48	–

Table 2. Descriptive statistics for perception of the meaning of life and affective state scores before and after inner temporal dialogue in the non-integration group.

	Non Integration Group					
	Before Dialogue		After Dialogue		Differences	
Variable	*M*	*SD*	*M*	*SD*	*t*	*p*<
Meaning of life	85.5	12.86	88.42	12.63	−6.002	0.001
Anxiety	16.86	5.40	18.28	5.14	−5.62	0.001
Curiosity	26.74	6.14	27.33	6.09	−2.08	0.05
Anger	16.87	4.13	16.36	4.49	4.21	–
Depression	16.55	4.16	16.66	4.18	−0.48	–

In addition to the quantitative analyses qualitative analysis was conducted. The main qualitative issue we investigated was the function of inner temporal dialogues. We analysed the form and contents of the dialogues participants produced. The participants (who were not patients or clients) were given the freedom to choose which moment from their past or future to use in the dialogues and they were assigned to groups on the basis of the topics they chose. The most common topics discussed in the dialogues were love and feelings (21%), family (27%), career or work (34%) and meaning of life (11%). The percentage distribution demonstrates that temporal I-positions are connected with values (love, family, career) and existential subjects. The qualitative analysis indicated that the different I-positions took various roles in such dialogue depending on the characteristic subject or plot of the dialogue.

Conclusion

The DTCT is based on Hermans's dialogical self theory and was inspired by mainstream psychotherapeutic techniques. The aim of this study was to explore how people construct temporal dialogues and what impact this process has on their perception of the meaning of life and their affective state. We investigated the relationship between the ability to integrate the various temporal perspectives and changes in perceived meaning of life and emotional states as well as exploring the functions of inner dialogues. Using the DTCT method allows the self to be expressed in space as well as in time. From a meta-position the individual is able to consider all the different temporal perspectives and reflect on them from a detached, outsider's perspective. Hermans and Hermans-Konopka (2010) claimed that a person who has an ability to take this act simultaneously is looking for 'bridges of meaning' for one's own experiences, thoughts and feelings. DTCT may promote a cognitive component of inner dialogicality. During counselling clients very often go back to past memories, they are often conflicted and unable to make sense of their past. But while activating future images, one's story may turn out to be completely different than the actual one. McAdams (2001) has claimed that constructing people's story lives chronologically is a way of making sense of them. It implicates the process of reconstruction of the past, evaluation of the present, making plans for the future. Our results show that activating temporal voices using the DTCT modifies the current psychological state and cognitive components such as perception of the meaning of life as well as affective states. Perception of the meaning of life is positively associated with dialogical ability. Oleś (2009) contended that the main form of autoreflection is the internal dialogue which is conducive to personal development. Confronting different points of view while using temporal dialogue gave an opportunity to look at a situation from various perspectives on chosen issues, where reflection can develop wisdom. It does not appear to matter if the participant is able to integrate the voices or not. It seems that the ability to integrate the voices may initiate the process of change but does not implicate the increase in it.

There is an interpretation of the role of integration. Individuals who are able to integrate two or more voices when constructing temporal dialogues tend to experience an increase in the intensity of positive affective states and perceived meaning of life. Participants who can achieve an internal integration via internal dialogue, and who are able to connect and unite different temporal voices, probably find such dialogues a way of resolving existential dilemmas. They clearly benefit from internal temporal dialogue. By activating their past, future and present selves, people clarify goals, values and desires. This process influences how they perceive the meaning of life. In this study we observed that temporal dialogues between past, present and future selves increased the perceived meaning of life and increased curiosity, whilst also decreasing anger. The different temporal positions also appear to be associated with different affective states. *Past-I* was often used to revisit negative experiences, *future-I* tended to be full of hope, making goals and plans, and the role of *present-I* seemed to vary according to the identity of its partner in the dialogue. Confronting the past or future causes individuals to view their present from a broader perspective (e.g. teenage values or the sum of life events). Present activities that seem urgent or important (e.g. completing school, one's first intimate relationship) may lose their importance when viewed from a broader temporal perspective or take on an entirely different complexion (e.g. undesirable rather than important). If the dialogue is between present and past positions, *present-I* is like an understanding friend/mentor in that it gives an emotional support at some distance. According to Puchalska-Wasyl's imagined dialogues research (2006) the function achieved in this dialogue would be called support and attachment. When there is confrontation between present and future positions, *actual- I* needs support and advice. On the basis of Hermans' theory we assumed that positions and their functions are changing with each other according to time and space dimensions.

The DTCT is an empirically validated technique. It may be useful for practitioners working with people dealing with inner conflicts, existential dilemmas or difficult decisions. The DTCT enables an individual to make sense of his or her present actions by juxtaposing at least two perspectives – the present perspective, which is often dominated by immediate needs, and a future or past perspective. The narrative voices allow interaction because they are directed towards a real or imagined receiver (here: past and future `I) and function as representative, because they communicate a personal and important message. Moreover, Sarbin (1995) argued that a story is not only a way of organising time and one's life, but also a way of determining one's goals and desires. It is even a cognitive and emotional perception of the future, therefore evoking and influencing motivational processes.

The dynamic and changing personality is formed by the existence of a person in time. A person can consciously develop an attitude towards their experience of the continuity of events and their endings. A temporal dialogue can influence the functioning of the 'self'. The dialogues which people construct reveal their motives and goals, their hopes and fears, and can help them to understand the implications of committing to or withdrawing from activities (Bruner, 1992). The DTCT is a tool that, because it activates a representation of one's past or future self, can influence how one perceives the meaning of life. Markova (2003) has claimed that dialogical relation of temporal positions has social character and that the process of assuming others' perspectives to resolve problems or dilemmas may support everyday relationships. When conflicts arise in relationships then a negotiator with a different, often more objective point of view is needed. In temporal inner dialogues the reflection process fulfils the negotiator's function, which in real life might be filled by a friend, partner or counsellor.

In conclusion, using the DTCT to compare one's current perspective with a specific past or future perspective through a dialogue process can prompt and facilitate personal development (Hermans, 1996).

Disclosure statement

No potential conflict of interest was reported by the author.

References

Baltes, P. B., & Staudinger, U. M. (Eds.). (1996). *Interactive minds. Life-span perspectives on the social foundation of cognition.* Cambridge: Cambridge University Press.

Bruner J. (1992). Życie jako narracja (life as narration). *Kwartalnik Pedagogiczny, 37,* 3–17.

Crumbaugh J. C., & Maholick, L. T. (1981). *Manual of instructions for the purpose in life test.* Munster, In: Psychometric Affiliates.

Hermans, H. J. M. (1996). Voicing the self: From information processing to dialogical interchange. *Psychological Bulletin, 119,* 31–50.

Hermans, H. J. M. (2001a). Conceptions of self and identity: Toward a dialogical view. *International Journal of Education and Religion, 1,* 43–62.

Hermans, H. J. M. (2001b). The dialogical self: Towards a theory of personal and cultural positioning. *Culture & Psychology, 7*(3), 243–281.

Hermans, H. J. M. (2003). The construction and reconstruction of a dialogical self. *Journal of Constructivist Psychology, 16,* 89–130.

Hermans, H. J. M. (2006). Moving through three paradigms, yet remaining the same thinker. *Counselling Psychology Quarterly, 19*(1), 5–25.

Hermans, H. J. M., & Hermans-Konopka, A. (2010). *Dialogical self theory. Positioning and counter-positioning in a globalizing society.* Cambridge: Cambridge University Press.

Linell, P., & Markova, Ą. I. (1993). Acts in discourse: From monological speech acts to dialogical inter-acts. *Journal for the Theory of Social Behaviour, 23,* 173–195.

Markova I. (2003). *Dialogicality and social representations. The dynamics of mind.* Cambridge: Cambridge University Press.

McAdams, D. P. (2001). *The person: An integrated introduction to personality psychology* (3rd ed.). Forth Worth: Hartcourt Brace College Publishers.

Oleś, P. K. (2009). Dialogowość wewnętrzna jako właściwość człowieka [Internal dialogicality as a feature of human being]. In J. Kozielecki (Ed.), *Nowe idee w psychologii* [New ideas in psychology] (pp. 216–235). Gdańsk: Gdańskie Wydawnictwo Psychologiczne.

Oleś, P. K, Brygoła, E., & Sibińska, M. (2010). Temporal dialogues and their influence on affective states and the meaning of life. *International Journal for Dialogical Science, 4*(1), 23–43.

Puchalska-Wasyl, M. (2006). Types and functions of inner dialogues. *Psychology of Language and Communication, 11,* 43–62.

Sarbin, T. R. (1995). *A* narrative approach to repressed memories. *Journal of Narrative and Life History, 5,* 51–66.

Sibińska, M. (2012). *Zmiana poczucia sensu życia pod wpływem dialogów temporalnych [Change in meaning of life following temporal dialogues]* (Unpublished dissertation). The John Paul II Catholic University of Lublin, Lublin.

Spielberger, C. D., & Reheiser, E. C. (2003). Measuring anxiety, anger, depression, and curiosity as emotional states and personality traits with the STAI, STAXI, and STPI. In M. Hersen, M. J. Hilsenroth, & D. L. Segal (Eds.), *Comprehensive handbook of psychological assessment, Vol. 2, personality assessment* (pp. 70–86). Hoboken, NJ: John Wiley & Sons, Inc.

Spielberger, C. D., & Reheiser, E. C. (2009). Assessment of emotions: Anxiety, anger, depression, and curiosity. *Applied Psychology: Health and Well-Being, 1,* 271–302.

Innovative career construction counselling for a creative adolescent

Jacobus Gideon Maree

ABSTRACT

This article reports on integrative career counselling provided to a creative young man selected purposefully. An explorative, descriptive, instrumental, single case-study approach was followed, and two recently developed questionnaires (one qualitative and one quantitative) were used to collect the data. A career construction counselling intervention comprising assessment and (meta-) reflective dialogues on the participant's elicited career-life story was conducted. The intervention involved elicitation of the participant's career-life story, authorisation of the story, and facilitation of action (forward movement). The participant's need was met for "different" career counselling. The intervention helped the participant to celebrate and draw on his sense of creativity. Multiple case and quantitative studies are needed on the topic as well as more longitudinal research.

Introduction

The career counselling theatre is changing irrevocably in a postmodern world and is characterised by globalisation, technological advances, downsizing, and organisational mergers in the aftermath of economic downturns (Reid & West, 2016; Savickas, 2011). Career counselling theory, research, and practice have to respond to the fundamental changes in the world of work brought about by successive waves in the economy, psychology, counselling, and the fourth industrial revolution over the past 100 years or more (Maree, 2013). According to Reid and West (2016), "[i]n the context of mass migration and unstable labour markets … traditional career guidance is no longer sufficient … the need for a paradigm shift is becoming more urgent" (p. 573). With the prospects of finding work or staying on in a single organisation for any length of time fast disappearing, the traditional "test-and-tell" counselling approach on its own no longer suffices to meet the changing career counselling needs of clients (Maree, 2018; Savickas, 2016). An innovative, flexible approach to change and its impact that takes global career trends and technological advances into account is required to help career counsellors adjust their praxis to meet the demand for new skills and attitudes (Pryor, 2008). While the career counselling field has experienced some innovation in European and North American countries over the past 30 years or so, the same cannot be said about many developing countries.

Doyle (2017) maintained that "[t]he era of employment (as defined in the first and second industrial revolutions) for life is long over" (p. 1). The new emphasis is on becoming "employable" because unless workers can think innovatively about how to manage the numerous barriers encountered in changing work contexts, they may simply stagnate (Savickas, 2005). Likewise, Van Vianen, De Pater, and Preenen (2009) have emphasised the importance of enhancing people's adaptive responses while addressing their non-adaptive responses (e.g. dysfunctional career thinking) in today's rapidly changing world of work (Maree, 2016a). Integrating people's career and comprehensive life themes in order to promote their ability to deal with work transitions has become an integral part of career development (Ebberwein, Krieshok, Ulven, & Prosser, 2004).

Krumboltz and Chan (2005) claimed that people who are open-minded and willing to keep on learning for the rest of their lives and to accept and in fact embrace change have the best chance of preparing themselves successfully for an increasingly unpredictable and uncertain future. Pfeiffer (2015) has argued that career counselling should also address people's socioemotional and spiritual needs. The development and implementation of innovative career counselling strategies should therefore take place in such a way that people can get in touch with their deepest emotions. People should be encouraged to learn how to retrieve these emotions, articulate them, and deal with them since they often reveal valuable personal information that can help them adapt to a rapidly changing world.

The career construction theoretical framework (Savickas, 2015a) that was used to analyse and interpret the research data is discussed below. The intervention described here is merely one way of applying the theories of self- and career construction in practice (Guichard, 2009; Savickas, 2011).

The career construction theoretical framework: general comments

In the twentieth century, career counselling endeavoured to establish people's "self-knowledge" and knowledge about "jobs" and to find an optimal fit between people's traits and different jobs (Hartung, 2011). In today's uncertain world, however, the aim is to help people improve their employability and become flexible, life-long learners (Savickas, 2016). Work is today seen as a channel to help people make meaning of their career lives and discover a sense of purpose through their narratives about themselves and about work. These new aims require a fundamentally different approach to career counselling (Savickas et al., 2009) based on, as discussed here, a narrative paradigm such as career construction theory.

Career construction theory (CCT)

Career construction theory (CCT) holds that people's multiple private and public roles contain meaningful experiences that can help with career choice making and career construction. CCT is a metatheory premised on three classic career counselling theoretical views (Savickas, 2011, 2016):

a. The differential (individual differences) view focuses on how people differ and emphasises the use of psychometric tests to yield "scores" that quantify personal traits to help counsellors determine an optimal person-environment fit between their clients and their work environments.
b. The developmental (psychology) or lifespan, life-space view holds that people develop over time. It also examines how people deal with career-related development tasks during different life phases and multiple career-related transitions and traumas. This view focuses on career adaptability, on people's readiness to enter a career, and on how individuals solve problems and adapt to changing environments by developing and drawing on certain attitudes, beliefs, and competencies (ABCs) (Savickas, 2005).
c. The dynamic or narrative (storied) view (Hartung, 2011; Savickas, 2005) investigates how key career-life themes add meaning to people's career-related behaviour. People are regarded as the authors of their own unique career-life stories. These stories, once elicited and examined, uncover key life themes that enable their authors to face a future that is becoming increasingly uncertain and difficult to predict. Numerous studies attest to the value of narrative methods (and career construction counselling in particular) to help people "coherently tell their life stories,

adapt to changes in themselves and their situations, and intentionally design their life careers" (Hartung & Santili, 2018, p. 318).

Some key aspects of CCT of relevance to the integrative counselling approach are discussed briefly in the following section.

Key aspects of career construction counselling

First, the success of self- and career construction counselling is dependent on counsellors' ability to create safe spaces (Savickas, 2011) or holding environments (Winnicott, 1964) that encourage clients to recount or narrate their career-life stories (narratability) and subsequently draw on these stories to advise themselves on key career choice and self-construction questions (auto-biographicity) (Savickas, 2009). By eliciting and reading these stories back to their clients so they can listen to and authorise them, career counsellors set the scene for forward movement (action by clients that can lead to clarifying their career identities and choices) (Krieshok, Black, & McKay, 2009). Therefore, identity formation is dependent on self-awareness, (critical) self-reflection (reflection about oneself prompted by questions by the career counsellor in the course of the counselling), and reflexivity (drawing on reflections to plan the future, which sets the scene for self- and career construction and, ultimately, life designing) (Savickas, 2011).

Career identity encompasses the "practice of articulating, performing and negotiating identity positions in narrating career decisions" (LaPointe, 2010, p. 2). When life stories are shared with others in an educational setting, the others become a "witnessing community" (Sliep, 2007, p. 122) or clients' "audience" (Di Fabio & Maree, 2013). Moreover, such sharing promotes career adaptability and career resilience. Career adaptability refers to people's concern about their future career-lives, taking responsibility for their career-lives (control), becoming curious about key facets of their future career-lives, and gaining confidence about what they want to achieve in their career-lives. Career adaptability promotes the ideal of employability. Resilience is "the capacity of a dynamic system to adapt successfully to disturbances that threaten system function, viability, or development" (Masten, 2014, p. 6). Career resilience refers to people's capacity to function efficiently in work-related contexts despite challenging or disabling circumstances (Rochat, Masdonati, & Dauwalder, 2017).

Much research has been conducted on the value of subjective (qualitative and storied or narrative) interventions and associated techniques in career counselling in addition to quantitative approaches (Maree, 2015, 2016a, 2016b; Watson, 2004). The use of integrative career counselling approaches (merging qualitative and quantitative approaches and interventions) has been growing in popularity globally (McMahon & Watson, 2015). Against this background, a practical solution for present-day career counselling challenges is discussed in this article. The research is integrative in multiple ways: it uses three paradigms (differential psychology, developmental perspective, and narrative identity) as well as a combination of qualitative and quantitative approaches as required by the three paradigms, typical of CCT.

An integrative qualitative + quantitative approach to career counselling

In this article I discuss the implementation of two newly-developed career counselling instruments, the *Maree Career Matrix* (*MCM*) (Maree, 2016c; Maree & Taylor, 2016a, 2016b) and the *Career Interest Profile* (*CIP*) (Maree, 2017a, 2017b).

Used in an integrative manner, the two instruments can identify clients' deep-seated strengths and motives and help clients first reflect on their career-life stories and then reflect on these reflections (meta-reflect). The meta-reflections provide the scaffolding for action and forward movement (Savickas, 2011). The integrative approach is based on the recognition of the need to draw on subjective and objective factors to help people facing a crossroads deal with a possibly traumatic past and rise above challenges by constructing, deconstructing, reconstructing, and co-constructing their life stories and converting challenges into opportunities, failures into success, and suffering into healing. The approach advocated here underwrites Duffy and Dik's (2009, p. 441) view that

> [o]nce clients have addressed the broad level of life purpose or meaning, a next step is for counselors to help clients connect what they view as their life purpose or role in the larger society with their activity within the work role.

Rationale for the study

Numerous case studies have been published on the use of either a quantitative or a qualitative approach to career counselling. Hartung and Santili (2018, p. 310) contended that "[r]ecognizing the power and prevalence of story in human life, career counsellors increasingly use narrative models and methods in practice". A relatively small number of case studies have also been done on the merits of merging quantitative ("objective") and qualitative ("subjective") methodologies to facilitate career counselling (Maree, 2017b).

Bimrose and Hearne (2012) and Blustein (2006) maintained that interventions that do not combine and merge quantitative and qualitative approaches seem to be less effective. The present article represents an attempt to contribute to this discussion. I conducted the study because I believed that research on implementing this approach to career counselling could help career counsellors meet the career counselling needs of a much wider audience (people seeking career counselling in general; the only exception would be some on the autistic spectrum). This article focusses on the particular needs of creative adolescents who were unwilling to be "tested and told what to do" ("fit the mould") and did not benefit sufficiently from "traditional" career counselling. I acknowledge that my personal views, preferred counselling style, possible bias towards creative people, and experience of "traditional", qualitative, as well as integrative approaches may have influenced me during the course of this career counselling intervention

Goals of the study

The goal of the study was to provide integrative career counselling using two recently developed questionnaires (one qualitative and one quantitative) to a creative adolescent who did not "fit the mould". The following questions guided the research: What is the impact of the style of career counselling intervention demonstrated in this article on a creative adolescent in search of "non-traditional" career counselling? Put differently: How can "stories" (qualitative approach) be elicited and "scores" (quantitative approach) obtained and then integrated to meet the career counselling needs of a creative adolescent who had difficulty deciding whether to stay true to his preferred identity and choose a "creative" field of study or to bow to societal pressure to conform and choose a "traditional" career?

Method

Participant and context

Dean (a pseudonym; the third of four children) was selected conveniently from a number of adolescents who had sought career counselling in July, 2017. A 17-year-old English-speaking adolescent in Grade 12, he was achieving excellent marks at school and was described by parents and teachers alike as highly creative, somewhat non-conformist, adaptable, flexible, able to think originally, able to make connections between seemingly unconnectable elements, and able to create "novel" order in the midst of "complexity" and "chaos" (Gyarmathy & Senior, 2018). Against this personal background, I asked him whom he considered the single biggest expert on him, and he immediately responded: "*I myself.*" Asked why he was seeking career counselling, he replied:

> I want to find out where my strengths lie and define my interests and what I can do with them one day as my career. Find out more about myself. Since I am unsure and it is late in the year already, I am considering taking a gap year. Is that a good idea?

He went on to explain that he had been assessed in Grade 9 but that he felt he had not benefited from the traditional ("test-and-tell") style of career counselling. Above all, he felt immensely frustrated by having had to complete questionnaires all day long without once having been given the opportunity to *"talk about my own needs, wishes, and feelings"*. After I had explained the essence of the integrative approach to Dean and his parents, we agreed that the assessment should be conducted using a combination of qualitative and quantitative approaches.

The counsellor

I am a lecturer, researcher, and psychologist with 30^{+} years of experience in individual and group career counselling.

Procedure

As Dean lived roughly 380 km from the town where the intervention was conducted, it was agreed that the intervention would be concluded in one day. In fact, it took about five hours (08:00 to roughly 1300), which included a number of breaks. I adopted a simultaneous approach, that is, the quantitative and qualitative assessment took place at the same time. In the "elicitation" phase (Phase 1; two and a half hours), the intake interview was conducted with the parents, after which they left the interview room. In the meantime, Dean had begun completing the *MCM* and the *CIP*, and, following this, his "My life story" as well as the reports written by his teachers were read to him and discussed with him. The session ended with the elicitation of his three earliest recollections. In Phase 2 (90 min), I read Dean's elicited "career-life story" back to him and his parents (Dean had agreed to his parents sitting in during the session) to clarify any uncertainties. Meta-reflection took place by asking Dean to reflect repeatedly on his own reflections (namely his responses to questions in the *CIP* in particular). I provided generalised career choice, psychosocial, and psychoeducational information and refrained from dispensing "advice". Instead, I helped him interpret key career-life themes that emerged from the qualitative outcomes ("stories") in particular (qualitative assessment). On the basis of these themes, and incorporating the interest-related outcomes obtained from the "scores" (quantitative assessment), Dean was helped to advise himself on what career to choose and also on how he could make meaning of and find a sense of purpose in his career-life. In Phase 3 (60 min), possible fields of study as well as action plans to help Dean move forward and obtain clarity regarding his tentatively chosen fields of study were finalised.

In line with Cardoso's (2015) belief in the need to educate clients about the goals of and the assignments associated with career counselling in order to strengthen the working alliance, whenever Dean or his parents asked me to "advise" him, I repeated my first question to him ("Who knows you better than anyone else in the world?") and encouraged him to reflect on his initial answers to the questions put to him. I scored the test (*MCM*) and identified career-life themes, while an external coder coded the data to ensure that the identified themes were in line with the data in order to enhance the reliability of the deductive process.

Mode of inquiry

Since there were no replicable studies, I implemented an explorative, descriptive, instrumental, single-case study approach. The study was "naturalistic" in that the participant was studied in a natural (real-life) context (Creswell, 2013).

Data-gathering instruments

Quantitative assessment

The *Maree Career Matrix* (*MCM*) (Maree, 2016c; Maree & Taylor, 2016a, 2016b). The *MCM* builds on Holland's interest theory and model and is related to (a) trait-and-factor theory, (b) developmental theory, and (c) social learning theory. The instrument was developed and standardised in South Africa between 2002 and 2015. It measures interests and self-estimates of confidence to follow certain careers. The *MCM* comprises a list of 152 occupations, each fitting one of 19 categories (with eight careers in each category). The psychometric properties of the *MCM* are considered good (Maree & Taylor, 2016a, 2016b). Rasch analysis showed that items in the *MCM* interest scales measured a single construct and all categories had reliability coefficients above .70. Moreover, test-retest reliability for career interests and self-estimates of confidence about aptitude exceeded .70 for all categories. Scores on the *MCM* provide career counsellors and their clients with a starting point for clarifying and discussing career profiles in greater depth.

Qualitative assessment

Developed from the developmental and the storied approaches, the *Career Interest Profile* (*CIP*) (Version 6) (Maree, 2017b) elicits information on career choice making over and above "traditional" (quantitative) information. The *CIP* reflects Adler (1958), Jung (1977), Savickas (2005), and other scholars' views on qualitative/narrative/storied (career) counselling. It was designed to extract clients' key career-life themes and advance reflection, reflexivity, and self-reflexivity (Hsiung, 2008) regarding core values and preferred interests to facilitate self-advising by clients in collaboration with the career counsellor. The *CIP* is consistent with the view that many micro- and meso-stories, autobiographies, and painstaking analysis of such information is needed to administer career counselling besides information obtained through quantitative questionnaires. The instrument was developed from the developmental, the storied (psychodynamic), and the differential perspective to elicit clients' career-life stories. It comprises four parts (see Table 1) purposefully designed to help learners and young adults identify their (a) key career-life themes, (b) career-related interests, issues and concerns, and (c) advice from within regarding how to turn "problems" and concerns into themes of hope that can promote their individual life projects. The *CIP* helps career counsellors listen for instead of to clients' career-life stories and story lines (Savickas, 2016; Welty, 1998). Dean was requested also to write an autobiographical narrative entitled "My life story" and to bring it with him on the morning of the intervention. Likewise, he was asked to obtain brief reports from his teachers on how they perceived him as well as from the person who (in his opinion) knew him best.

Rigour of the study

I repeatedly asked Dean to reflect on and let me know whether he was happy with the intervention (conducted in English, his mother tongue) and noted all his comments. The simultaneous use of qualitative and quantitative techniques promoted triangulation, and, in addition, sufficient information was obtained to enable replication of the case study in other settings. Crystallisation was promoted by asking different qualitative questions (Janesick, 2000).

Table 1. Description of the *CIP* (Maree, 2017a, 2017b).

Part	Information elicited	Associated processes (Savickas, 2011, 2015b)	Paradigm (Savickas, 2015b)
1	1a Family influences and work-related information	1b Guiding, advising	1c Career development
2	2a Five most and least preferred career preferences	2b Guiding, advising	2c Vocational guidance
3	3a Six career-choice questions	3b Educating, facilitating	3c Vocational guidance/ Career development
4	4a 15 career-life story narrative questions	4b Designing, healing	4c Life designing

Data analysis

Qualitative data

I followed the steps listed below to analyse the *CIP* data (Maree, 2013; Savickas, 2011):

a. words and phrases that might "uncover" Dean's central life themes were recorded,
b. Dean was repeatedly asked to reflect on his responses to questions,
c. repeated words and phrases were noted, and
d. Dean's own words were read back to him and he was urged to listen carefully to himself. In addition, he was prompted to say these words out loud to make sure that he experienced them as valid and trustworthy. Together we used Dean's responses to the question about his three earliest recollections in conjunction with his responses to other relevant questions in the *CIP* as a basis for examining and uncovering his key career-life themes. These themes were subsequently used to help him choose fields of study and decide on strategies to promote his career development, including his career adaptability (co-construction).

Quantitative data

The quantitative results were studied carefully to help us identify common interest patterns. The identified patterns were reflected on by Dean and me to see if they aligned with his career aspirations and the related responses from his interest profile (triangulation).

Ethical issues

Written informed consent from Dean's parents and assent from Dean were obtained for the analysis of the data and the reporting of the findings, which was approved by the University of Pretoria' Institutional Review Board. The research was conducted in Pretoria.

Outcomes

Outcomes of the quantitative part of the assessment

According to the *MCM* and Part 2 of the *CIP*, Dean's highest preferred interest categories were Arts (painting, sculpture, and decorating); Practical-creative and consumer science; Adventure, plants, animals and the environment; Medical and/or paramedical services; Word artistry; Marketing; Entrepreneurship; and Tourism. All of these fell in the *MCM*'s "Go for it!" quadrant. Categories in this quadrant indicate definite, clearly defined interests and confidence levels, which means that Dean not only displayed an interest but also believed he would succeed in careers associated with these categories.

Outcomes of the qualitative part of the assessment

Dean's responses to questions in Part 4 of the *CIP* appear below (due to space constraints, only selected responses are discussed).

"What are your greatest strengths?" (Dean's answers are reported verbatim with only very light editing to preserve the authenticity of the responses.)

"I am creative, adventure seeking, friendly, and accepting of others. I have a good sense of humour and I am curious."

"What are your areas for growth?" (Dean was reminded that his [perceived] areas for development or growth [formerly referred to as "weaknesses"] could and should be converted into strengths.

"Lack of self-discipline, unfocused, lazy. I do not like going out of my comfort zone even though I want to."

"How do other people (for instance, teachers and friends) see you?"

"Dean is a dreamer who knows there is a better, bigger life to be lived. He believes that his dreams may very well happen in the future."

"His biggest enemy may be himself – he has a cautious nature despite his drive for excellence in his creativity."

"He is an enigma – an unreadable, deep well of complex thoughts and emotions. Sometimes displays a slightly nihilistic way of looking at things."

"What do you value most?"

"Relationships, creating things, making a difference in the lives of people around me and closest to me, and being unique."

What do or did you enjoy most?

"Designing and being given freedom to make up my own mind; make choices myself."

What do or did you not enjoy?

"Having had to make new, close friends all the time."

"Enduring the monotony of high school."

"Whom did you admire or who were your role models when you were young and why?" (Dean's sense of who he is or wants to be or become)

"Vincent van Gogh. He was different, he had his own style, and he went against conventions."

"Diogenes. He was relaxed; went against society's accepted norms. He lived in a barrel in a performance-based society; he saw the superficiality in philosophy; spoke against them."

"Nelson Mandela. He was forgiving, he had an ability to focus on the future and what needs to be done to change the world."

"What are your favourite quotations?" (Dean's advice to himself.)

"It is not the years in the life that count, it is the life in your years." (*"Life is too short to spend time doing things that 'are not you'."*)

"An eye for an eye makes the world blind." (*"Doing whatever without having considered the long-term consequences is risky."*)

"Creativity is more important than logic." (*"It is more important to create or design than to wonder whether it makes 'logic sense'."*)

The most hurtful experiences in his youth that he doesn't want others to suffer or go through (his "deepest secrets"; what he had to suffer passively in early life and needs to undo actively now)

"I had only a few friends when I was young. At the end of Grade 5 my closest friends left to go to different countries. The insecurity that brought has always been a pattern in my life … people closest to me leaving me." (Moving around so often meant that he struggled to establish long-term friendships, leading to feelings of insecurity.)

"I home-schooled for a year. I struggled with being the only child at home."

"I always wanted to make things; like creating tortoises on paper. However, I was not allowed to do so." Recurring themes included his loneliness, his inability to establish long-term friendships, and denial of enjoyment he derived from being allowed to satisfy his need to be creative.

Dean's earliest recollections (Dean's central life themes [preoccupations] and his advice to himself regarding how to deal with these preoccupations).

(Interestingly, these recollections also feature in the "My life story" narrative. We analysed these recollections in the manner prescribed by Adler (1958), Hartung (2015), Maree (2013), Savickas (2011), and Watkins (1984).

Freedom to design leads to fulfilment

a. *"This happened at home, when I was between three and four years old. (SMILES HAPPILY). I was in my room, drawing on a piece of paper. (PUZZLED LOOK APPEARS IN HIS EYES). I do not know why I am telling you this story! I was drawing a tortoise on paper and subsequently making a paper tortoise."*

Performing own script pleases and rewards

b. *"I was five to six years old. My sisters and I performed a play at home. It was a play about some Christmas story. I was Father Christmas while my sisters were a reindeer and a mouse. We wrote the story for our parents, and we charged them to watch it!"* (Dean spontaneously reflected on his reflections – meta-reflection thus occurred.)

Unplanned "trip" satisfies curiosity but leads to confusion and insecurity

c. *"When I was four or five years old, our parents took us to a little country town where we walked around. At some stage I suddenly walked on and wandered off; walked around by myself. While it was exciting to explore the interesting little town, I remember feeling insecure and confused.* (SIGHS SOFTLY). *Someone eventually brought me back to my parents."*

I then asked Dean to suggest an inclusive heading for all three earliest recollections. After staring into the distance for a while, he replied: *"I learnt about the power of creativity, entertainment, curiosity … and peril."* Together, we crafted the following headline: *"Freedom and creativity satisfy and reward but can also be dangerous."* Dean's overall heading summarises his approach to life.

Analysing Dean's earliest recollections enabled us to uncover his central career-life themes. The first "story" reveals his deep-seated need to be given the freedom to express himself artistically. The tortoise (which carries its own "home" around) sheds light on his need to design structures but also his subconscious need to create something that will last for a long time. This experience sets the tone for his career-life story. He realises that, for him, satisfaction and fulfilment occur when he is given the opportunity to create and design something "timeless" (a key life theme).

The first verb Dean uses is "(draw[ing])". A bright, introverted child, he had always felt "different" from his peers, and, believing that he did not "fit in", he expressed himself by drawing and making things. Moreover, his father's work entailed the family moving around often and even spending time abroad. He consequently struggled to make friends and retain friendships. The action (drawing/designing/creating) indicated here is consistent with the themes depicted in Story 2 (performing) and in Story 3 (eagerness to explore). Dean displays a propensity for artistic expression and exploring. All three recollections are also consistent with the themes revealed by his responses to many of the *CIP* questions (e.g. his main strengths and his role models (creativity) and his loneliness (question about those things that hurt him most). Asked about his mentioning three animals, Dean replied: *"In addition to my love for freedom and creativity, I have always loved animals and the outdoors."*

Lastly, I asked Dean how he had experienced the intervention.

a. "What did you enjoy?"

"The conversations; talking about myself. Not being 'told' who I am but, instead, being assured that I am the expert on myself and that I will be helped to listen to my own advice" (Reflexivity).

b. "What did you not enjoy?"

"Sitting still for such a long time … I hate monotony!" (SMILES).

c. "Is there anything else that I need to know about you?"

"There is something about the creative freedom of art that I really enjoy; especially that it's not defined by set rules you have to follow slavishly. (LOOKS DOWN). *Inside, I am not as self-assured as some might think."*

Dean's answers to the questions asked in the *CIP* (coupled with his meta-reflections on his answers) shed light not only on his interests and other personality traits, on his career preferences and dislikes, but especially on his key career-life themes, on how he makes meaning of his life, and on his sense of purpose (Savickas, 2005). Together, we drew on the integrated data (co-construction) to distinguish certain fields of study that would not merely help him find a job and start his career journey but, especially, help him make meaning of his career-life and acquire a sense of purpose in his career-life.

We compiled a rough table in which we put the quantitative "results" (scores) side by side with the many qualitative "career stories" and themes. Dean then reflected repeatedly on the intersection or crosswalk between the "scores" and "career stories" to triangulate these two sets of data. A strong, positive association between the "stories" and "scores" emerged, as can be seen in Table 2.

Table 2. Integrated career-life themes and related study fields.

		Data sources	
Identified career-life themes	Associated study fields	Qualitative	Quantitative
A. Interest patterns	Information or Interior Design	*CIP*	*MCM*
1. Arts (painting, sculpture, and decorating)	Textile Design	"My life story"/ reflections/	
2 Practical-creative and consumer science	Architecture	meta-reflections	
3. Medical and/or paramedical services	Landscape Architecture	Earliest recollections	
4. Adventure, plants, animals and the environment	Interior Architecture		
	Construction Management		
5. Marketing	Industrial Design		
6. Word artistry	Veterinary Science		
7. Information Communication Technology	Photography		
	Film and Media Production		
	Digital Art (Game Design)		
	Performing and Visual Art (Game Design)		
B. Artistic inclination			
1. Creativity			
2. Sense of being different			
3. Dreamer			
4. Love for drawing			
5. Rejection of set routine			
6. Exceptional sense of humour			
C. Inquisitiveness	Journalism		*MCM*
1. Exploring nature	Law		
2. Curiosity			
3. Sense of fairness			
D. Unconventionality	See (A)	*CIP*, "My life story"	
1. Own style (uniqueness)			
2. Desire for "freedom"			
3. Hatred of monotony, "set rules"			
4. Self-sufficient			
5. Future orientation			
E. Insecurity			
1. Grew up protected			
2. Was often left alone ("*A common theme in my life*")			
3. Unwilling to leave comfort zone			
4. Moved around often, having to make new friends repeatedly			
5. Hesitant			
6. Overcautious			
F. Brightness		School reports; teacher comments	
1. Academic excellence			
2. "Unreadable"; deep thinker			

Dean could also consider enrolling on short courses in one or more of the following fields to help him make meaning of his career-life.

- Designing
- Film and Video Technology
- Song Writing
- Photography
- Creative Writing
- Copywriting
- Project Management and Marketing
- Tourism Management (eventually purchase his own lodge)

Near the end of the third session, I asked Dean to formulate his vision and mission statement to help him make meaning of his career (make sense of why he decided on a few possible fields of study) and inspire him to decide what his purpose in life was (Why do I live? Why am I here?). Somewhat hesitant at first, he eventually wrote:

> *"I will take time to ensure that I pursue one of the fields of study agreed upon that will enable me to help and inspire others who are creative and want freedom to just be who they really are, become who they want to become* (social meaning) *and in the process* (personal meaning) *meet my need to achieve, work on my own, be free, creative, secure, and not overly bound by monotonous rules.*

Follow-up

Wrapping up the third session, I asked Dean how he had experienced the intervention. He smilingly replied that he was still not "*100% sure about my career choice*" but that he had received sufficient information ("*from myself*") to help him make up his mind. Because he had not applied to any university, I said that his idea of perhaps taking a gap year to give him more time to decide on a university course made sense. He undertook to peruse the list of options we had agreed upon, do a thorough job analysis, and think about his options for finding a career that would meet his need to be creative, to inquire, to be unconventional, to deal with his deep-seated insecurity, and to be bold and daring. He was told that he could come back to me if and when he was ready and willing to do so.

Five months later, Dean informed me that although he was more or less certain about his preferred field of study, he had decided to take a gap year to allow him more time to make a considered decision. He was "*careful not to make an inappropriate decision*".

Discussion

The study discussed in this article investigated the provision of integrative career counselling to a creative adolescent who refused to "fit in". The following question guided the research: What is the impact of integrative career counselling using two recently developed questionnaires (one qualitative and one quantitative) on a creative adolescent in search of "non-traditional" career counselling? Essentially, the strategy comprised eliciting, interpreting, and integrating the research participant's "subjective" career-life stories and "objective" test results (Savickas, 2015a). The aim was to help him not only choose a career but also make meaning of his career life, find purpose, design a successful life, and make meaningful social contributions (Duarte, 2017; Maree, 2018; Savickas, 2013). The participant's response to the question as to why he was seeking career counselling confirms Arnett (2000) and Benjamin, Domene, and Landine's (2014) contention that young people's reasons for seeking career counselling revolve around their search for (career-life) identity.

The research study was a response to global calls for innovation in career counselling (Hughes, Law, & Meijers, 2017; Subich, 2011). The specific methodology used in the study yielded the envisaged outcomes. First, consistent with the first of the traditions associated with career construction theory (CCT) (the differential approach; vocational guidance), the *MCM* (quantitative) outcomes in conjunction with/triangulated with the information obtained from responses to Part 2 of the *CIP* elicited useful information about different careers and fields of study, including a number of preferred interest patterns, but also strong dislikes. Second, some of the questions in the *CIP* (e.g. on the narrative entitled "My life story", and questions about the participant's main strengths and areas for development) yielded useful qualitative information relating to the developmental approach; career education. Third, questions on his three biggest challenges when he was young, as well as his three earliest recollections, relate strongly to the third theoretical orientation of the CCI, namely the storied or narrative or psychodynamic approach.

Consistent with the views of Cochran (2011), McAdams (2013), and Savickas (2011), the qualitative part of the assessment succeeded in uncovering central life themes, such as the participant's deep-seated insecurity, as well as his need to "validate" his emergent worldview, and his need to be given the freedom to express himself artistically. Reading his career-life story, it became clear that his sense of insecurity, uncertainty, and hesitation in finalising his decision stemmed from a number of factors.

They included the fact that his family had moved around extensively resulting in his losing good friends and having to establish new relationships on a regular basis. Little wonder that he needed additional time to decide on the direction of his career-life journey. Reluctant to embark on a journey that might result in his having to change direction again, he would rather spend another year doing job analyses and trying to deal with his insecurity than run the risk of making an inappropriate choice. This part of the intervention confirms Lengelle, Meijers, and Hughes (2016) view that

> [n]arrative counselling (i.e. career construction) is founded on the idea that in order to survive and thrive on the labor market of the 21st century, individuals must reflexively construct their identities in a process of meaning making, where identity is co-constructed in the form of a narrative: a story about who one is that provides both meaning and direction (p. 60).

Analysis of the earliest recollections, too, yielded useful information (Hartung & Vess, 2016; Watkins, 1984) that confirmed Adler's (1958) contention that "in vocational guidance, first memories should be considered very important" (p. 245). Dean's preferred interests (gleaned from his responses to the questions posed from a "differential" orientation) suggested that he might be interested in artistic and design-related careers, for example careers such as architecture, landscape architecture, and interior architecture. His reflections confirmed his interest in creative endeavours. In addition, his uncertainty and insecurity when he attempted to satisfy his curiosity (Story 3) shed light on the reasons behind his decision to take a gap year. The "advice" he subconsciously offered himself (Savickas, 2009) seemed clear: you made an ill-advised decision that left you confused and insecure; therefore, you should guard against repeating the mistake. His decision to take a gap year rather than risk making an overhasty decision is consistent with this "advice" and confirmed his increased level of self-awareness.

The case study demonstrated the value of the methodology used to implement self- and career construction theory (Savickas, 2015a) in a one-on-one context. This could be seen in the participant's enhanced sense of self, his increased self-awareness, and his willingness to put his studies on hold for a year to avoid making an inappropriate career choice. This indicated also his increased career readiness and confirmed Arnett's (2000) view that societal and other changes can give rise to protracted identity uncertainty in adolescents. After the intervention, the participant could accept responsibility for his career-life story and adapt his future plans in accordance with his newfound self-insight (Savickas et al., 2009). Narrating his career-life story helped him identify key career-life themes and gain increased self-insight and acceptance of who he was – a creative, unconventional young man who was unwilling to be "boxed in" by others and circumstances beyond himself.

Novel aspects of the intervention

Two newly developed career counselling instruments were administered to elicit the participant's career-life story "to create a productive equilibrium between a constructivist approach ... and a 'traditional' [approach]" (Hughes et al., 2017, p. 133). The two instruments yielded complementary data that were integrated to help the participant clarify his career-life identity (Who am I?) and uncover central life themes such as his need to be given the freedom to express himself artistically as a precursor to facilitating authentic self- and career construction and, ultimately, life designing.

The approach described here shows how career construction theory can be converted into a practical intervention to help people choose careers and construct their career-lives. This was achieved through the construction, de-construction, re-construction, and co-construction of the participant's career-life story. Lengelle and Meijers (2014) (after Law, 1996) have described narrative career counselling as a four-stage process of "sensing, sifting, focusing, and understanding" (p. 67). Whereas, in Stage 1, emotions and cognitions are expressed, in Stage 2 a number of central career-life key themes are identified, after which (in Stage 3) a particular theme (in this instance, the participant's inability to reframe the disjunction caused by the repeated disruption of his interpersonal relationships) is identified that needs to be focussed on. In Stage 4, a "new" story, built on respect and dignity, is crafted. The approach is consistent with McAdams and Cox's (2010) view that people as the "authors" of their narrative identities are capable of reflecting themselves as "actors" with unique characteristics (as uncovered by the narration of their career-life stories) but also as "agents" with a number of plans and goals for the future. Summarised, the approach and intervention described here provides a framework for understanding and addressing the career counselling needs of an "unconventional" participant and probably of other young people as well – in line with other research pointing to the value of career construction counselling for adolescents (Hartung, 2015).

Guidance for counsellors intending to conduct this type of intervention

First, understanding and accepting the rationale for this approach to career counselling is crucial as is, second, training in the procedure/strategy. Third, the number of sessions is negotiable. Three or four sessions spread over a number of weeks should be sufficient to complete the entire intervention (unless, of course, the parents wish it to be concluded in one day). Fourth, minimal "advice" should be given to clients – rather, they should be allowed to make decisions on their own, under the watchful eye of the counsellor. Lastly, support for clients who are not so used to reflecting in the way demonstrated in this article or responding so directly and eloquently to the questions asked include giving them adequate time for reflecting on and responding to their questions and clarifying their own questions and responses in a meticulous manner. Since reflection and meta-reflection allow insights, clients should be guided to reflect and reflect on their own reflections (Rogers, 1952).

Limitations

Although care was taken to ensure rigour of the research, I realise that the insights may be coloured to some extent by my own worldview. As the principal data collection and analysis "instrument" (Merriam, 2009), I had to rely largely on my own feelings, observations, and proficiencies (and, to an extent, on the proficiencies of the external coder). Moreover, the language of the young person and ability to engage in meta-reflection of the participant was exceedingly high.

Recommendations for future research

Future research should focus on multiple case studies, quantitative studies, and more longitudinal research. Tracing the long-term progress of clients is needed as is determining the value of the approach for diverse clients in individual as well as group-based contexts. Lastly, consideration should be given to using auto-ethnography as a conceptual framework for illustrative case studies that demonstrate the approach advocated here.

Conclusion

The research reported demonstrated the value of addressing the particular participant's career counselling needs in an integrated manner. The holistic approach followed in the intervention blended his "career and personal-emotional issues" and enabled the career counsellor to focus not only on his "problems" but also on helping him "develop [a] more resilient, open attitude" (Lee & Johnston, 2001, p. 184). The career construction, qualitative-cum-quantitative approach described in this article offered a viable theoretical and practical strategy for achieving these goals in the case of the research participant (a creative young man).

Disclosure statement

No potential conflict of interest was reported by the author.

ORCID

Jacobus Gideon Maree http://orcid.org/0000-0002-9492-8445

References

Adler, A. (1958). *What life should mean to you.* New York: Capricorn.

Arnett, J. J. (2000). Emerging adulthood: A theory of development from the late teens through the twenties. *American Psychologist, 55,* 469–480.

Benjamin, A., Domene, J., & Landine, K. (2014). Constructing the future in the liminal spaces between adolescence and adulthood: Responsibilities, careers, and social contexts. *The Canadian Journal of Career Development, 13*(1), 2014.

Bimrose, J., & Hearne, L. (2012). Resilience and career adaptability: Qualitative studies of adult career counselling. *Journal of Vocational Behavior, 81,* 338–344. doi:10.1016/j.jvb.2012.08.002

Blustein, D. L. (2006). *The psychology of working: A new perspective for career development, counseling, and public policy.* Mahwah, NJ: Lawrence Erlbaum.

Cardoso, P. (2015). Integrating life-design counseling and psychotherapy: Possibilities and practices. *The Career Development Quarterly, 64,* 49–63.

Cochran, L. (2011). The promise of narrative career counseling. In K. Maree (Ed.), *Shaping the story – a guide to facilitating narrative counselling* (pp. 7–19). Rotterdam: Sense.

Creswell, J. W. (2013). *Qualitative inquiry and research design. Choosing among five approaches* (3rd ed.). Thousand Oaks, CA: Sage.

Di Fabio, A., & Maree, J. G. (2013). Effectiveness of the career interest profile. *Journal of Employment Counseling, 50,* 110–123.

Doyle, A. (2017). *How often do people change jobs?* Retrieved from https://www.thebalance.com/how-often-do-people-change-jobs-2060467\

Duarte, M. E. (2017). *Sustainable decent work.* Invited public lecture at University of Pretoria. Pretoria: Pretoria University Printers.

Duffy, R. D., & Dik, B. J. (2009). Beyond the self: External influences in the career development process. *The Career Development Quarterly, 58,* 29–43.

Ebberwein, C. K., Krieshok, T. S., Ulven, J. C., & Prosser, E. C. (2004). Voices in transition: Lessons on career adaptability. *The Career Development Quarterly, 52,* 292–308.

Guichard, J. (2009). Self-constructing. *Journal of Vocational Behavior, 75,* 251–258.

Gyarmathy, E., & Senior, J. (2018). The creative being and being creative: Human and machine neural networks. In B. Wallace, D. Sisk, & J. Senior (Eds.), *Handbook on gifted and talented education* (pp. 538–552). London: Sage.

Hartung, P. J. (2011). Career construction: Principles and practice. In K. Maree (Ed.), *Shaping the story: A guide to facilitating narrative counselling* (pp. 103–120). Rotterdam: Sense.

Hartung, P. J. (2015). Life design in childhood: Antecedents and advancement. In L. Nota & J. Rossier (Eds.), *Handbook of life design: From practice to theory, and from theory to practice* (pp. 89–101). Göttingen: Hogrefe.

Hartung, P. J., & Santili, S. (2018). My career story: Description and initial validity evidence. *Journal of Career Assessment, 26* (2), 308–321.

Hartung, P. J., & Vess, L. (2016). Critical moments in career construction counseling. *Journal of Vocational Behavior, 97,* 31–39.

Hsiung, P. C. (2008). Teaching reflexivity in qualitative interviewing. *Teaching Sociology, 36,* 211–226. Retrieved from http://www.biomedcentral.com/1471-2288/11/100

Hughes, D., Law, B., & Meijers, F. (2017). New school for the old school: Career guidance and counselling in education. *British Journal of Guidance & Counselling, 45*(2), 133–137. doi:10.1080/03069885.2017.1294863

Janesick, V. J. (2000). The choreography of qualitative research. In N. K. Denzin & Y. S. Lincoln (Eds.), *Handbook of qualitative research* (2nd ed., pp. 390–396). London: Sage.

Jung, C. G. (1977). *Two essays on analytical psychology*. Princeton, NJ: Princeton University Press.

Krieshok, T. S., Black, M. D., & McKay, R. A. (2009). Career decision making: The limits of rationality and the abundance of non-conscious processes. *Journal of Vocational Behavior, 75*, 275–290.

Krumboltz, J. D., & Chan, A. (2005). Professional issues in vocational psychology. In W. Walsh & M. L. Savickas (Eds.), *Handbook of vocational psychology* (3rd ed., pp. 347–370). Mahwah, NJ: Lawrence Erlbaum.

LaPointe, K. (2010). Narrating career, positioning identity: Career identity as a narrative practice. *Journal of Vocational Behavior, 77*, 1–9.

Law, B. (1996). Careers education in a curriculum. In A. G. Watts, B. Law, J. Killeen, J. M. Kidd, & R. Hawthorne (Eds.), *Rethinking careers education and guidance: Theory, policy and practice* (pp. 210–232). London: Routledge.

Lee, F. K., & Johnston, J. A. (2001). Innovations in career counseling. *Journal of Career Development, 27*(3), 177–185.

Lengelle, R., & Meijers, F. (2014). Narrative identity: Writing the self in career learning. *British Journal of Guidance and Counselling, 42*, 52–72.

Lengelle, R., Meijers, F., & Hughes, D. (2016). Creative writing for life design: Reflexivity, metaphor and change processes through narrative. *Journal of Vocational Behavior, 97*, 60–67.

Maree, J. G. (2013). *Counselling for career construction. Connecting life themes to construct life portraits: Turning pain into hope*. Rotterdam: Sense.

Maree, J. G. (2015). Research on life design in (South) Africa: A qualitative analysis. *South African Journal of Psychology, 45*, 332–348.

Maree, J. G. (2016a). Career construction counseling with a mid-career black man. *The Career Development Quarterly, 64*, 20–34.

Maree, J. G. (2016b). Using interpersonal process during career construction counselling to promote reflexivity and expedite change. *Journal of Vocational Behavior, 97*, 22–30.

Maree, J. G. (2016c). *Maree Career Matrix (MCM)*. Randburg: JvR Psychometrics.

Maree, J. G. (2017a). *The Career Interest Profile (CIP) (version 6): Obtaining, qualitatively, a profile of personal career-life themes and interests*. Randburg: JvR Psychometrics.

Maree, J. G. (2017b). *Career interest profile (version 5)*. Randburg: JvR Psychometrics.

Maree, J. G. (2018). Contextualisation as a determining factor for career counselling throughout the world. In J. A. Athanasou & H. N. Perera (Eds.), *International handbook of career guidance* (2nd ed.). New York: Springer.

Maree, J. G., & Taylor, N. (2016a). Development of the *Maree Career Matrix*: A new interest inventory. *South African Journal of Psychology, 46*(4), 462–476.

Maree, J. G., & Taylor, N. (2016b). *Manual for the Maree Career Matrix (MCM)*. Randburg, SA: JvR Psychometrics.

Masten, A. (2014). Global perspectives on resilience in children and youth. *Child Development, 85*(1), 6–20.

McAdams, D. P. (2013). The psychological self as actor, agent, and author. *Perspectives on Psychological Science, 8*(3), 272–295.

McAdams, D. P., & Cox, K. S. (2010). Self and identity across the life span. In R. Lerner, A. Freund, & M. Lamb (Eds.), *Handbook of life span development* (Vol. 2, pp. 158–207). New York: Wiley.

McMahon, M., & Watson, M. (Eds.). (2015). *Career assessment: Qualitative approaches*. Rotterdam: Sense.

Merriam, S. B. (2009). *Qualitative research and case study applications in education: Revised and expanded from case study research in education*. San Francisco, CA: Wiley.

Pfeiffer, S. I. (2015). *Essentials of gifted assessment*. Hoboken, NJ: Wiley.

Pryor, R. (2008). Does career counselling matter? A personal reflection. *Australian Journal of Career Development, 17*(2), 55–58.

Reid, R., & West, L. (2016). Negotiating professional and personal biographies in a liquid world: Creating space for reflexive innovation in career counselling. *British Journal of Guidance & Counselling, 44*(5), 562–575. doi:10.1080/03069885.2016.1145014

Rochat, S., Masdonati, J., & Dauwalder, J.-P. (2017). Determining career resilience. In J. G. Maree (Ed.), *Psychology of career adaptability, employability, and resilience* (pp. 125–144). New York: Springer.

Rogers, C. R. (1952). *Client-centered therapy*. Boston, MA: Houghton Mifflin.

Savickas, M. L. (2005). The theory and practice of career construction. In S. Brown & R. W. Lent (Eds.), *Career development and counseling: Putting theory and research to work* (pp. 42–70). New York: Wiley.

Savickas, M. L. (2009). Career-style counselling. In T. J. Sweeney (Ed.), *Adlerian counselling and psychotherapy: A practitioner's approach* (5th ed., pp. 183–207). New York: Routledge.

Savickas, M. L. (2011). *Career counseling*. Washington, DC: American Psychological Association.

Savickas, M. L. (2013). The theory and practice of career construction. In S. D. Brown & R. W. Lent (Eds.), *Career development and counseling: Putting theory and research to work* (2nd ed., pp. 147–186). Hoboken, NJ: Wiley.

Savickas, M. L. (2015a). *Life-design counselling manual*. Rootstown, OH: (n.p.).

Savickas, M. L. (2015b). Career counselling paradigms: Guiding, developing, and designing. In P. Hartung, M. Savickas, & W. Walsh (Eds.), *The APA handbook of career intervention* (Vol. 1, pp. 129–143). Washington, DC: APA Books.

Savickas, M. L. (2016). Reflection and reflexivity during life-design interventions: Comments on career construction counseling. *Journal of Vocational Behavior, 97*, 84–89.
Savickas, M. L., Nota, L., Rossier, J., Dauwalder, J.-P., Duarte, M. E., Guichard, J., ... Van Vianen, A. E. M. (2009). Life designing: A paradigm for career construction in the 21st century. *Journal of Vocational Behavior, 75*, 239–250.
Sliep, Y. (2007). Waving a learning community by the telling, deconstructing and retelling of life stories. In J. G. Maree (Ed.), *Shaping the story* (pp. 138–151). Pretoria: Van Schaik.
Subich, L. M. (2011, August). *Tracing the evolution of career counseling theory.* Paper read at the 119th annual meeting of the American Psychological Association, Washington, DC.
Van Vianen, A. E. M., De Pater, I. E., & Preenen, P. T. Y. (2009). Adaptable careers: Maximizing less and exploring more. *The Career Development Quarterly, 57*(2), 298–309.
Watkins, C. E. Jr. (1984). Using early recollections in career counseling. *Vocational Guidance Quarterly, 32*, 271–276.
Watson, M. B. (2004). Post-modern (narrative) career counselling and education. *Perspectives in Education, 22*, 169–170.
Welty, E. (1998). *One writer's beginnings.* Cambridge, MA: Harvard University Press.
Winnicott, D. W. (1964). *The child, the family and the outside world.* Cambridge, MA: Perseus.

The philosophy of self-care, individuation and psychodrama: exploring creative means to encountering the "unknown other" in self

Barbara A. Schellhammer

ABSTRACT

In this article I investigate creative means to encounter otherness in oneself as a prerequisite for intercultural education. Firstly, I look at ancient Greek philosophy and the concept of self-care. Secondly, I draw from C. G. Jung's individuation as a process of incorporating shadow parts in the self and thirdly I explore psychodramatic methods. The article is concluded with the example of a concrete application of the "Inner Team" model in a workshop on intercultural competence for caregivers in the context of elderly care.

Introduction

I have been working in the field of conflict resolution, restorative justice and peace building as a philosopher and social worker for a long time. In particular, I have dealt with conflicts that occur when people from diverse cultural backgrounds have to get along with each other. Teaching "intercultural education" for working professionals, my intuition gained momentum that *knowing* about a foreign culture and gaining *competencies* are not enough to be able to openly engage with otherness: People may know a lot about another culture and they may have learned many communication tools, but they still get angry if the other person is not behaving in a way they anticipated.

Offering professional training programs on cross-cultural skills is still a growing field in Germany (Dreyer & Hößler, 2011; Mecheril, 2013; Weidemann, Straub, & Nothnagel, 2010). Many universities and private companies offer courses and workshops promising to help people to effectively deal with differences. These offerings often rely on "experts" to teach Germans about cultural peculiarities using specific typologies to get a better grasp of what seems alien by fitting the unknown into familiar categories. Recently I delivered a workshop in a residential home for the elderly in Munich. The group of participants, a team of caregivers who have been working together for several years, came from different regions in Europe, some were Muslims, others Christians, Baha'i or agnostics. When I was asking the group for their expectations of the workshop, one person said that she would like to know more about Muslims, how they think and "what makes them tick". I was quite surprised by this comment as it dawned on me that it may never have occurred to her to actually approach and engage with one of her Muslim colleagues directly. It seems to be much more comfortable and less risky to have somebody else explain foreign customs and beliefs. Being taught about a different culture helps to ease the uncomfortable discrepancy; it sorts the "alien otherness" into one's own knowledge system. As Waldenfels (1990) has explained, it takes away the awkward or frightening 'sting' of the unknown other.

In times of worldwide migration movements and a continuing influx of refugees seeking asylum in Europe, intercultural training and other educational efforts to equip people with "intercultural competencies" will most likely continue to boom. However, I would argue that to learn just one-sidedly how to manage the "strangeness *of the stranger*" is not enough to create common ground and a reliable base for intercultural dialogue and integration. Rather, we ought to develop what I call "alien-ability" (*Fremdheitsfähigkeit*) by encountering *our own* discomfort and fear, by engaging with the "stranger *within us*". Instead of trying to "fix" and "integrate" the other, we ought to turn to ourselves and honestly face and be attentive to what we experience.

This thought is, however, by far, not new. In philosophy as well as in psychology several scholars have emphasized the concept and practice of *self-care* (Greek: *epimeleia heautou*) as a prerequisite for an ethical and meaningful encounter with the other. Self-care practices focus on the importance of reflecting on experiences that exceed a primarily rational approach of the Delphic "know thyself" (Greek: *gnothi seauton*). Here, *creative methods* become important, because they are able to take into account the fact that we always experience otherness on several levels with our body, mind and spirit. In Western philosophy, especially during the Enlightenment, we lost this holistic approach of engaging with ourselves and the world around us.[1] Although it may be uncomfortable for some philosophers and scientists who think that people can grasp and handle the peculiarities of life through rational concepts and universal formulas, it is essential to enter the less predictable realm of multi-level dialogue. Elberfeld (2017b, p. 440) argued that we have to be courageous enough to venture out into "philosophical taboo-zones" if we want to practice philosophy in a globalizing world. One of these "unthinkable" and largely repressed zones deal with the unconscious, an area on which philosophy ought to engage with psychology and psychoanalysis. Conversely, creative methods in guidance and counselling may also benefit from a wide variety of "spiritual exercises" practiced in ancient philosophy (Foucault, 2015; Gödde & Zirfas, 2016; Hadot, 1991; Mortari, 2016). Hadot (1991) claimed that these exercises transform the whole being. Interpreting Greco-Roman texts, he argues that philosophy is best pursued in actual dialogue as it also pursues *therapeutic* goals (see also Cushman, 1958; Elberfeld, 2017b, p. 395; Foucault, 2015, p. 75; Nussbaum, 1994).

In the following, I would like to (1) present some key themes regarding the *philosophy of self-care* as therapy and creative practice. (2) I draw from Jung's *process of individuation*, particularly emphasizing venturing into our "shadow" in order to tap into its vast source of inspiration and creativity. In (3) I focus on the creative method of drama-therapy, particularly on Moreno's *psychodrama* as an experiential way to explore and develop oneself. Lastly (4), in order to concretize the application of this method, I refer to my experience of using the "Inner Team" model (Schulz von Thun, 2003). Whereas (1) and (2) lay the theoretical foundation and overall rational for the importance of self-care, (3) and (4) present concrete methods that attest to the importance of artistic expression, symbolic forms of communication and embodied knowing.

The philosophy of self-care as therapy and creative practice

In her book *Therapy of Desire* Nussbaum (1994, p. 3) maintained that "Hellenistic philosophical schools in Greece and Rome – Epicureans, Skeptics, and Stoics – all conceived of philosophy as a way of addressing the most painful problems of human life". She goes on to explain:

> They saw the philosopher as a compassionate physician whose arts could heal many pervasive types of human suffering. They practiced philosophy not as a detached intellectual technique dedicated to the display of cleverness but as an immersed and worldly art of grappling with human misery. They focused their attention, in consequence, on issues of daily and urgent human significance – the fear of death, love and sexuality, anger and aggression – issues that are sometimes avoided as embarrassingly messy and personal by the more detached varieties of philosophy. (Nussbaum 1994, p. 3)

Before Nussbaum, Cushman (1958, p. xv) similarly explained that Plato regarded philosophy as a way of life that helps people to cope with chaos and confusion. "Its root impulse is man in trouble with unresolved contradiction in his spirit, a contradiction which manifests itself in calamitous social derangements. As called forth by a destructive distortion in human life and experience, philosophy offers itself as a therapy". Socrates described thinking as a dialogical activity that occurs between me and myself, as an inner dialogue. A person who lives responsively is somebody who is able to listen and respond to oneself, creating inner harmony and peace. In *The Life of the Mind* Hannah Arendt (1978, p. 185) stressed that Socrates's quest for personal congruency is directly linked with morality.

As long as we pay attention to what is happening inside of us and we are able to *respond* to it, we are less likely to simply react and "snap" at things that trigger us on the outside. Thus it is less important to be in harmony with the people around me and more important to speak the "truth" as I *experience* it.[2] Quite the contrary is happening for people who experience personal uncertainties and who struggle within as they try to solicit recognition by pleasing the people around them (Satir, 1998). Similarly, Seneca (1786, p. 21) wrote in his *Moral Letters to Lucilius*:

> These, my Lucilius, are the things which I would have you treasure up in your mind, that you may despise the vain pleasure, that accrues from the approbation of the world. Many praise thee: but are you satisfied with yourself, if you are what they take you for and applaud? Let your goodness be approved within.

Referring to Epicurus, Seneca uses the *metaphor of a theatre* for what is going on in a person: "I write to the many, but to you alone [...], for we are to each other a theatre large enough" (Seneca, 1786, p. 21). In antiquity, people used a number of creative practices to cultivate the "inner theatre", the "arts of the self" and the "aesthetics of existence" (Foucault, 2015, p. 60; Foucault, 2007). All of them employed experiential techniques which encouraged a person to work on him or herself like on a piece of art. The chief goal of this lifelong work was to gain the ability to govern oneself instead of being ruled by one's passions, appetites and emotions. The "art of living" manifested itself in the freedom of oneself as *sine qua non* for ethical conduct.

Following Socrates, Plato and Aristotle, the Greek philosophy believes strongly in the *rational capacity* of human beings. Based on the *knowledge* of the "good life" being the ultimate goal to strive for, we ought to practice mastering ourselves. It is our *thinking* that should control irrational impulses. Foucault (2015, p. 75) mentioned that the term *pathos* (perceived as the malfunction of the body or an involuntary slip of the soul) is central for ancient philosophy as well as for therapy and medicine. Self-care practices should address this "dysfunction" through *paideia* (education), which ought to direct people towards the ultimate "idea of the good".

However, with Nietzsche and Freud, we must accept that we are never fully in charge, we are not the "masters of our own house". Waldenfels (2016, p. 42) also used the term *pathos* to describe something that happens to us that we can never fully control or "fix". In such situations, we experience something beyond comprehension and order, something that is *alien* to us – although it is part of who we are; we are *patients* (from Latin *patiens*, to suffer), not actors. All we can do is to *respond* to what is happening, knowing that our response depends on *what we are responding to*. What we say, is not solely determined by us, but also through our responding to something or somebody else. What we respond to exceeds what we answer. Waldenfels (1997, p. 53) wrote: "We encounter the paradox of a creative response through giving what we don't have." It was not before the eighteenth, nineteenth and mostly twentieth century that the unknown, stranger or alien started penetrating the core of rationality (Waldenfels, 1997, p. 17).[3]

This was also the time when the arts and aesthetic practices, especially the visual arts, began playing a more significant role in philosophy (Elberfeld, 2017a, p. 173). Thus, practices of self-care widened their repertoire: Not just our mind ought to be engaged in self-reflective, spiritual exercises, also our body and "irrational" phenomena became part of self-exploration and self-transformation. Bodily sensations help us to understand ourselves and our relationship to the world around us.[4] Creative practices open a pathway to our embodied knowing that is otherwise often suppressed by our inclination to explain things rationally. In the process of expressing oneself bodily, "we view the body not as the visible, touchable and sentient physical body but first and foremost as our capacity to see, touch, sense" (Fuchs, 2011, p. 91).

One way to discover the unknown other in our self is through *theatrical expression*: We act out what we experience in our inner drama. Waldenfels (2010, p. 241) referred to the "theatre as the showground of the alien". However, the performance of the alien is a paradox: It affects us before we even know it. We become aware of something that we cannot fathom. It shows itself as *pathos* and through its play, it plays with us – from ancient times this play has been part of the effects of drama and tragedy. In the theatre of ancient Greece, the stage was called "*skene*" (Greek for "tent" or "hut") which means "shadow-place" (Waldenfels, 2010, p. 244). The actors would go to this back-stage or "hidden stage" to change their masks and clothes. In some scenes, the actors would speak or make noises from this hiding place in the back and leave the audience to themselves to make sense of what was going on. Like a whispering, we realise something that is "absence in presence", that is "unperceived in the perceived" (Fuchs, 2011, p. 101). It is this tension that ties us to our seats: "One does not know something and does not want to know it; one does not see something and does not want to see it" (Waldenfels 2010).

Jung relates to the metaphor of the theatre using the term *persona* as a mask which we use to impress others and to hide the true nature of ourselves (Jacobi, 1984, p. 36). Part of our true nature lives in the "shadow-place" hiding at the "backstage". Without going there and attuning ourselves to what is going on in this trembling "field of dark perception" (Kant, 1977, p. 419), we tend to reject and despise others. This brings me to me to my second point, the process of individuation as a self-care practice that seeks to explore and develop the creative sources in our shadow to become more of who we are.

Individuation as a pathway to the creative sources in our shadow

> In his book, *The Stranger within Us*, Gruen (2014) encourages us to embrace what we fear, dislike and even hate about us. We suppress what we learned to be ashamed of when we were small children (Gruen, 2014, p. 7). The source of our violence and cruelty towards others stems from an anxiety which is deeply rooted in ourselves, in parts that belong to us, but became alien (Gruen, 2014, p. 18). "Strangely, the foreigner lives within us", writes Kristeva (1991, p. 1), "he is the hidden face of our identity, the space that wrecks our abode, the time in which understanding and affinity founder. By recognizing him within ourselves, we are spared detesting him in himself".

The process of individuation seeks to explore the alien shadow regions of our self to get back what we once lost in order to become more complete or whole. Jacobi (1983, pp. 117–118) explained, that individuation does not aim at perfectionism, but at helping a person to develop towards his or her true being, "and not to hide behind the ideal mask which is so easily mistaken for his true essence, although by so doing he makes it all the more likely that the evil repressed behind it will break out". The more we try to become perfect, the greater the chances are of subjugating parts of us that represent failure. The harder we try to control and suspend these parts, the likelier it gets, that they will burst out and make us feel miserable. This results in endless inner fights that rob us energy, we act angry and agitated with the people around us.

For Jung, the creative resources to grow and develop the self in its unique way rest, oddly enough, in what we consider as deficient or inadequate. To be whole means to be full of contradictions, ambiguities and paradoxes (Jung, 1933, p. 131). It is, however, a scary endeavour to confront our past injuries, disappointments, and rejections, because we are afraid of feeling the pain and helplessness that we felt when we were little.[5] And yet, Jung encourages us to face our shadow by pointing out that our creative potential lies not in perfection, but in difference:

> There is no light without shadow and no psychic wholeness without imperfection. To round itself out, life calls not for perfection but for completeness; and for this the "thorn in the flesh" is needed, the suffering of defects without which there is no progress and no ascent. (Jung, in Jacobi, 1983, p. 119)

In Jungian terms, the shadow resembles the antithesis of the persona, our adjustable masks through which we try to find recognition by adapting and conforming to social expectations. It may even happen, that we habitually start identifying with one of our masks which results in self-loss through alienation. The more we live our persona, the stronger our shadow grows. The shadow stands in sharp contrast to the conscious ego, it is rebellious and full of energy. Instead of repressing that energy, individuation aims at drawing from it to create inner balance. For Jung, our psychological life balance rests on a continuous tension between opposing counterparts which tend to fall into problematic exaggerations, if we avoid or fight parts of us that are needed to cultivate stability. Jacobi explained:

> Since the psyche is built on polar opposites which complement each other, but also stand in glaring contradiction to each other, it must of its very nature exist in a state of tension and suffer this. One can even say that the confrontation with these opposites lies at the heart of the individuation process. (Jacobi, 1983, p. 120)

Jung found what he calls "natural law of self-regulating opposites' in Heraclitus" principle of *enantiodromia*, the tendency of everything to transform itself into its opposite in the process of becoming (Jacobi, 1984, p. 58). What appears to the conscious has a corresponding opposite principle that dwells in the unconscious. However, not the conversion of a perceived negative trait in its opposite, not the negation of differences, but rather the preservation of its inherent value or quality and its sincere appreciation is the goal to aim for. "To confront a person with his shadow is to show him his own light", Jung (in Jacobi, 1983, p. 122) stated and went on to say:

> Anyone who perceives his shadow and his light simultaneously sees himself from two sides and thus gets in the middle. He knows that the world consists of darkness and light. I can master their polarity only by freeing myself from them by contemplating both, and so reaching a middle position. Only there I am no longer at the mercy of the opposites. (Jung in: Jacobi, 1983, p. 122)

Yet, to become aware and to honestly relate to one's shadow is not only important to gain inner balance and congruence, but also to avoid dreadful projections and intergenerational transmissions of hatred and antagonisms. In projections, we fight everything we don't want to see and dislike in ourselves in the outside world. This combat shapes our personal and collective identity and reinforces the battle lines between ourselves and others and between our conscious ego and our unconscious shadow. In *The "Others" within Us* the Israeli psychologist Bar-On (2001) showed how the Israeli identity transitioned from a monolithic phase (where the "other" and the "self" seemed black and white or evil and good), through the disintegration of the monolithic self, to the first signs of internal dialogue accepting and integrating the conflicting parts of identity. A key factor in this process was to not only recognize and attend to the victim in oneself, but also to the perpetrator and to move toward reconciliation between both of them.

Similar to Jung, Bar-On realised that a person whose identity starts crumbling and "softening" by becoming aware of his or her inner contradictions, is considered to be weak and fragile. Yet, it is this very "weakness" which enables a person to encounter otherness, it is the precondition for the development of "alien-ability".[6] However, Jung cautions that when making people aware of their dark sides, one has to be prepared to deal with great resistances as they cannot bear to accept the shadow as part of themselves. They are afraid of seeing the arduously erected structure of their conscious self-collapse (Jacobi, 1984, p. 115). Therefore, Bar-On (2001, p. 22) noted, "the urge for the monolithic phase never really vanishes".

We become aware of our personal unconscious through emotionally charged *complexes* and we realise our collective unconscious through *archetypes* (Jung, 1976, p. 12).[7] Both complexes and archetypes, present themselves in *symbolic forms* that are often incomprehensible for our conscious mind. Thus, we have to find other ways to decipher their messages: We have to learn to respond to bodily reactions with our body, and to emotional sensations with emotions. Exploring our shadow with our whole being, we will tap into a deeper knowledge system. Here, creative methods are essential as they allow for a dialogue with symbolic forms and hidden meanings. Since "good theatre is always archetype"[8] (Scategni, 2002, p. x), psychodrama seems to be the most suitable way to explore unconscious truths by acting out what we experience.

Psychodrama and the importance of experience

The originator of the psychodrama, Jacob Levi Moreno, never met Jung, although they lived almost at the same time (Moreno 1889–1974 and Jung 1875–1961). Many sharp differences divide the two men in their approach to healing and psychology. However, one could also argue, that they were complementing each other like positive opposites. Therefore, it is not surprising, that Scategni (2002, p. 14) pointed out:

> In fact, when analysts with Jungian training applied psychodramatic techniques, these techniques were the concrete expression of their reciprocal interest in Jung and Moreno as well as the evidence that there was a developing sense that their different typologies were complementary.

Jung and Moreno sided in their harsh criticism of Freud's bias for the natural sciences, biologism and positivism. Both emphasized the religious and spiritual yearnings of human beings and claimed that it is impossible to illuminate and explain intrapersonal dynamics without supposedly "irrational" truths (Buer, 1989, p. 143). Also, both of them saw the unconscious as a reservoir of creative energy, not as a destructive force as Freud did. During his second year of studying medicine, Moreno was invited by Professor Wagner, a well-known psychoanalyst in Vienna, to join his research staff. Here, he also met Freud personally. Moreno (1953, pp. xxvii–xxviii) wrote about this experience:

> I did not think that a great healer and therapist would look and act the way Wagner and Freud did. I visualized the healer as a spontaneous-creative protagonist in the midst of the group. My concept of the physician as a healer, and that of theirs were very far apart. To my mind, persons like Jesus, Buddha, Socrates and Gandhi were doctors and healers; for Freud they were probably patients. [...] Freud's psychoanalysis was the natural opponent of play techniques and play psychotherapy, except as they yielded "material" for analysis.

In this quote two of the key features of the psychodrama are clearly articulated: *spontaneous-creative play* and the *group setting*. Moreno (1953, p. 81) defined the psychodramatic method "as the science which explores the 'truth' by dramatic methods". Moreover, he explains that it employs mainly five instruments: "the stage, the subject or actor [the protagonist], the director [the facilitator of the psychodrama], the staff of therapeutic aids or auxiliary egos, and the audience" (Moreno, 1953, pp. 81–82). Although Moreno clearly refers to classical forms of theatre (Petzold, 1978, pp. 13–38), for his "impromptu theatre" he proclaims the ultimate freedom of expression, the "art of the moment", instead of following a predefined screenplay. The stage "provides the actor with a living space which is multi-dimensional and flexible to the maximum" (Moreno, 1953, p. 82). Moreno argued that in actual life, people find themselves often restrained and therefore out of balance. On the stage, however, they may find their equilibrium again "due to its methodology of freedom – freedom of unbearable stress and freedom for experience and expression" (Moreno, 1953, p. 82). They become the ultimate, "God-like" creators of their own lives again.

In a psychodramatic play, "auxiliary egos", members of the group who play various roles in a particular scene, could play parts of the protagonist's[9] inner self. What used to be confusing and emotionally draining becomes clearer. By naming parts, assigning roles and listening to their arguments, the protagonist realises that his or her identity is not set in stone, rather, it is dialogical and dynamic. Moreover, experiencing different parts of oneself helps to escape horrific "I-prisons" (Hermans & Hermans-Konopka, 2010, p. 197), constraining perceptions of oneself, often accompanied by very strong and sometimes overpowering emotions.

Putting Jung's enantiodromic principle in psychodramatic practice, people are able to play and actually experience their "other side", shadow-parts they once lost – parts, which they would need to feel and act in balance. They can step into the "stranger in themselves" and act out what he or she stands for or struggles with. Slipping into the antagonist's role helps to understand their positive intention, which is essential in order to integrate them as valuable members of their own inner drama. Realising that some of the frightening shadow parts are actually needed to become "whole" again helps to "reframe" (redefine and reimagine) them, it helps to see them in a new, more positive light. Through role-playing protagonists can practice "being" that new, more integrated self.

In psychodrama, multidimensional *experiences* and *creative processes* are key factors for the development or healing process of the self. A mere rational understanding of inner dynamics or the explanation of certain laws is not enough. Also, our language is often not able to capture what we experience. Moreno (1953, pp. 86–87) explained:

> According to psychodramatic theory a considerable part of the psyche is not language-ridden, it is not infiltrated by the ordinary, significant language symbols. Therefore, bodily contact with subjects, if it can be established, touch caress, embrace, hand shake, sharing in silent activities, eating, walking or other activities, are an important preliminary to psychodramatic work itself.

The group generates a safe place for the actors to enter a creative process that provides the protagonist with a new and more intensive experience of reality, a "surplus reality" (Moreno, 1953, p. 85). A sense of security and confidence are necessary for him or her to let go of limiting belief-systems and move into an open space for something to happen that he or she hasn't anticipated or experienced before. Elberfeld (2017b, p. 334) mentioned that creative processes are characterized through their beginning at a distinctive form of "nothingness" which transforms itself into something new, something that wasn't prompted, expected or foreseen. For creativity to transpire, we have to allow and release our ego to play spontaneously and unintentionally. For Moreno this cannot happen in the isolated and artificial setting of the Freudian "Couch Container" (Buer, 1989, p. 133), it needs the dialogical dimension of reality.

In summary, the psychodramatic play offers its participants creative ways to engage with their shadow parts. They enter a field of experience that opens itself up between intrapersonal dialogue and interpersonal encounters. Instead of controlling and repressing themselves, participants learn to appreciate and incorporate neglected and ostracized parts of their identity. The spontaneous play helps to cultivate inner balance which enables people to congruently encounter otherness. A great tool to apply psychodramatic principles in regular inter-cultural training and workshop settings is the "Inner Team" (Schulz von Thun, 2003).

The "Inner Team" as concrete application of the psychodramatic play

The method of the "Inner Team" follows several stages which I will briefly outline using an example from my professional practice. It uses the metaphor of a team that works together on an "intrapersonal stage" with some members acting at the forefront, others as supporting actors and some hiding behind the curtain, at the backstage or even underneath the stage like the Phantom of the Opera (Schulz von Thun, 2003, p. 181).

In the first phase, I let the participants tell me a story where they experienced inner conflict and dysfunctional communication on the outside. I ask them to associate with this moment and have them describe how it felt like. I then (secondly) have them draw a big torso on a piece of paper (their inner stage) and ask them who they think appeared on their stage in this situation: Who showed up first? Who followed? Who was the loudest? Who was frustrated and holding back his or her anger? Schulz von Thun (2003) suggested that participants think of a message of the inner team members first and then to give them a suitable name. It sometimes takes a while to attend to all of the parts that played a role in the difficult situation. Especially the ones who are silently hiding in the back because they are used to being avoided, disregarded or perceived to be shameful take a while to come out. Once the core inner team is identified, we can (third phase) look at their interactional dynamic: Who is working well together with whom? Who is in conflict? Where are allies and adversaries? Who got out of balance and where could we potentially find positive opposites in order to respond to the conflict on the outside with "one voice" instead of just reacting to the most dominant voice? The fourth and last step is to have the participants think of concrete possible action steps to develop inner parts in order to (re-)gain balance. A key question here is: "How would you know that you are moving towards a more congruent response?"

I would like to illustrate this with an example: In one of my workshops in an elderly care home one of the nurses shared a recurring situation with a Muslim stewardess who keeps aggressively complaining about the quality of care given to her mother. She yells loudly at several staff in the hallway and then disappears again for several weeks. One of the workshop participants volunteered to work with her inner team and first identified two dominant inner team members who appeared on her inner stage in that situation: the *Proud Professional* saying "I know that we are doing our job well" and the predominant *Harmony Seeker* saying "Just swallow it, don't make a fuzz". After talking a bit more about the situation and what is happening on her inner stage, she also "hears" another voice which she calls *Empathy* giving her the message: "It must be hard for her to leave her mother with us" – knowing that in her Muslim tradition elders are supposed to be cared for at home. After digging a bit deeper asking her if there might be somebody on her inner stage who may reside in the background, she tells me that every time the stewardess is leaving after her outburst, she feels being treated like a doormat and hates the fact that she didn't say anything which makes her very angry. Once I asked her what this inner team member's message could be and how she could call her, she took quite a while to think about it and then responded warily that it could be *Self-regard* saying "Stand up for yourself".

After a short silent pause, she continued to tell me that her dad left her mother with four small children and she being the oldest had to take care of her three younger siblings. *Self-regard* had to withdraw. Back then she already experienced inner conflict between *Harmony Seeker* (who allied with *Empathy*) and *Self-regard* who was silenced and yet very alive in the background, mostly as a vague feeling of sadness and anger.

Through looking at her inner team she realised that *Harmony Seeker* essentially needs *Self-regard* to create the positive tension relationship that is necessary for her to respond to the stewardess congruently. She explained that she would know that she responded well if she were able to stand up for herself, maybe working together with *Proud Professional* making sure that she shows empathy and yet assertively sets boundaries.

Asking her for possible action steps towards this envisioned response, she said that she would take a deep breath to be able to express compassion by saying that it must be hard for her (the stewardess) to work so much and to assure her that her mother is well taken care of. She continued to say that *Self-regard* can help her not to take the frustration of the stewardess personally, but to become aware of the concerns and needs which stand behind it.

The Inner Team model works well because it is easy to comprehend and in my experience people coming from different cultural backgrounds can quickly relate to it. It is a playful method to talk about difficult intra- and interpersonal conflicts and it can be combined with other methods, e.g. the "chair technique" from Gestalt therapy where people can "sit" on a particular inner team member consciously identifying with it. However, in regular workshop settings one has to be careful not to move too deep into therapeutic issues. It can also be time-consuming. Still, people take away a lot for themselves and it is worthwhile to trust the creative process of engaging with the unknown other in the self.

Conclusion

The philosophy of self-care has been pushed to the background, to the "hidden stage", of academic philosophy. The demand to look at the vast "field of dark perceptions" seems to be counterintuitive and philosophically irritating (Elberfeld, 2017b, p. 441). The same is true for educational endeavours that aim to explain cultural differences and deliver recipe-like communication techniques. However, without engaging in "spiritual exercises", accessing the "wisdom of our body" (Nietzsche, 1960, pp. 28–29), listening and responding to the *pathos* of the alien within ourselves, we fall prone to the most dominant voices in us, to reactive behaviour and spiteful habits of reoccurring patterns that establish monolithic forms of identity. In order to practice self-care in this holistic manner, creative methods are indispensable. They complement our inclination toward analytic explanations and help to establish intrapersonal congruency. Here the ancient notion of the "aesthetics of existence" or the "art of life" materializes itself in concrete practices. We ought to work on ourselves as a "piece of art" – a task that never comes to and end and always needs otherness as source of creative inspiration.

Notes

1. Michel Foucault (2004, p. 31) called this the 'Cartesian Moment', when *knowing* oneself became a necessity for truth. However at the same time it suppressed *practices of self-care* as means to the "art of life" which dominated the Classical and Hellenistic philosophies.
2. Foucault (1996) referred to this form of 'truth-speaking' as *parrhesia*, a crucial part of the practice of self-care. Instead of the Cartesian model of evidential truth and the use of rhetoric finesse, *parrhesia* expresses a person's intimate relationship to the truth. This expression may even place the *parrhesiastes* (a person who exercises *parrhesia*) in a position of danger if he or she stands up against the opinion of the majority.
3. Waldenfels (1997, p. 16) talked about the 'shattering of rationality' and the 'decentralization of the subject' as the great adventures of Western modernity. Explorers discovered new continents and slowly realised that there are other *logoi* and other cultures. In German the plural of the word culture, cultur*es*, was first introduced by Burckhardt in 1968. Before that it seemed obvious: only Europeans had 'culture'. (Elberfeld, 2017b, pp. 222–224) With Freud (1991, p. 60) this experience of otherness invaded our self as we experience within us an 'inner foreign country'. Even Kant (1977, pp. 417–419) warily wrote about 'perceptions we have without being consciously aware of them' saying: 'The field of dark perceptions is the largest in man'. It tends to play with us although we try to hide unwanted parts in the shadow. However, unlike Freud, Kant wasn't prepared to go there and explore this realm. Instead, he focused on the human ability to reason.
4. Here, Merleau-Ponty's (1966) work on the *Phenomenology of Perception* is of great importance. For him it is obvious that we 'know' through our body. Moreover, we experience our relatedness with the world through our bodies. Our bodies resonate with each other when we enter the realm of 'intercorporeality' or 'interaffectivity'. Merleau-Ponty argues that philosophy is not just finding the truth of a reality that already exists, rather, it realises truth *like the arts*. (Merleau-Ponty, 1966, p. 18) To observe and describe reality in *statu nascendi* (in the process of becoming) is the philosopher's task as well as the artist's. Both have to trust the process.
5. Gruen (2014, pp. 23–24) explained: 'As children we were helpless and at the mercy of our parents. Our survival depended on our complying with them. The inner terror accompanying victimisation is therefore profoundly existential. That is why fear of losing our job, our social position, or our role in society can shake the foundations of our being. If our self-esteem is based primarily on success, status, and material gain, then the potential loss of these external achievements must be experienced as existentially threatening because the old feeling of terror – at being helpless, at the mercy of others, and ashamed – is reawakened.' This, he believes, is the true reason that in times of great uncertainty the phenomenon of xenophobia upsurges (Gruen, 2014, p. 24).
6. Welsch (1991, p. 36) confirmed this by saying: 'Whereas the strong subject is characterised by authority and domination, the weak subject doesn't concentrate on producing itself and at the same time mastering and controlling the other, rather it is willing to open itself up for the other, to letting itself become alienated.'
7. A 'complex' is a repressed, unconscious part of self that finds its way to consciousness through acting out what it stands for – often against our will. 'Archetypes' are universal, archaic patterns that originate from our collective unconsciousness. They express themselves in dreams, stories, images, methodologies or art.
8. Jacobi (1984, p. 111) mentioned that the shadow is a reoccurring and popular motive in the arts. In her creative process, the artist draws from the depths of her unconscious and in turn touches with what she creates, the unconscious of her audience. Herein lies the secret of her impact – even if her audience doesn't understand where their emotional reactions came from.
9. The *protagonist* is the 'subject' or 'actor' who is also the narrator and scenarist in charge of setting the stage. 'The subject is enabled not only to meet parts of himself, but the other persons who partake in his mental conflicts. These persons may be real or illusions' (Moreno, 1953, p. 83). The protagonist can opt to have an 'auxiliary ego' to play the role of him- or herself to be able to look at his scenario from outside themselves.

Disclosure statement

No potential conflict of interest was reported by the author.

References

Arendt, H. (1978). *The life of the mind (Vol. 1)*. New York, NY: Harvest Book.
Bar-On, D. (2001). *Die „Anderen" in uns. Dialog als Modell der interkulturellen Konfliktbewältigung* [The "Others" within us. Dialogue as Model of Intercultural Conflict Resolution]. edition Körber Stiftung: Hamburg.
Buer, F. (Ed.). (1989). *Morenos therapeutische philosophie* [Moreno's therapeutic philosophy]. Opladen: Leske & Budrich.
Cushman, R. E. (1958). *Therapeia. Plato's conception of philosophy*. Chapel Hill: University of Carolina Press.
Dreyer, W., & Hößler, U. (eds.). (2011). *Perspektiven interkultureller kompetenz* [perspectives of intercultural competence]. Göttingen: V&R.
Elberfeld, R. (2017a). Philosophie und ästhetische praxis [philosophy and aesthetic practice]. In R. Elberfeld & S. Krankenhagen (Eds.), *Ästhetische praxis als gegenstand und methode kulturwissenschaftlicher forschung* (pp. 171–189). Paderborn: Wilhelm Fink.
Elberfeld, R. (2017b). *Philosophieren in einer globalisierten welt. Wege zu einer transformativen phänomenologie* [Philosophizing in a globalized world. Ways towards a transformative phenomenology]. Freiburg im Breisgau: Karl Alber.
Foucault, M. (1996). *Diskurs und wahrheit. Berkeley-vorlesungen 1983* [Discourse and turth. Berkeley-lectures 1983]. Berlin: Merve.
Foucault, M. (2004). *Hermeneutik des subjekts* [The hermeneutics of the subject]. Frankfurt a.M.: Suhrkamp.
Foucault, M. (2007). *Ästhetik der existenz. Schriften zur lebenskunst* [Aesthetics of existence: Writings of the art of life]. Frankfurt a.M.: Suhrkamp.
Foucault, M. (2015). *Die sorge um sich. Sexualität und wahrheit 3* [The care of the self. History of sexuality 3] (12th ed.). Frankfurt a.M.: Suhrkamp.
Freud, S. (1991). *Neue folge der vorlesungen zur einführung in die psychoanalyse*. Frankfurt a.M.: Fischer.
Fuchs, T. (2011). Body memory and the unconscious. In D. Lohmar & D. J. Brudzinska (Eds.), *Founding psychoanalysis. Phenomenological theory of subjectivity and the psychoanalytical experience* (pp. 86–103). Dordrecht: Kluwer.
Gödde, G., & Zirfas, J. (2016). *Therapeutik und lebenskunst. Eine psychologisch-philosophische grundlegung* [therpeutics and the Art of life. A psychological-philosophical groundwork]. Gießen: Psychosozial.
Gruen, A. (2014). *Der fremde in uns* [The stranger within us] (10th ed.). München: dtv.
Hadot, P. (1991). *Philosophie als lebensform. Geistige Übungen in der antike* [philosophy as a Way of life. Spiritual exercises from socrates to foucault]. Berlin: Mathias Gatza.
Hermans, H., & Hermans-Konopka, A. (2010). *Dialogical self theory. Positioning and counter-positioning in a globalizing society*. Cambridge: Cambridge University Press.
Jacobi, J. (1983). *The Way of individuation*. New York, NY: Meridian.
Jacobi, J. (1984). *Die psychologie von C.G. Jung. Eine einführung in das gesamtwerk* [The psychology of C.G. Jung. An introduction in the complete works]. Frankfurt a. M.: Fischer.
Jung, C. G. (1933). *Die beziehungen zwischen dem ich und dem unbewussten* [The relationship between I and the unconscious] (4th ed.). Zürich: Rascher.
Jung, C. G. (1976). *Bewußtes und unbewußtes* [Conscious and unconscious] (16th ed.). Frankfurt a.M.: Fischer Taschenbuch.
Kant, I. (1977). *Schriften zur anthropologie, geschichtsphilosophie und pädagogik* 2 [Writings about anthropology, historical philosophie and pedagogics 2]. Frankfurt a.M.: Suhrkamp.
Kristeva, J. (1991). *Strangers to ourselves*. (L. Roudiez, Trans.) New York, NY: Columbia University Press.
Mecheril, P. (2013). „Kompetenzlosigkeitskompetenz". pädagogisches handeln unter einwanderungsbedingungen. In G. Auernheimer (Ed.), *Interkulturelle kompetenz und pädagogische professionalität* [Intercultural competence and pedagogical professionalism] (4th ed.) (pp. 15–34). Wiesbaden: Springer.
Merleau-Ponty, M. (1966). *Phänomenologie der wahrnehmung* [Phenomenology of perception]. Berlin: Walter de Gruyter & Co.
Moreno, J. L. (1953). *Who shall survive? Foundations of sociometrie, group psychotherapy and sociodrama*. Beacon: Beacon House.
Mortari, L. (2016). *Die sorge um sich* [The care of self]. Würzburg: Königshausen & Neumann.
Nietzsche, F. (1960). *Also sprach zarathustra* [Thus spoke zarathustra]. München: Goldmann.
Nussbaum, M. (1994). *The therapy of desire. Theory and practice in hellenistic ethics*. Princeton: Princeton University Press.
Petzold, H. (1978). *Angewandtes psychodrama in therapie, pädagogik und theater* [Applied psychodrama in therapy, pedagogics and theatre] (3rd ed.). Paderborn: Junfermann.
Satir, V. (1998). *Selbstwert und kommunikation. Familientherapie für berater und zur selbsthilfe* [Self-esteem and communication. Family therapy for counselors and self-help] (13th ed.). München: Pfeiffer.

Scategni, W. (2002). *Psychodrama, group processes and dreams. Archetypal images of individuation. (V. Marsicano, trans).* New York, NY: Taylor & Francis.

Schulz von Thun, F. (2003). *Das "Innere Team" und situationsgerechte kommunikation* [The inner team and context specific communication] (11th ed.). Reinbek: Rowohlt.

Seneca. (1786). *The epistles of seneca (Vol. 1).* London: Woodfall.

Waldenfels, B. (1990). *Der stachel des fremden* [The sting of the alien]. Frankfurt a.M.: Suhrkamp.

Waldenfels, B. (1997). *Topographie des fremden* [Topography of the Alien]. Frankfurt a.M.: Suhrkamp.

Waldenfels, B. (2010). *Sinne und künste im wechselspiel. Modi ästhetischer erfahrung* [Senses and arts as interplay. Modes of aesthetic experience]. Frankfurt a.M.: Suhrkamp.

Waldenfels, B. (2016). *Grundmotive einer phänomenologie des fremden* [Main themes of a phenomenology of the alien] (5th ed.). Frankfurt a.M.: Suhrkamp.

Weidemann, A., Straub, J., & Nothnagel, S. (eds.). (2010). *Wie lehrt man interkulturelle kompetenz? Theorien, methoden und praxis in der hochschulausbildung. Ein handbuch* [How to teach intercultural competence? Theories, methods and practice of the university education. A handbook]. Bielefeld: transcript.

Welsch, W. (1991). Subjektsein heute. Überlegungen zur transformation des subjekts [Being subject today. Thoughts of the transformation of the subject]. *Deutsche Zeitschrift für Philosophie, 39*(4), 347–365.

Standards of performance and aesthetics in counselling and beyond

Morten Nissen

ABSTRACT
In this article I discuss how drug counselling can be transformed through "aesthetic documentation": a hybrid of art with narrative practice. After outlining the concepts of performance and standards, and a critique of "customising" counselling through formalised feedback, five claims are made about "aesthetic documentation": The art works are prototypes rather than rigid standardisations; they represent collaboration rather than individualised performance; they both display and enact substantial meaning; they objectify and achieve recognition of clients and professionals; they facilitate flexible, diverse and transformative attributions of meaning and value; they address social problems rather than individualised malfunctions. This may help overcoming stigmatisation, and suggest a kind of trans-disciplinary knowledge that is different from the dominant scientific forms.

Introduction

In November, 2013, I attended a conference on *The Subject of Addiction* in Nottingham, UK, together with two counsellors and an artist who worked at municipal services for young people with drug problems in Copenhagen and Elsinore, called *U-turn* and *HelsingUng*, respectively. We presented our collaboration partly in the form of a *gallery* that displayed art work – images, poems, song, videos etc. – made as a way of performing and expanding drug counselling. In one such art video, a young man called Sebastian is filmed close-up singing karaoke to the song "You Ruined Everything" which he seems to hear in his headphones, in the middle of a street festival with noisy rhythms and intoxicated people dancing[1]. Another sample is the song "Time Passes", about love and trust, written and performed by Louie, a very young woman, assisted by Halberg, her psychologist[2].

Our hope was that this collaboration of counsellors, artists, clients and researchers could be modelled as a *prototype* at several levels. First, and most importantly, the art works were a kind of portraits and self-portraits that would represent personal narratives of value and worth, struggle and hope, for a public; as such, they provided models for youth life, as strong alternatives and corrections to the often derogatory and stigmatising ways the young clients had otherwise been depicted. Building on and expanding the methodologies of narrative practice that were important inspirations (White, 2007), the counselors called it *"aesthetic documentation"*. Second, the gallery – along with internet sites[3] and articles in counselling and social work journals (Halberg, 2013; Nielsen & Kofod, 2013; Nissen, 2014) – provided vivid illustrations of this way of (not quite) doing counselling and of working with young drug users. Third, this was one expression of a "relational aesthetics" that pushed the limits of art to include outsider artists and dialogues on its social relevance and implications. Fourth, and finally, the whole infrastructure of activities, artifacts and standards would make out a form of knowledge and competence that could serve as a much needed alternative, not only to traditional academic and professional disciplines, but also to their dominant current successors: Evidence-based practices. In particular, it would represent a way of engaging expert professionals in dialogue with users, which did not predefine their service as a commodity, whether pre-packed and labelled, or customised.

This text is an edited version of my own contribution to our presentation at the conference. At the time, I was leading a research project on standards and subjects, of which one part was about "user-driven standards in social work" (Nissen, 2016)[4]. The project connected research on standards and standardisation with the rising recognition and power of the user in public services, in particular in drug treatment and counselling. This was the angle from which I approached matters and took part in the collaboration (although, it should be noted, this specific project was only one phase of a much longer history of collaboration, which stretches back to the 1980s). Accordingly, this article will focus on the fourth aspect: *Articulating the concepts of performance, standards, and aesthetics implied in the practices and models displayed.*

The reader should thus not expect an empirical study, presentation and assessment of a therapeutic method, for two reasons. *First*, since the articulations that I propose render these practices as a way of overcoming, of going beyond therapy. Performance or aesthetics, as I propose to conceive of these practices, do not fit into therapy, as means to the cure of "addiction". The very idea, the framing standards, of therapy – and the ways of imagining such standards as "user-driven" – are being problematised fundamentally if we think of aesthetics and performance in this way. Second, the point in this is *theoretical* – yet hopefully relevant to such a radical rethinking of some of the *practices* in which we currently deal with young people whom we would consider diagnosing as dependent or addicted.

Still, my academic role, then at the conference and now as author, is not to sanction conceptual clarity, nor is it to provide foundations. Mine is a specialised practice in dialogue with those of the counsellors – it is not above them, nor underlying them. It is better to think of the articulations that I propose as a conceptual *repertoire*, even if part of what they are for is to reshape commitments and rethink relevances (on the methodology of such dialogue, see e.g. Mol, 2008; Nissen, 2009, 2012). Finally, I should emphasise that neither I, nor the counsellors I collaborate with, would claim that "aesthetic documentation" or even "performance" as such would work as the only approach to multidimensional social problems such as young people's excessive drug use. On the contrary, the approach to performance and standards that I argue here is meant to remind us of a humility that is sometimes forgotten in the quest for "best practice": Social problems require broad and varied interventions, where multiple disciplines contribute to a social change that includes care, cure, and growth of individuals, families, communities etc.

State – not of the – art, but as multiple references

In their work with young drug users, the counsellors are interested in creatively modelling ways to change performances, ways to perform inspiring and convincing narratives about *how life could be*[5]. But of course, looking to possible futures does not mean disregarding experience. As mentioned, their "clinical" references are mostly from "narrative therapy" (White, 2007). This tradition has its own approach to performative and aesthetic elements, centred on the ways that re-/presentations of persons can work to challenge and replace powerful oppressive narratives and identities, including those implied in "therapy" (Linnell, 2010).

In addition, performance has been important in the traditions of social youth work in these Copenhagen communities for decades. Thus, street happenings and shows were a key ingredient of the grassroots youth work community "The Crew" which I studied in the 1990s (Nissen, 2012). Variously drawing on political traditions and theories of theatrical performance (Boal, 2000; Høgsbro & Nissen, 2014; Jameson, 1998), performance arts and relational aesthetics (Bourriaud, 2002; Groys, 2016), this is a local tradition, though it connects to attempts, for instance, in New York (Newman & Holzman, 1996), London (Sloan, 2014), and Sao Paulo (Liberali, 2000). Social youth work is a conceptual hotchpotch, a trading zone of a wide variety of professional traditions, and so, this kind of local, trans-disciplinary mingling of global ideas is not uncommon.

The traditions of using elements of (theatrical) performance in counselling, such as psycho-drama or gestalt therapy, have not been taken up much here. The same is true of the great many clinical uses of (other) aesthetic practices such as art or music, apart from those within the narrative tradition. The reason for this is that the clinical literature generally takes for granted that art or performance are "means to therapeutic ends" (as in the title of White & Epston's early articulation of narrative therapy, 1990), that is, ways of exploring, expressing and curing pathologies. When aesthetics is about challenging the very notion of pathology, it is a different project altogether. Of course, many forms of art or performance therapy can be seen to point or move beyond that clinical framework, for instance by evoking a political, spiritual, or social emancipation through sensuous registers, even if they perhaps do not themselves question the clinical framework (e.g. Brooke, 2009); and so, the present argument can be said to suggest a rearticulation of what is at stake also in some forms of performance or art therapy. It would be interesting to establish this in detail in another article. But first of all, this rearticulation proposes a set of questions to ask that is different from the set derived from clinical standards. These questions come from other research traditions, such as science studies and theories of aesthetics. The first of these questions is about performance itself.

Performance and standards

Performance is a key term in current social theory, to the point that some even refer to a "performative turn" (Martin, 2007; Turner, 1995). To state this approach very simply, the things we are are mostly things we do. We can often change by doing otherwise. Sometimes, of course, that is not easy – many kinds of resources and premises must be in place for a performance to succeed; performance is not (at least not *literally*) magic. But *part* of why it isn't easy is often that we can't imagine other performances; and so we don't set out looking for ways to provide the right conditions for them. An important way to encourage performative imagination is to show it. Performing is doing, but it is also showing, displaying; repeating acts, and through that, directing attention to them, facilitating reflection and possible change. This may be done in the flow of activities, for instance as humour, but it can also be specialised as "performance" activities. Further, it is much amplified by modelling – by creating artifacts that serve to make acts present again – thus, to re-present them[6].

But performance is also a key term in *standardisation*: Performance standards. Here, the meaning is much narrower: To perform means here only to enact, to do something which is stipulated in advance – for instance, to run a 100 m dash in no more than 10 s. The quality (what it is) is fixed, and so the focus is on the only variable, which is some quantity (how fast, how much etc.). This matches the idea of standardisation: of standards described and prescribed, using models of practices to regulate them. And it matches the idea that performing reproduces certain cultural patterns that already exist.

Figure 1[7] is a cartoon version (by B.E. Kaplan) of Judith Butler's theory that gender is performed and only thereby reproduced (Butler, 1993). The boy *always* gets to be the boy ... Yet we can already see that maybe the girl has had enough of it. What would happen if *she* got to be the boy? This may sound weird, or even queer, but it is a bit like: What if a young drug user got to be an artist? Butler, too, is preoccupied with performance as enactment of given subjectivities; but her point is that it could be otherwise. Once we see that gender, or addiction, or singer-songwriting, is something that is performed, we can see other possibilities. This opens to a different approach to performance: not as the enactment of a pre-given pattern, but as creative acts.

In fact, this is not only the case when something new and unheard of is performed. Even reenacting something is already a remaking of it, opening it to debate and possible change. This is one way to understand the magic of theatre and art in general. And standards, too: Standards are modelled to

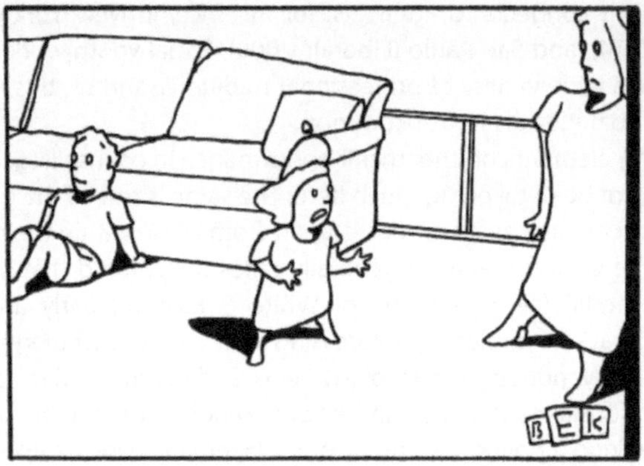

"Why does he always get to be the boy?"

Figure 1. Cartoon by Bruce Eric Kaplan. Reprinted with permission.

stipulate and regulate, but they still have to be performed in each instance, and that is itself a creative act that opens to possibilities of transformation, of setting new standards (Nissen, 2016).

Standards of counselling

In counselling, we can see similar approaches. Many are busy defining performance standards for counselling that works (e.g. Rowland & Goss, 2013). Evidence-based counselling is counselling that is performed in a way that meets certain performance standards – and is then said to lead to certain desired results. But they run into a problem, since it takes at least two to do counselling. There is no direct and immediate causality from the counsellor's performance to the more or less curative effects on the client. At the end of the day, the client is the one who has to cash in any gains achieved in counseling. The counsellor may do all the right things and still the client neglects to change. The subjectivity of the client is inescapable.

This has been known and discussed all through the twentieth century in different vocabularies since Freud. The history of psychotherapy is a history of the ways in which client subjectivity has been objectified, colonised, fenced off, and otherwise handled, once given over to the therapist. But in recent decades, an important cultural-historical transformation has occurred. People are no longer expected to surrender to the authority of the therapist, not even if they are diagnosed with diseases, and not even if those diseases are psychological or psychiatric; not even addicts. Users have been mobilised in governance, under various catchwords, in the general framework of New Public Management.

Although the mobilisation of user experience, user assessment etc. appears the opposite, it really works in tandem with the trend toward governance through standards. This is because a meta language is needed. User experience was no great epistemological problem in the twentieth century because experts were trusted with the authority to interpret and translate it. But now that users are pitted against experts, trust in expertise is replaced with trust in standards and numbers (cf. Porter, 1995). The subjectivity of the client is still pivotal, but in a new way: not as objectified in the expert's language (as denial, anxiety, automatic thoughts, resistance etc.), but in a *logic of choice* (Mol, 2008), as the user or customer who choses, evaluates and decides about the service provided.

In a word, counselling is being based on evidence that is made and treated as valid in the encounter with clients (and other stakeholders). For this reason, performance standards tend increasingly to prioritise collaboration, measure effect as self-reported, and often settle pragmatically for client retention (Norcross, 2011). But to do this, you must apply a very conservative, common sense version of what counts as counselling. This is because the logic of choice requires a well-defined standard intervention or service. If you are to measure effects, in a way that is accountable to users and managers, you have to define the service in a way that bases directly on common sense. The boy must *always* get to be the boy. This leads to the paradox that these quite radical changes in practices and their governance and epistemologies are effected with surprisingly traditional concepts. This may be one reason that these developments are often hard to decipher, for clients, practitioners and researchers alike.

This is in large part why Cognitive–Behavioral Therapy (CBT) is becoming *the* standard form of counseling. It is immediately recognisable as a service directed at solving predefined problems or diseases understood in a common sense framework. It matches well with the ICD and DSM, the international diagnostic manuals, in which the disputes over ontologies and metaphysics have long been declared passé – and diagnoses are instead supposedly based purely on empirical data and description. CBT also stages a kind of collaboration. It was originally associated with the classic Modernist ambition to a unified scientific body of knowledge, but it has moved toward a more pragmatic epistemology, and is often mixed with some version of client-centred counseling, as in the most widespread drug counseling method, Motivational Interviewing (Miller & Rollnick, 1991).

Clients can indeed be met on the basis of descriptive diagnosis. Many users, clients and patients – not to mention relatives – declare diagnosis a relief; and no doubt, it is less stigmatising now than it used to be. Yet, given that psychiatric diagnoses – even those with a massive prevalence, such as depression, ADHD, or dependence – still imply some measure of self-deceit, and thus some weight attributed to expert judgment, there remains a tension between diagnosis and user experience (cf. Martin, 2007). Even if CBT is collaborative, it still rests on the authority of the expert counsellor. This is perhaps most clearly expressed in the practice of "psycho-education", which assumes and performs an almost caricatured traditional idea of teaching as the channelling of authoritative information about a given disease and the workings of the brain. The authorised knowledge remains unchallenged and only has to be chopped up and fed to the individual client.

This process of chopping up standards for the individual client was always, in principle, required in evidence-based counselling, and treatment more generally (Sackett et al., 2000). Typically, this aspect has been acknowledged, but given very limited attention. However, this may be changing, since it matches a version of user-driven standards that is becoming widespread in many other spheres of our lives: *Customisation* (cf. Busch, 2011). We might compare such customised counselling with a smart-phone: It is made to be customised to each individual user's specific habits and preferences. But it is also a framework that is the same all over the world, and over which the smartphone company rules with absolute authority, once you've chosen the product.

If such customisation is taken to its full implications, does this not challenge the authority of the counsellor? That question is raised by the idea of *Feedback-Informed Treatment* (FIT; cf. Duncan, Miller, Wampold, & Hubble, 2010). FIT is the ultimate in customised counselling. A continuous and systematic formal feedback from the client – in the form of simple scales on how she thinks she is doing and what she thinks of the sessions – is used to modify the counselling. This, way, the counselling is no longer adapted to meet a generalised performance standard, but rather to what works for the individual client – as measured by herself. That appears to correlate with client retention (cf. Wampold, 2001). This is called "practice-based evidence". It is no coincidence that FIT has branched off from the *Solution-Focused Brief Therapy* (SFBT) which boasts a complete rejection of psychological explanation and claims to always take what the client says at face value (De Shazer, 1991). Here we find one current example that numbers are used pragmatically when expert interpretation is given up or denounced. Both SFBT and FIT have attracted the attention of the counsellors I work with, for their radical deconstruction of psychological expertise and for recognising the voice of the user, drawing on Wittgenstein and Derrida. For this reason, we have discussed it intensely and critically (Nissen & Barington, 2016).

Ideally, the user gets exactly what she wants. The customer is always right. This is in fact a well-known standard in commercial relations. Except for one thing: What does she in fact buy – a conversation with a salesperson? A reflection of her preferred self-image? As we know from many other spheres of life, when recognition is reduced to immediate preferences, it is emptied and turned around to its opposite.

Neither SFBT nor FIT challenges the form of treatment and its concomitant stigmatisation and power differentials. Metaphorically, the hardware of therapy has not really been touched by the customisation of its software and all its apps. Even the most radical deconstruction of the language games of diagnosis and healing, *within* the therapeutic space, only leads back to the common sense that defines what the customer has come to buy in the first place. It is still a performance standard in that sense, a regulating model that remains within the given, even if the details are left to each client to choose. The counsellor becomes the actor, performing the version of counsellor that best matches the client's imagination. But the basic act remains the same.

In fact, even customisation is itself standardised. It is really only that a unique (or quasi-unique) combination of equally predefined standards has emerged, within the framework, just as all the apps and settings on the smartphone are defined in advance and all that is left to the customer is to combine them. Customisation appears different from standardisation, but in fact it is a continuation of the ongoing proliferation of formalised standards.

All this is relevant, as mentioned, because FIT suggests itself in the same communities of practitioners that I discuss here. And I want to oppose it to an alternative articulation of their practices of "aesthetic documentation" (drawing on, among others, an alternative reading of Wittgenstein and Derrida), as an expanded prototype for how performance standards can be user-driven.

Five claims

I am going to make five claims about the gallery that I and my collaborators presented, and about the "aesthetic documentation" practices that produced it – to make the case that they represent a much more radical way to develop and problematise performance standards in counselling. I suggest that they should be articulated in terms of a deeper and wider way of addressing the classic qualities of scientific knowledge: Generalisation, abstraction, and objectivity – since this is more fruitful than attempting to disregard those qualities.

Again, these claims are not authoritative. They remain debatable. It is not just that, inevitably, the subjectivity of my experience, position and projects limit the data and the theories I refer to and shape the relevance of what I propose. This "bias" is what is usually controlled with standardising scientific procedures, which feed on standardised data and apply knowledge in standardised practices. That works well where such standardisation is deemed possible and desirable. But in some areas and with some issues it isn't, and those procedures won't help us judge whether it is or not. What is more, they do not lend themselves to transforming or creating standards – as we are out to do here. Here, instead, we must reflect and discuss *qualities* with reference to (historically situated) singular instances and to theoretical traditions, and we must reflect on ourselves and on the texts we write. Such "qualitative" work never leads to authoritative claims, only to prototypes.

Prototypes

My first claim, then, is that the performance standards provided here are *prototypes*. Prototypes are artifacts that hold some generalising promises or hopes, but in visibly contingent and precarious ways, and without hiding their singularity and the situations of their emergence and use. As the word suggests, they are not yet and not quite types (Jensen, 1987; Nissen, 2009; Suchman et al., 2002). Anyone who listens to the song that Halberg the counsellor produced along with Louie the client and posted on the internet (cf. note 1 above), will realise that this models a unique event with unique persons in unique situations. Or take a look at the "Give a Story" art videos posted by U-turn in Copenhagen, such as the one mentioned above with "Sebastian".

That uniqueness doesn't mean we can't learn from all this; far from it, the whole point about it is that it speaks to us, it generalises. And to be sure, we can only learn from it and bring it home by focusing on some aspects and forgetting others – to generalise is to perform abstraction. But with prototypes it is clear that we leave other things behind when we do take something with us. It is clear that we take different things from it, and it is clear that when we do, we transform it on the way. We know that if we want to learn more, we have to engage with the specifics of Copenhagen or Elsinore municipality, as well as with certain elements of youth subcultures etc. And we know it's not going to be quite the same in Glasgow or Sydney. Perhaps, there we would have to change the model slightly, or we need to build an infrastructure around it for it to work. That's basically how people have always learnt from great educational or social experiments, such as those of Paulo Freire in Brazil, Anton Makarenko in Ukraine, or Sigmund Freud in Austria. But it is very different from the medical format that reigns in psychotherapy, which seems to imply a much more rigid and simplistic standardisation.

The concept of prototype points to the historicity of standards – which, incidentally, could draw on a reading of Wittgenstein (2010) that emphasises how language games are historically situated life forms, rather than discrete patterns that can be manipulated for more or less concealed therapeutic purposes, as in SFBT. It also highlights how values and hopes are part of the story, and how standards always, as embedded in historical circumstance, guide evolving dramas. If we take up that emphasis, we can call them *prototypical narratives* (Nissen, 2015). This way of thinking speaks to the fertile tradition of narrative anthropology (Mattingly, 2010) as much as to the narrative therapy from which the counsellors have taken inspiration.

Collaboration

My second claim is that these are prototypes of *collaboration*. They do not separate what the professional does from what the client does, as it is the case with typical performance standards in counselling, including the ever so feedback-informed treatment. They highlight this aspect in that they are hybrid activities that lead to tangible products; but it is a general characteristic of counselling. The client is not just a user, but also and probably first of all a participant. This is crucial because that is how people really learn, and because the whole approach to activities like counselling or teaching should start from the assumption that they are first of all collective. This was a main point in my book *The Subjectivity of Participation* (Nissen, 2012). The most fertile question for the participant to ask is not "what's in this for me?", or "am I doing the right thing?", but "who are we, what are we doing, what comes of it, and how does that make sense?" Even when a crucial point is that such collectives are made up of very different people with diverse power and premises – and very different positions, contributions, and gains.

Jean Lave, the anthropologist, once said that "social practice is a dance" (personal communication; but see Lave, 2011). I take that to mean that we continuously create it together, sometimes loving, at other times fighting, but always together. Of course, this is easy to state in general, but hard to practice and govern counselling by, even as both professional accountability and user self-care are cherished. The ways that responsibility is currently split up and shifted around between providers and users of public services do not encourage a reflexive collective approach that allows users to grow as participants. In the final analysis, this requires a revitalisation of the "gift economy" that was emerging precariously in the era of the welfare states (Hart, 2006).

Staging

But the "dance" could also be a metaphor for the reflexivity or self-consciousness of social life that led Shakespeare to have a character suggest that "all the world's a stage", and many social theorists – such as Goffman (1986) – to agree centuries later. This is my third claim. The activities of counsellors and clients are always also *staged performances* of how it is possible to act; how life could be. We display standards as we act together. Performing is acting, and acting is showing. That is an important part of how we learn when we learn by doing, by participating.

Setting standards is more than just going through the movements. It is also confirming values. The meaning of who we are and what we are doing is *immanent* to our practices, as when for instance it makes sense quite directly to record a song for people to hear. But it is also constantly being displayed, as we modify and adjust our actions to address that meaning. Those two aspects should not be thought of as two separate things. The meaningfulness of songwriting and of being someone who can write and perform songs is at once enacted, displayed, and confirmed. The different "laminations" of performance (Goffman, 1986) – layers of reference and meta-reference – are dynamically interwoven and mutually defined in our activities; this is what endows reflection with meaningful substance and vice versa.

This is very important because performance standards so easily become parodic (Stenner, 2016). That is to say, they are detached from the point of the whole thing, and become ends in themselves. Signs that were supposed to refer to meaning, but which take over the whole show as hyper-real signs that are more important than what they refer to (Baudrillard, 1994; Hanson, 1993). That is in fact the story of much governance by standards and accountability today. Yet, this danger of alienation should not lead us to reject the modelling of standards altogether. In fact, my fourth claim is that a key to how aesthetic documentation works is that it externalises and objectifies what is meaningful. This is basically what creativity means, and it has two dimensions.

Objectification

The first is the simple fact that these are artifacts made by us – the clients, the counselors, and the researchers – for a public. When performance, and its sense and meaning, are turned into artifacts, they are objectified: made into objects – as in the art videos, or as in the videos and texts that document performance art (Groys, 2016). They become something solid over time, and something for other people to witness. And thus something to which power and recognition can be attached, through which they get to be mediated.

This was already in a sense the case with gestures and winks of the eye on the dance-floor or in group therapy – especially if those movements are rehearsed and become habits – but it is more visible and gets to be more important when it is built into things. At this level it makes a huge difference whether the things that are made by users and counsellors in places like HelsingUng or U-turn are case files with words about "anamnesis", "diagnosis", "social action plan", etc., circulated among professionals, or rather, music and works of art for a general public. Not only in the direct sense of the recognition attributed to the participants – that e.g. Sebastian is seen as someone who took part in making an interesting art video – but also in more roundabout ways, for instance through the ways it mediates connections and relations between different communities, and the ways it invites a public into the discussions about what goes on at HelsingUng or U-turn.

The case file and the recorded video are two very different ways to learn about Sebastian, for himself, for us, and then again for him because he knows how he presents himself to us. As already mentioned, just as we could claim that the videos are prototypes of counselling or youth work, we can also see them as prototypes of self-hood. He recognises himself in that prototypical narrative, not least because of the horizon of hope that is built into it (Mattingly, 2010). This is who he is, then: He can use it to remind himself that he is, among other things, a budding video artist, and also a participant in the making of a new kind of youth work that people study even in Nottingham because they are looking for ways to work with the subject of addiction.

Creativity

Each time, he sees the same images and hears the same song, but he sees and hears something different each time. Because the reservoir of meaning in artifacts like that is endless, and Sebastian is constantly developing and finding himself in new situations. This leads to the second aspect of my claim about creativity. Even though meaning is frozen into things, producing artifacts is always in some sense innovative. This idea goes back to Hegel's (1969) notion of the "cunning of reason": Means are made for ends, but they always tend to go beyond them and even prompt us to rethink our aims, purposes, and values[8]. Inviting an unpredictable future, which Derrida (2005) calls *l'avenir* – that which is to come. The reason for taking up art, and for talking about aesthetic practices, is just this. Art is when artifacts are made that are, we might say, paradoxically specialised in this becoming, in l'avenir.

Innovation is at the heart of science and theory, too, but in a different way. In theory, although we know that the meaning of our texts keeps changing through history, we always try to keep track of it, we always discuss what it means. In art, the point is just the opposite, to open up to multiple, contradictory ways to make sense of it – to create *dissensus* (Rancière, 2009). And tradition is mainly used as inspiration and material, never as a way to establish and sanction meaning. You can always ask *me* to unfold and explain; conceptual accountability is at the core of my job, even if I hope to create new understandings; but don't ask the poet what the poem means – just read the poem!

This is important here because it implies that art is "proposals of shared worlds" (Bourriaud, 2002, p. 9): If we use our senses and imagination, we can find ways to create prototypical narratives that work with people who are very diverse, and whose ways of engaging with cultural tradition we perhaps don't recognise at first. This doesn't mean there are no standards, as some critics of modern or post-modern art would perhaps claim. The standards that are taken up, performed, and recreated, as Halberg and Louie at *HelsingUng* produce the song, or Kofod, Larsen and Sebastian at U-turn make a video, are *aesthetic* standards. They want to create something that is somehow beautiful and appealing, but first of all intriguing, captivating, worth spending time pondering over. Something that is recognisable, alludes to some kind of known tradition, while at the same time doing that in a way that takes off from that tradition, perhaps visibly quotes it, paraphrases it, mocks it, etc., or perhaps just puts it into a new context.

This implies a recalcitrance that takes it beyond the simple mirroring of preferred self-images. A nice example of this was the production of the video with Sebastian. They recorded several "takes", some of which featured a Sebastian who sang much more confidently and more in tune; but Kofod and Larsen, the artists-counsellors, persuaded him that this first take was far better, precisely with the tangible fragility of his trembling voice. The success of this educational process was in Sebastian's submission to this augmented aesthetic value – and in our appreciation of it – as much as in how it achieved an expression and recognition of his idiosyncratic experience, and of his courage in exposing it.

But this could not have been predicted. Aesthetic value is the paradoxical value of *l'avenir*, of the setting of new standards to come. Aesthetics, then, is what finally takes these performance standards beyond the idea of just going through movements, reproducing acts – without resting on the dubious assumption of therapeutic effect regardless of client subjectivity.

In sum, they can be user-driven in a way that is quite different from FIT because they are prototypical narratives, made in a collaborative practice that enacts and displays how life could be, objectified for a diverse and heterogeneous audience, with recalcitrant and dissensual aesthetic artifacts, and with a view to the value of transforming values.

The social problem

This could all be simply the story of why we should forget about addiction and social problems and focus instead on creative activities. But if all this were done while just bracketing our "certain" knowledge that it's *really* methods applied at a drug treatment facility, and *really* about addiction and therapy, it would not amount to much more than refusing accountability. And all the points I've made here would be about a surface performance, with something quite different going on behind the stage. In fact, in education and social work there is a long history of just that move – pretending to be something else.

Rather, my fifth and final claim is that this should all be articulated as ways to address the suffering, the drama, the trauma, the doubts and fears, and the hopes and dreams, that we *share* with those people whom we now call clients. In other words, a way to perform and construct *addiction as a social problem*, a problem for the community, and even perhaps for our culture as a whole, rather than as a problem for designated individuals.

If we zoom out, it becomes obvious that this is how it is with addiction. In our modern individualised cultures and communities, it is so easy to get lost in habits, to lose control; in particular, perhaps, to lose control of our self-control (Alexander, 2008). This is a problem for all of us. One reason to take inspiration from Michael White is just that he realised this and took the whole narrative practice beyond an instrumental version of therapy that would ironically reproduce the instrumentalism of addiction itself (White, 1997). The paradox of the therapeutic "fix" is, in fact, one possible dead end of a purely pragmatic approach to user-driven standards (Nissen & Barington, 2016).

It is also easy to forget that our bad habits typically reflect social, ethnic, gendered or other inequalities. It is no coincidence that clients – or at least the target group population who *ought* to be helped – overwhelmingly represent the disadvantaged; those who have experienced trouble in school, those from poor families and so on. That is basically why we should overcome the idea that it is all about addiction as a diagnosed individual pathology. That is the only way we can create prototypical narratives in this field that challenge our diagnostic culture without simply tabooing addiction and its social conditions and consequences.

This can be expressed in terms of equality of health, and in terms of how public services can help cultivate our communities on a large scale. But it can also be expressed in aesthetic ways, with stories and pictures and songs of real people whom we can recognise and who can recognise themselves as part of communities rearticulated to make sense in new ways.

Conclusion

These claims about the practices of aesthetic documentation represent aspects of my standpoint and contribution to an ongoing dialogue with counsellors, managers and users around the facilities *U-turn* and *HelsingUng*, and in the wider fields of youth work, social work, and drug treatment. In terms of content, they articulate how, while what they do may be referred to and governed as "counselling drug users", their performances *also* take it beyond that standard. They break up and expand the *hardware* of therapy – with its individualising and stigmatising implications – that otherwise would frame any "language game" regardless of how radical a deconstruction and customisation to individual users. In terms of their form, they circumscribe an emergent infrastructure of practices, communities, and competences, which could be thought of as another bid for the currently evolving transdisciplinary forms of knowledge demanded in a post-industrial world. But, in contrast to the mainstream bid – the emerging apparatus of evidence-basing – this is one that does not itself contribute to the instrumentalist culture with which we are losing control of our self-control, and one that allows a place for philosophy, arts and humanities as forms of self-reflection, at a time when religion seems otherwise to regain its grip on our imagination in all the holes and cracks and blind spots that the standardising sciences keep producing.

Notes

1. See https://player.vimeo.com/video/98728123 (May, 2018).
2. See http://www.stuffsite.org/tiden-gar/ (May, 2018).
3. The portal http://www.stuffsite.org/ emerged from this collaboration (May, 2018).
4. Note that 'social work' in a Danish context is different from its UK version. For one thing, it is a generic term for a range of professions, including – as is mostly the case here – academically trained psychologist. See, to this Nissen (2012).

5. One 'aesthetic documentation' project was called *'Could Life Be ... '*. This is discussed in Nissen (2014).
6. We use the Danish term *'fremstilling'*, which means enacting, rendering, and displaying, but even also creating. Those with an interest in Heidegger's approach to technology will perhaps note an etymological connection with his concept 'Gestell' and its derivatives; in fact, "fremstilling" is at once Darstellen (rendering) and Herstellen (production), and thus the practical root of Vorstellen (imagination).
7. Reprinted from https://condenaststore.com/featured/why-does-he-always-get-to-be-the-boy-bruce-eric-kaplan.html
8. In recent science and technology studies, this is an important point; Bruno Latour coined it nicely in the title of his article "The end of the means" (2002).

Disclosure Statement

No potential conflict of interest was reported by the author.

ORCID

Morten Nissen http://orcid.org/0000-0003-4001-9163

References

Alexander, B. K. (2008). *The globalisation of addiction. A study in the poverty of the spirit.* New York, NY: Oxford University Press.
Baudrillard, J. (1994). *Simulacra and simulation.* Ann Arbor: University of Michigan press.
Boal, A. (2000). *Theater of the oppressed.* New York, NY: Pluto Press.
Bourriaud, N. (2002). *Relational aesthetics.* Dijon: Les presses du reel.
Brooke, S. L. (Ed.). (2009). *The use of the creative therapies with chemical dependency issues.* Springfield, IL: Charles C Thomas Publisher.
Busch, L. (2011). *Standards - recipes for reality.* Cambridge, MA: MIT Press.
Butler, J. (1993). *Bodies that matter. On the discursive limits of Sex.* New York, NY: Routledge.
De Shazer, S. (1991). *Putting difference to work.* New York, NY: W.W. Norton & Co.
Derrida, J. (2005). *The politics of friendship.* London: Verso.
Duncan, B. L., Miller, S. D., Wampold, B. E., & Hubble, M. A. (Eds.). (2010). *The heart and soul of change: Delivering what works in therapy* (2nd ed.). Washington, DC: American Psychological Association.
Goffman, E. (1986). *Frame analysis. An essay on the organisation of experience.* Boston: North Eastern University Press.
Groys, B. (2016). *In the flow.* London: Verso Books.
Halberg, M. (2013). Skriften på væggen - gruppesamtaler som værdsættende ceremoni. [The writing on the wall: Group conversations as appreciating ceremony]. *Stof* (22): 63–75.
Hanson, F. A. (1993). *Testing testing: Social consequences of the examined life.* Berkeley, CA: University of California Press.
Hart, J. T. (2006). *The political economy of health care: A clinical perspective.* Bristol: Policy Press.
Hegel, G. W. F. (1969). *Hegel's science of logic.* London, New York, NY: Prometheus Books.
Høgsbro, K. K., & Nissen, M. (2014). Narrative, substance, and fiction. In J. R. Z. Zontou (Ed.), *Addiction and performance* (pp. 151–177). Newcastle upon Tyne: Cambridge Scholars Publishing.
Jameson, F. (1998). *Brecht and method.* London: Verso.
Jensen, U. J. (1987). *Practice and progress: A theory for the modern health care system.* Oxford: Blackwell.
Latour, B. (2002). Morality and technology. The end of the means. *Theory, Culture & Society, 19*(5/6), 247–260.
Lave, J. (2011). *Apprenticeship in critical ethnographic practice.* Chicago: University of Chicago Press.
Liberali, F. (2000). Developing argumentative processes for critical reflection. *Research And Teacher Development SIG Special Joint Issue, 21*(1), 62–66.

Linnell, S. (2010). *Art psychotherapy and narrative therapy: An account of practitioner research.* Melbourne: Bentham Science Publishers.

Martin, E. (2007). *Bipolar expeditions: Mania and depression in American culture.* Princeton: Princeton University Press.

Mattingly, C. (2010). *The paradox of hope: Journeys through a clinical borderland.* Berkeley, London: University of California Press.

Miller, W. R., & Rollnick, S. (1991). *Motivational interviewing: Preparing people to change addictive behavior.* New York, NY: Guilford Press.

Mol, A. (2008). *The logic of care. Health and the problem of patient choice.* New York, NY: Routledge.

Newman, F., & Holzman, L. (1996). *Unscientific psychology: A cultural-performatory approach to understanding human life.* Westport, CT: Praeger.

Nielsen, S., & Kofod, K. (2013). Æstetisk dokumentation af unges selv-fortællinger. [Aesthetic Documentation of young pepole's self-narratives]. *Stof,* (21), 33–37.

Nissen, M. (2009). Objectification and prototype. *Qualitative Research in Psychology, 6*(1), 67–87.

Nissen, M. (2012). *The subjectivity of participation. Articulating social work practice with youth in Copenhagen.* London: Palgrave MacMillan.

Nissen, M. (2014). Could life Be ... producing subjectivity in participation. In A. Blunden (Ed.), *Collaborative projects* (pp. 69–84). London: Brill.

Nissen, M. (2015). Meeting youth in movement and on neutral ground. *Dialogic Pedagogy: An International Online Journal, 3.* doi:https://doi.org/10.5195/dpj.2015.34.

Nissen, M. (2016). Standards and standpoints: Why and how standards, and studying them, imply critique. *Theory & Psychology, 26*(2)), 163–181.

Nissen, M., & Barington, K. (2016). Numbers: Manageable nothingness or user- driven standards? In D. A. Winther-Lindqvist, & J. Bang (Eds.), *Nothingness* (pp. 251–286). New Brunswick, London: Transaction Publishers.

Norcross, J. C. (2011). *Psychotherapy relationships that work: Evidence-based responsiveness.* Oxford: Oxford University Press.

Porter, T. (1995). *Trust in numbers. The pursuit of objectivity in science and public life.* Princeton: Princeton University Press.

Rancière, J. (2009). *The emancipated spectator.* London: Verso.

Rowland, N., & Goss, S. (eds.). (2013). *Evidence based counselling and psychological therapies: Research and applications.* London: Routledge.

Sackett, D. L., et al. (2000). *Evidence-Based medicine - How to practice and teach EBM.* Toronto: Churchill Livingstone.

Sloan, C. (2014). From substance misuse: The musical To double whammy: The affect Of outside edge theatre company. In J. Z. Reynolds & Z. Zontou (Eds.), *Addiction and performance* (pp. 214–233). London: Cambridge Scholars Publishing.

Stenner, P. (2016). On standards and values: Between finite actuality and infinite possibility. *Theory & Psychology, 26*(2)), 144–162.

Suchman, L., et al. (2002). Working artefacts: Ethnomethods of the prototype. *British Journal of Sociology, 53*(2), 163–179.

Turner, V. (1995). *The ritual process: Structure and anti-structure.* London: Transaction Publishers.

Wampold, B. E. (2001). *The great psychotherapy debate: Models, methods, and findings.* Mahwah, NJ: Erlbaum.

White, M. (1997). Challenging the culture of consumption. Rites of passage and communities of acknowledgement. In M. Raven (Ed.), *New perspectives on addiction.* Adelaide, AU: Dulwich Centre.

White, M. (2007). *Maps of narrative practice.* New York, NY: W.W. Norton.

White, M., & Epston, D. (1990). *Narrative means to therapeutic ends.* New York, NY: WW Norton.

Wittgenstein, L. (2010). *Philosophical investigations.* London: John Wiley & Sons.

Transforming career stories through poetry: a group-based career counselling intervention

Esther Wafula

ABSTRACT

Contemplating the school to work transition in the insecure and unpredictable twenty-first century world of work can be anxiety inducing for college students. Consequently, college students may develop disempowered career stories in which they feel ill prepared to explore career prospects or engage with the world of work. This paper describes a career counselling intervention aimed at transforming the disempowered career stories of college students into more empowered versions. Grounded in career construction theory and designed as a group modality, the intervention employs poetry therapy to enhance the development of internally defined and motivated career stories among the group participants. Although this paper highlights the Kenyan context, the intervention itself can easily be adapted to other contexts.

Introduction

Developmentally, most college students fall within the young adulthood stage (also called emerging adulthood), which refers to the life period between ages 18 and 25 (Berger, 2014). Young adulthood provides an opportunity for college students to develop their self-concept in relation to their careers (Hartung, 2013). However, this stage is also rife with anxiety, uncertainty and self-questioning (Arnett, 2015), conditions that are only compounded by globalisation and information saturation in the twenty-first century (Del Corso, 2017). As they contemplate their transition from school to work, college students cannot avoid the realities of the twenty-first century world of work. The current career landscape is increasingly unpredictable (Di Fabio & Maree, 2013), highly insecure and complex (Lengelle, Meijers, & Hughes, 2016) – a situation some have termed "a career management nightmare" (Callanan, Perri, & Tomkowicz, 2017, p. 362). In the Kenyan context, many students are the first, and often the only members of their families to attend college. Such students must confront the challenge of fulfilling their own career aspirations in a competitive employment market. They also bear the additional burden of family expectations that they will secure well-paying jobs to support themselves and their extended families. All these realities, pressures and expectations can make college students develop disempowered career stories in which they feel overwhelmed and ill prepared to explore career prospects or engage with the world of work. Disempowered career stories among college students may also emerge in the form of career related anxiety, which has been described as affective distress in relation to career decision making (Germeijs, Verschueren, & Soenens, 2006). Such distress can adversely affect self-exploration and information seeking about careers.

This paper describes a career counselling intervention aimed at transforming the disempowered career stories of college students into more empowered versions. Grounded in career construction theory and designed as a group modality, the intervention employs poetry reading and writing tasks to enhance the development of internally defined and motivated career stories among the group participants. The proposed intervention innovatively leverages the inherent power of both narrative career counselling and poetry therapy. The intervention responds to the frequent calls for career counsellors to develop dynamic programmes that address twenty-first century career challenges (Callanan et al., 2017) and foster career adaptability and resilience in their clients (Busacca, 2007; Del Corso, 2017; Maree, 2017; Rehfuss, 2013; Savickas, 2005; Savickas, 2011; Savickas & Hartung, 2012).

After outlining the career guidance needs of college students, the paper introduces the My Career Story (MCS) workbook (Savickas & Hartung, 2012), a tool based on career construction theory, which will act as the guiding framework while poetry will be used as an ancillary tool. Thereafter, an overview of poetry therapy and its practical application, especially in a career counselling context is provided. The therapeutic rationale for using poetry in 5 successive group sessions is highlighted. Finally, a practical application guide detailing the overall goals of the intervention, objectives and tasks of each group session is also provided.

The need for career guidance in higher education settings

The need to guide college students as they navigate young adulthood and its attendant challenges is widely acknowledged. A study by the American College Health Association found that over half the college students surveyed had experienced overwhelming anxiety during the previous year (2015). In a phenomenological study among college students, Pisarik, Rowell, and Thompson (2017) found that lack of career guidance was one of the seven themes that emerged as a contributor to career anxiety. It has also been noted that the complexity of the contemporary world of work makes parents ill-equipped to support their children in making suitable career choices (Lengelle, Meijers, Poell, & Post, 2014). Furthermore, for young people to thrive in the twenty-first century, they must develop complex identities, which are internally defined and not dependent on external forces such as authority figures like parents, teachers and the wider society (Baxter Magolda, 1999). Various writers have also underscored the fact that higher education settings provide unparalleled opportunities to help students navigate the developmental challenges of young adulthood (Baxter Magolda, 1999, 2004; Chireshe, 2012; Evans, Forney, Guido, Patton, & Renn, 2010).

According to Donald Super's life-span, life-space theory of careers, young adulthood coincides with the exploration stage (Hartung, 2013). During this stage, young adults develop their self-concept in an occupational role by clarifying what they want to do (crystallization), specify a career choice (specification) and begin working (implementation) (Hartung, 2013). In addition to the concerns that Donald Super associated with the exploration stage, Arnett (2015) has characterised young adulthood, which he refers to as emerging adulthood, as a period of anxiety, uncertainty, self-questioning and insecurity. This sense of self-questioning and insecurity among young adults is compounded by globalisation and information saturation, especially from social media which create unrealistic expectations incongruent to the realities of the twenty-first century career landscape (Del Corso, 2017). In the meantime, it has been argued that thriving in the twenty-first century world of work requires skills such as openness to multiple careers and lifelong learning (Van Vianen, De Pater & Preenene, 2009). Furthermore, many students find the college to work transition a challenging experience because of the significant changes it entails (Domene, Landine, & Stewart, 2015; Wendlandt & Rochlen, 2008).

In view of these challenges, Del Corso (2017) has argued that career counsellors must foster the career adaptability and resilience of young adults by helping them enhance their own agency and self-construction. Narrative career counselling approaches, which emphasise client stories, enhance client reflexivity and clarify identity (Busacca, 2017), are highly recommended for this task.

In designing the intervention proposed in this paper, I take the view that helping college students develop an internally defined career identity is one of the most effective ways to enhance their career adaptability and resilience. To that end, use of the MCS workbook process, enhanced through poetry for a group career counselling modality is proposed. Although the use of poetry in the context of career counselling is applicable anywhere in the world, the proposed intervention has been designed with Kenyan college students in mind. As such, several poems prescribed for the third group session specifically target concerns pertinent to the Kenyan context. Some of these concerns include gender and vocational stereotyping (Osoro, Amundson, & Borgen, 2000; Suda, 2002; USAID, 2014). However, the intervention can be applied in other settings with slight modifications, for example, to the poems selected for readings during the group sessions.

Overview of twenty-first century career guidance and the my career story workbook

Career guidance in the twenty-first century

Career counselling aims at improving work behaviour or preventing work related problems. On the other hand, career guidance is typically offered in educational settings to enhance students' awareness about self-attributes and planning in relation to the world of work and different career options (Lent & Brown, 2013). The career counselling and career guidance practices of the past presumed predictable career trajectories where competent individuals were almost assured of job security and career advancement up the organisational ladder. However, deindustrialisation, globalisation and technological advancements have raised the level of precarious work (Busacca & Rehfuss, 2017), underemployment and anxiety in the twenty-first century (Blustein, 2017). In this context, career counsellors are required to enhance the career adaptability of their clients and to help them become more employable and resilient in the face of multiple career transitions (Maree, 2017). Career counsellors must therefore employ dynamic approaches responsive to the current realities in the world of work (Callanan et al., 2017).

Career construction theory

Career construction theory, formulated by Mark Savickas (Savickas, 2002, 2005, 2006, 2013), has emerged as one of the promising theories in the context of a rapidly changing career landscape. The theory explains the "interpretive and interpersonal processes through which individuals give meaning and direction to their vocational behaviour" (Di Fabio & Maree, 2013, p. 5) and emphasises the notion of career as story (Maree, 2017). Furthermore, career construction theory asserts that individuals drive their career development by adapting to their environment, rather than through maturation, and as such, even career related traits are considered strategies for adapting rather than as fixed categories (Savickas, 2006, 2013). This attention to how clients adapt to their contexts in developing their careers is referred to as "self-construction" and is central to the career construction theory (Savickas, 2013, p. 147). Various career counselling tools have been developed based on career construction theory. One of these tools, the My Career Story workbook, is described briefly below.

My Career Story workbook

My Career Story: An Autobiographical Workbook for Life-Career Success (MCS; Savickas & Hartung, 2012) is a workbook containing a series of questions designed to facilitate clients' reflection on their life stories or autobiographies, and by so doing to deepen their life-career planning and to add meaning to those career plans and choices. The MCS is grounded conceptually in career construction theory, developed by Mark Savickas at the turn of the century (Savickas, 2002, 2005). The MCS is accessible free of charge from www.vocopher.com and is suitable for use in group or educational settings.

According to its authors, the MCS aims at helping an individual tell, hear and author their own life story (Savickas & Hartung, 2012). This narrative or qualitative character of the MCS is considered one of the tool's greatest strengths since it elicits self-reflective questions and facilitates individuals, alone or with the help of others, gain a clearer sense of direction about the future (Rehfuss, 2017). The central idea of the workbook is that an individual's life-story has the capacity to empower them, but, "the power is in its telling" hence the need to give it voice and clarity (Rehfuss, 2017, p. 95). This paper proposes to enhance the articulation of the life stories of the career counselling group participants through poetry reading and writing in addition to the regular MCS workbook tasks. The section below will first outline the procedural and technical features of the MCS. Thereafter, the historical background of poetry therapy in general and then, more specifically, the utility of poetry reading and writing in career counselling will be explained.

Procedural and technical features of the my career story workbook

The MCS workbook is designed for use with individuals completing it alone, or in group settings. Thoughtfully responding to the questions in the MCS could take 1–2 h, or longer depending on the number of sections that one decides to address in a single sitting (Rehfuss, 2017). When used in a group setting, the participants complete the different sections of the workbook individually, then meet to share their responses and stories with other group members during career counselling group sessions (Rehfuss, 2017). Group settings are preferred because they provide an audience that listens and offers an opportunity for the individual to tell and enact their stories (Savickas & Hartung, 2012). The importance of audience in narrative therapy is underscored by Briddick and Sensoy-Briddick (2013), who describe it as "a means of supporting new, preferred and more favourable life stories" (p. 79).

The MCS workbook comprises three sections to guide the user in telling their life-story. In Part 1, "Telling My Story," clients describe the transition they currently face and how they hope the workbook will be useful to them; list occupations they have considered pursuing; identify and describe role models they admired when growing up, including favourite magazines and television shows, their current favourite story (from a book or movie) and a favourite saying or motto. In Part 2, "Hearing my story," the client creates a portrait of their life by pulling together the small stories from Part 1 into a larger, more cohesive life-career story (Savickas & Hartung, 2012, p. 3). This is done by responding to questions like "Who am I/Who am I becoming?" (the self) (Savickas & Hartung, 2012, p. 10), and "Where do I like to be?" (the settings one likes to work in) (p. 11). By clarifying the client's life story, Part 2 makes the story more easily accessible to the client as they try to make sense of the changes they are facing and the choices they must make (Savickas & Hartung, 2012). Part 3, "Enacting my story," involves creation of a detailed, three-part plan to facilitate a client's movement from the story into action. First, under "Reflect" the client is prompted to select a goal that will enable them to enact and bring their career story to life. Secondly, under "Tell" the client is encouraged to share their story and the conclusions they have drawn from the workbook with trusted others, such as family members, friends, mentors, or teachers. Finally, under "Perform," the client is urged to identify two to four specific objectives or steps they will take to help move them forward toward the goals they have set.

Proposed use of poetry with the my career story workbook for career counselling in a group modality

An overview of poetry therapy and its practical application

Poetry therapy has been variously defined as "the application of poetry to the therapeutic process" (Lerner, 1982, p. 229); or "the use of language, symbol and story in therapeutic, educational and community building capacities" (Mazza, as cited in Mazza, 2017, p. 3). Poetry therapy can be applied in different modalities, for example, with individuals, families, groups and communities (Mazza, 2017). Historically, poetry was used by healers in ancient societies such as the Greeks and indigenous people in America (Mazza, 2017). The potency of the word is also noted in the belief systems of major ancient civilisations, for example in Biblical literature, the Egyptian Book of the Dead, and among pre-Islamic Arabs (Reiter, 2000). In the 1970s, poetry therapy was described as being "in a state of flux" – it lacked a central guiding theory or rationale (Lerner, 1978, p. xv) and the associated literature was mainly anecdotal (Schloss & Grundy, 1978). More recently, however, poetry therapy has become an increasingly recognised approach. This is evidenced by the establishment of a National Association for Poetry Therapy in 1980 (NAPT, n.d.), publication of numerous books on the subject, its inclusion in key reference books and the inclusion of the *Journal of Poetry Therapy* in major research databases such as PsychINFO (Mazza, 2017).

Theoretically, poetry therapy has been associated with analytical psychology (Ansell, 1978; Mazza, 2017). Like dreams, poems are believed to tap into the unconscious in a manner that can facilitate an "epiphany of the self" (Edgar, 1978, p. 24). According to Edgar, clients project their unwanted emotions (or "parapathy") in their early poems while growth and recovery can be noted as the client's intense emotions are "assimilated" through analysis of the client's own poems (Edgar, 1978, p. 25). The therapeutic benefits of writing are also noted by researchers Pennebaker and Seagal (1999). Their study demonstrated improvements in the mental and physical health of participants who wrote about significant personal experiences in an emotional way for as little as 15 minutes during the course of three days.

Poetry therapy has been used with adolescents and young adults in different settings such as schools, colleges, at spoken word poetry workshops and at correctional facilities. Some counsellors and social workers have leveraged the growing popularity of hip hop and rap music in their work with the adolescent and young adult population (DeCarlo & Hockman, 2004; Grace, Smith, & Hinchman, 2004; Levy, 2012; Olson-McBride & Page, 2012; Xerri, 2017; Yücesan & Şendurur, 2018). According to Candy Royalle, an Australian poet who works with youth, spoken word poetry

> is a potent means by which to combat the voice poverty that young people are prone to experience. It helps to empower them to express themselves in a language they can understand, and enables them to explore their own vulnerability and build resilience (Xerri, 2017, p. 269).

In their work with at-risk youth, most of whom are in correctional facilities, Gold and his colleagues in the Pongo Teen Writing project focus on helping their clients to write their own poetry, a process that offers an effective way to help youth and also learn from them (Gold, 2014). Although some of the group members may have an affinity to reading literature and / or listening to music, an inclination to poetry reading or writing is not a prerequisite to joining a group where poetry therapy is used. Moreover, as Gold (2014) has argued, expressive writing which can include poetry writing is based on the lived experience of the writer, not only from the past and present but also the imagined future. As such, no special knowledge is required to qualify one to participate in a group that employs expressive writing for healing and personal development.

The practical application of poetry in therapy has been described in different ways. Reiter (2000) states that poetry therapy is typically practiced in one of two ways. First, a therapist brings in, or imports, metaphors and symbolism relevant for the client(s) through carefully selected words or literature; or secondly, the therapist draws out, or exports, the personal metaphors or symbolism of the client(s) through structured writing (Reiter, 2000). The methodology is described somewhat differently by Mazza (2017) whose RES framework consists of three components. These are (i) (R) the receptive or prescriptive component where literature is introduced; (ii) (E) the expressive or creative component where the client's own writing is used and (iii) (S) the symbolic or ceremonial component which employs metaphors, rituals and storytelling (Mazza, 2017).

The use of poetry reading and writing in career counselling

The utility of therapeutic writing, including the use of poetry, in healing is well articulated by Lengelle and Meijers (2009) in their transformation-through-writing model in which a painful "first story" is re-written to become a more life-giving "second-story" (p. 57). According to Meijers (2002), the transformation or identity development that occurs as one moves from their first story to their second story is triggered by a "boundary experience," which he defines as "an experience in which the individual experiences the boundary of his existing self-concept" (p. 158). A boundary experience can be a condition, such as a chronic illness or an event like sudden job loss; or a disempowering attitude that compromises the person's ability to cope, challenges their sense of identity and limits their ability to act with confidence (Lengelle, 2014). The boundary experience may manifest itself as a cognitive problem where the individual feels they do not understand the situation or have the necessary knowledge and skills to resolve it (Meijers, 2002). However, boundary experiences more often emerge as an emotional problem whereby a person's identity structure is incongruent to the situation they are facing (Meijers, 2002) because their earlier identification inhibits an appropriate response to the situation at hand (Lengelle, 2014). For growth or transformation to occur, the individual would have to be freed from the trap of the "fight, flight or freeze mode" of their first story (Lengelle, 2014, p. 25), by working toward a more empowering second story. According to Lengelle and Meijers (2009), counsellors can facilitate this movement from disempowered first stories to more empowered second stories by guiding their clients through therapeutic writing which can include poetry reading and writing.

Lengelle and Meijers argued that therapeutic writing facilitates healing through a "transformative and dialogical-learning process" (2009, p. 57) that occurs in four cognitive stages, namely sensing, sifting, focusing and understanding originally borrowed from career researcher Bill Law. Later, Lengelle and her colleagues demonstrated that this model of transformation-through-writing, referred to as "Career Writing" when applied to career concerns, can facilitate the construction of a career identity (Lengelle et al., 2014, p. 75). In Career Writing, the client's past (the "first story") is brought into the present through creative, expressive and reflective writing, with the aim of developing "a more empowering perspective" or "second story" (Lengelle, 2014, p. 25).

Lengelle posits that as clients explore, describe and write down their emotions in the sensing stage, they "open up to what is happening inside" and by so doing useful initial images and transformative metaphors emerge (2014, p. 27). Poetry writing is recommended for the sensing stage because it uses words sparingly thereby helping focus the client's attention to the most salient themes (Lengelle, 2014). In the sifting stage, clients explore questions of causality (Lengelle & Meijers, 2009); compare their circumstances with those of their peers, develop analogies and attend to the emerging constructs and concepts. In the focusing stage, the client attempts to "string together feelings, ideas and life themes" (Lengelle, 2014, p. 28), which enables them to connect the fragments of their life and to observe patterns (Lengelle & Meijers, 2009). Poetry is also considered useful at this stage since it provides structure through which feelings can be expressed and contained (Lengelle & Meijers, 2009). Finally, the insights gained in the focusing stage are consolidated into a second story in the understanding stage (Lengelle & Meijers, 2009). This involves the client formulating their own theory or hypothesis to explain what has happened in their life so far. By so doing, the client can notice what the first story they have been telling themselves is, and how they need to develop a more empowering second story. This swath of literature provides a sound basis for the proposed intervention. Further details on the therapeutic rationale for the use of poetry in the career counselling contexts are provided in the section below.

Therapeutic rationale for use of poetry in the transforming career stories intervention

This section provides the rationale for the poetry therapy tasks proposed for each of the career counselling sessions in the Transforming Career Stories through Poetry intervention. For purposes of this paper, the boundary experience facing college students is considered both an event and an attitude. The event is the imminent transition from college into a complex, uncertain and insecure employment market (Callanan et al., 2017; Di Fabio & Maree, 2013; Lengelle et al., 2016). The attitudinal aspect of the boundary experience is the overwhelming anxiety that college students experience as they contemplate their career prospects (Pisarik et al., 2017) and their potential lack of internally defined identities (Baxter Magolda, 1999).

Writing about career assessments in African contexts, Mkhize (2015) has argued that the social and ethical understanding of what it means to be human ("Ubuntu") should be considered (p. 247). The African concept of Ubuntu is expressed in one language as: "a person is a person through other people" (Bolden, 2014, p. 799). The positive aspects of the Ubuntu philosophy include collaboration, cooperation and community (Bolden, 2014). In other words, the Ubuntu philosophy places more value on the interdependence and mutual responsibility of individuals in the family and community setting than on the individual's independence and self- interest. Nevertheless, Mkhize (2015) contends that the resulting tension from communal, family and personal demands on individuals must be considered when conducting career assessments in the African context. Similar considerations must be borne in mind when delivering career counselling interventions to African clients in an African context (Watson, McMahon, Mkhize, Schweitzer, & Mpofu, 2011). In Kenya, many college students are often the first members of their respective families to attend college. As such, they bear the burden of familial expectations that when they graduate, they will secure good jobs to support themselves and their extended families. In the meantime, youth unemployment in Kenya has been cited at rates as high as 55%, and even higher (62%) among women (Awiti & Scott, 2016). Competing and often unrealistic family expectations, the discouraging employment situation and lack of career guidance can create a disempowered first story in a Kenyan college student. Consequently, many Kenyan college students are unlikely to have internally developed career identities or the confidence necessary to explore career prospects in the complex and competitive employment market.

The career counselling intervention proposed here aims to help such college students to move from the disempowered first story, to a second story in which they have internally defined career identities, with concrete steps to pursue toward their desired career paths. As the students go through the different sessions of the intervention, the process will help them examine, more consciously, the internalised social commitments they are pressured by within a context where the Ubuntu philosophy is still dominant. The poetry writing tasks will help participants tease out the career related expectations that are based on family and community concerns vis á vis personal career interests that may or may not have been considered so far. Table 1 below outlines how the sessions of the proposed intervention correspond to the cognitive stages described in Lengelle and Meijers' (2009) transformation-through-writing model. Also highlighted is how poetry will facilitate the participants' transformation from their disempowered first career stories to their second more empowered versions.

Rationale for use of a group modality in career counselling

Use of a group modality for career counselling interventions is especially advantageous when working with young adults in educational settings. Compared to working with individual clients, the group format is more time and cost effective, in addition to providing a peer environment of support where recognition of shared difficulties offers relief and a context where participants can try out things they may later enact in the 'real-world' (Lengelle & Meijers, 2018). In Kenya the counselling profession is still in its formative phase (Masambia, 2014) and many students do not have access to career guidance services (USAID, 2014). The group modality would therefore be an efficient approach to provide career counselling services in Kenyan colleges. The modality also leverages therapeutic factors such as the building of social skills, instillation of hope, interpersonal learning and insight (Goldstein, 1989; Yalom & Leszcz, 2005).

Table 1. Therapeutic rationale of using poetry at each stage of the intervention.

Career counselling session	Corresponding cognitive stage	How poetry will facilitate transformation from the "first" to the "second" career story
1. Orientation 2. Telling my story	Sensing	• One's "parapathy" (Edgar, 1978, p. 25) or career concerns are projected in the initial poem (s). • Salient images and metaphors are surfaced. • Catharsis through poems that describe early recollections.
3. Hearing my story	Sifting and Focusing	• Causes and patterns of disempowered first story e.g. gender stereotyping, a dangerous "single story" (Adichie, 2009) are explored. • Potent life themes and negative aspects of one's disempowered story are identified and documented in a "dead-end-circle" poem (Gustavson, 2006, *p.* 20). To do this, the participant starts writing the poem near the top of the page in a circular format going clockwise. This creates a circle that winds in on itself and gets tighter as one nears the centre of the circle, which is the dead-end. Writing the dead-end circle poem will help demonstrate how negative life themes and disempowered stories constrict people's perspectives and lead to dead ends or blockages with no way out. • An alternative, more positive story is developed by noting affirmations, promises, prophesies (including those by the self) and documented in a "reverse circle" poem (Gustavson, 2006, p. 21). A reverse circle poem is formed as one starts writing words or phrases at the centre of the page and working outward in an anticlockwise direction to create an ever- expanding circle. This type of poem illustrates how affirmations, promises and a new more positive narrative can help one work their way out of the dead-end circle of their first disempowered story. • External dialogue is facilitated through reading one's poems to the group.
4. Enacting my story	Understanding	• Consolidate insights gained from the previous sessions through a new motto / mantra and creation of a collaborative poem. • Emphasise a more agile, receptive and intentional posture toward one's career through reading and discussion of the prescribed poems.

Participation in the group will be limited to undergraduate students enrolled at the college where the intervention will be implemented. Students interested in exploring their career stories will be encouraged to participate. However, no limitation in terms of age, gender, year of study or affinity to poetry will be imposed on those interested in joining the group.

The proposed career counselling group consisting of between 10 and 12 participants is expected to meet once a week for 5 successive sessions only. As such, the group can be considered a closed-ended, short term group (Brabender, Fallon, & Smolar, 2004). The design of the proposed intervention has considered the lifecycle of groups (Brabender et al., 2004; Corey, 2012). Hence, the first session will involve orientation and exploration tasks such as establishing trust, defining goals and clarifying expectations (Corey, 2012); building a sense of cohesion and developing group norms to support the overall group goals (Brabender et al., 2004). The working stage of the group will encompass the second, third and fourth sessions. These sessions will involve in-depth exploration (Corey, 2012) of the group members' career concerns through the MCS workbook framework, enhanced with poetry reading and writing tasks. The termination of the career counselling intervention will be done in the fifth session. This stage will involve consolidating the gains made by members during the previous group sessions, identifying future goals and deciding how to pursue those goals (Brabender et al., 2004). It will also be an opportunity for group members to review their experience in the group, give and receive feedback (Corey, 2012), and to share what has been most meaningful to them personally from participating in the group. Table 2 outlines the tasks typically performed through the MCS workbook, as well as the poetry therapy tasks designed to enhance the development of career identities for individuals who participate in the proposed intervention. The poems listed for reading during the intervention were selected based on their potential to evoke reflection on themes pertinent to career identities. However, different poems could be used, as long as they too are carefully selected by the career counsellor to facilitate reflection on similar themes.

Table 2. Practical application guide for the "transforming career stories through poetry" career counselling group.

General goals The "Transforming career stories through poetry" career counselling group will help participants to: (1) Understand the relationship between their personal interests and career interests; (2) Explore how their self- identity and career identity are influenced by personal stories and narratives; (3) Identify emerging life and career themes; (4) Learn how the emerging themes can be used to address their career decisions. Adapted from Rehfuss (2017).	
Session 1- (Lasting 60 min) Orientation Objective: Group member introductions; group orientation to the My Career Story workbook and the poetry therapy components; and setting of group norms.	
Group process and My Career Story Work book orientation	Proposed poetry therapy task
The group members introduce themselves and state why they joined the group, what they expect to gain from it, and their feelings about poetry.	Warm up exercises to help break the ice and facilitate introductions and cooperation between group members (Schloss & Grundy, 1978): (i) Read a poem suggesting an introduction e.g. Emily Dickinson's "I am nobody, Who are you?" (Schloss & Grundy, 1978, p. 83). (ii) ii. Each group member picks one of the natural elements that they most identify with: Earth, Water, Wind and Fire. Group members who identify with the same element collaborate on a poem describing the common element; then the collaborative poem is read aloud to the wider group. This exercise is adapted from Jones (1996).
With guidance from the Facilitator, the group members agree on the group norms (Johnson & Johnson, 2014). The Facilitator documents the group norms so that a copy can be shared with each group member at the start of the next session. The Facilitator briefs the group members about: (1) The therapeutic factors of group therapy (Brabender et al., 2004; Yalom & Leszcz, 2005) and how to leverage these during future group sessions; (2) Career counselling using the My Career Story workbook process (Savickas & Hartung, 2012). Copies of the MCS workbook are distributed. (3) Enhancement of the career counselling process through poetic creativity (4) How forthcoming sessions will be structured.	To inform the group norms, each group member writes a short poem, of four to six lines describing conditions in which they feel safe to be themselves. Individual group members read these poems to the rest of the group. End the session with a reading of the poem "Meditation" by Laurie Beth Jones which describes the four elements (Jones, 1996, p. 31).
Session 2 (Lasting 2 h including a 15-minute break) Part 1- Telling my story Objective: Group members identify the key influences in their lives and reflect on their life stories.	
Typical My Career Story workbook task (45 min)	Proposed poetry therapy task (60 min)
Group members identify their current career concern or transition.	Each group member writes a poem expressing what they feel right now about their career transition or concern. Based on Stekel's argument that clients tend to "displace symptoms into the poetry" (as cited in Edgar, 1978, p. 24), these initial poems will facilitate an assessment of each member's concerns, and a baseline from which growth and evolution following the career counselling process can be monitored.
Group members list possible occupations	No poetry related activity to be undertaken here.
Each group member responds to four questions about: (1) Role models they admired when growing up (these can be real or fictional characters) (2) Their favourite magazines or television shows (3) Their current favourite stories (4) Their current favourite saying or motto (Savickas, 2015)	To emphasise how role models may have influenced group member's lives, group members perform an adapted version of the Past Personality Influences (PPI) exercise from Jones, 1996, p. 37 as follows: (i) Group members imagine themselves receiving a gift e.g. a vase with flowers or a goblet from each of their 3 role models- and write words to describe the 3 gifts (e.g. incorporating items such as traits, attitudes, values and problem solving strategies) (Stoltz & Barclay, 2015); then

	(ii) Each group member writes a poem based on the above exercise and shares it with the group. Individuals can write a poem about one of the gifts or a composite of the various gifts from their role models.
Group members describe 3 of their earliest recollections of what they recall happening when they were between 3 and 10 years old. These should be actual memories of events, not stories that were reported to them by others (Mosak & Di Pietro, 2006; Stoltz, 2017). Note: although the early recollections task is not part of the My Client Story workbook, it is one of the most significant tasks in Savickas' original Career Construction Interview (Savickas, 2015). The use of early recollections helps identify how clients view problems, including their thinking, behavioural and attitudinal patterns (Stoltz, 2017).	Each group member is requested to create a composite prose poem based on their 3 earliest recollections. The poems will explore: (i) Captions for each of the early recollections (such as headlines for newspaper stories) (Mosak & Di Pietro, 2006; Stoltz, 2017); (ii) The most important scene and most salient moments (Clark, 2013; Stoltz, 2017); (iii) The most prominent emotions experienced; (iv) The prominent striving force, movement or posture (using verbs) (Stoltz & Barclay, 2015); (v) The prominent moral (s) of the stories in the early recollections (Stoltz & Barclay, 2015); (vi) The predominant thinking, behavioural and attitudinal patterns or themes (Stoltz, 2017). Group members willing to share their prose poems will be invited to read them to the rest of the group.
Session 3 (Lasting 2 h, including a 15-minute break) Part 2- Hearing my story Objective: Group members draw together the separate stories from Part 1 to create larger, more cohesive narratives of their life-careers and have an opportunity for clients to hear their own stories.	
Review of typical My Career Story workbook tasks (45 min)	Proposed poetry therapy task (60 min)
Self: Group members identify words and phrases used in Part 1 that describe who they are and who they want to become.	No poetry related activity to be undertaken here.
Setting: Group members identify the plots they relate to and link those to the RIASEC model for more descriptive words relating to work setting. Using the identified words, clients determine the type of environments they would like to work in. Note: RIASEC stands for Realistic, Investigative, Artistic, Social, Enterprising and Conventional. This framework of grouping vocational interests was developed by John Holland (Holland, 1997). According to Holland, individuals look for work environments that are congruent to their interests, and such congruence enhances persistence, performance and satisfaction at work (Stoll et al., 2017).	No poetry related activity to be undertaken here.
Summary Portrait: Individual group members develop a single summary page of their story including: (1) Self. (2) Setting. (3) Script/plot: group members apply the plot from their favourite story or movie to what they want to do in the setting described in point 2 above. (4) Success formula: Drawing from the first 3 summaries above (Self, Setting, and Script) group members create a one sentence personal life-career mission statement. (5) Self-advice: Group members write the best advise they can give to themselves (or motto) to help them resolve their current career concern.	No poetry related activity to be undertaken here.
Rewriting My Story: Group members rewrite their initial career concern using the success formula and self- advice they developed under the task above.	The whole group watches Chimamanda Adichie's Ted talk titled: "The Danger of a single story" (Adichie, 2009). Thereafter, poems highlighting gender stereotypes in the African context are read to the whole group. For example, on women read: "Freedom Song" (Oludhe-Macgoye, n.d); and about men read "Trousers of wind" (an Amharic traditional from Ethiopia in Heywood, 1983, p. 129). Then each group member:

(i) Identifies the "single story" that he or she (or other people) have been telling about them.
(ii) Identify any negative/ disempowering connotations/ descriptions of that single story, including gender stereotypes where relevant;
(iii) Write a "Dead-end circle" poem (as in Gustavson, 2006, *p.* 20) using the most striking words from that single story.
(iv) Then, each group member will list positive words, affirmations or positive prophecies (Jones, 1996) that others have said to them, including self-affirmations and positive promises they have made to themselves.
(v) Each group member will create an alternative story by writing a poem in a "reverse circle" (Gustavson, 2006, *p.* 21) using the positive words, prophecies and affirmations listed in the previous step.

Group members will be invited to show and read their Dead-end circle and Reverse circle poems to the wider group.

Exploring Occupations: Group members review the initial occupations they had considered at the start of the intervention and based on the summary portrait developed earlier, outline a list of occupations they are now considering.	No poetry related activity to be undertaken here.

Session 4 (Lasting 2 h including a 15-minute break)

Part 3- Enacting My Story

Objective: Group members develop action plans to put their story into action.

Review the typical My Career Story workbook task (45 min)	Proposed poetry therapy task (60 min)
Reflect: Group members focus on their career story and use it to set specific goals for the next part of their lives.	Read a poem to the group to emphasise on decision making. For example, the poem: "The road not taken" by Robert Frost (from https://www.eduplace.com/activity/pdf/frost.pdf).
Tell: Group members identify important individuals with whom they want to share their story and explain the conclusions they have drawn from the My Career Story workbook.	Each group member shares their new career story with fellow group members. For example, through a prose poem describing how he or she plans to bring the new career story to life. Visuals or film could also be used when presenting the new career stories. Each group member draws a "Hand of Support" (adapted from Lowenstein, 2011, p. 7) identifying people he/ she trusts enough to share their career story with.
Perform: Group members list two to four objectives or steps they plan to take to move toward the goals they have developed.	End the session with a reading of some poems on: (i) Contrast between passive fatalism as suggested in the poem "Destiny" by Philippa Namutebi Barlow (in Amateshe, 1988, p. 20) and a more proactive approach as suggested in the poem "After a while" attributed to Veronica Shoffstall (in McNally, 1990, p. 65). (ii) Hope that plans can go well e.g. "Sometimes" by Sheenagh Pugh (cited in Benson, Chernaik, & Herbert, 1998, p. 131). (iii) The unknown future e.g. "What if this road" by Sheenagh Pugh (n.d.).

Session 5 (Lasting 60 min)

Final group session

Objective: To consolidate lessons learnt during the group sessions and facilitate forward movement after termination of the group (Brabender et al., 2004; Corey, 2012).

Proposed poetry therapy tasks for the debrief and termination session

In small groups of 3–4 people, group members share:

(i) Their most memorable experiences and lessons learnt since the group sessions began (previous 4 sessions).
(ii) A motto, or mantra they have created for themselves based on the lessons they have learnt to guide them going forward.
(iii) Create a collaborative poem (Thompson, 2006) based on the experiences of the small group members.

A representative from each small group reads their collaborative poem to the wider group.

To emphasise the need for openness to lessons life might proffer to each group member as they prepare to/as they transition from the group and from college to the world of work, the following poems are read and discussed in the group:

(i) "To an English Friend in Africa", by Ben Okri (Okri, 1997, p. 82).
(ii) "Finistere" by David Whyte (Whyte, 2012); and

Conclusion

The current world of work demands career adaptability, resilience and employability from workers. To foster development of such qualities in their clients, career counsellors must use dynamic counselling approaches that are responsive to the twenty-first century context. The Transforming Career Stories through Poetry intervention developed and presented in this paper is one such approach. Not only does it focus on clients' career stories; it is also innovative in its proposed use of poetry to facilitate the transformation of career stories from disempowered to more empowered versions in addition to being founded on well-established principles of career construction. At a time when the use of poetry in different therapeutic contexts is being applied widely already, this paper demonstrates how poetry reading and writing can be incorporated into career counselling settings in higher education as well. The proposed intervention could introduce both Kenyan counsellors and clients to the transformative power of poetry in counselling contexts. The intervention will also capitalise on the strong oral tradition common in African settings, and young people's growing interest in spoken word poetry, hip hop and rap music to attract potential participants.

In Kenya, poetry therapy is virtually unheard of and in order to make such interventions possible and available, counsellors and educators would need training (e.g. in Career Writing; principles of poetry therapy). As these ideas are so new in the Kenyan context, some scholars and counselling practitioners may also doubt their potential utility in career guidance and counselling. This is why, prior to implementing the intervention, I have presented it here as a detailed proposal for a workshop, giving the reader opportunity to see its strong theoretical foundation. Piloting the intervention in several higher education institutions in Kenya along with a systematic measurement of its outcomes would be necessary and would allow researchers to evaluate its usefulness. I propose two instruments to measure the effectiveness of this intervention. First, the Future Career Autobiography (Rehfuss, 2009) because it enables a researcher to identify participants' current occupational desires before a career intervention, and to measure change or stability of the participants' occupational narratives after the intervention. Noted changes could include movement from general to more specific occupational themes, and from hindered to more hopeful themes subsequent to the career intervention. Second, the Linguistic Index Word Count (Pennebaker, Booth, Boyd, & Francis, 2015) as it allows researchers to examine text samples and see if progress had been made towards a beneficial narrative (i.e. indicating a movement towards a second story). Both analysis methods have been cited in the literature and used as instruments to measure the effectiveness of career counselling interventions (Lengelle, 2014; Rehfuss & Di Fabio, 2012). I intend to pilot the Transforming Career Stories through Poetry intervention in Kenya in the near future in collaboration with colleagues.

Disclosure statement

No potential conflict of interest was reported by the author.

References

Adichie, C. N. (2009, July). *The danger of a single story* [Video file]. Retrieved from https://www.ted.com/talks/chimamanda_adichie_the_danger_of_a_single_story.

Amateshe, A. D. (1988). *An anthology of East African poetry*. Harlow, UK: Longman.

American College Health Association. (2015). *National college health assessment: Spring 2015 reference group executive summary*. Retrieved from http://www.acha-ncha.org/docs/NCHA-II_WEB_SPRING_2015_REFERENCE_GROUP_EXECUTIVE_SUMMARY.pdf

Ansell, C. (1978). Psychoanalysis and poetry. In A. Lerner (Ed.), *Poetry in the therapeutic experience* (pp. 12–23). New York, NY: Pergamon Press.

Arnett, J. J. (2015). *Emerging adulthood: The winding road from the late teens through the twenties* (2nd ed). New York, NY: Oxford University Press.

Awiti, A. O., & Scott, B. (2016). *Kenya youth survey report*. Nairobi: The Aga Khan University.

Baxter Magolda, M. B. (1999). Constructing adult identities. *Journal of College Student Development, 40*(6), 629–643. Retrieved from https://search-proquest-com.tcsedsystem.idm.oclc.org/psycinfo/docview/619436124/8B6AF2350FE14556PQ/4?accountid=34120

Baxter Magolda, M. B. (2004). *Making their own way: Narratives for transforming higher education to promote self development*. Stirling, VA: Stylus Publishing.

Benson, G., Chernaik, J., & Herbert, C. (1998). *London poems on the Underground* (7th ed.). London, UK: Cassell.

Berger, K. S. (2014). *The developing person through the life span* (9th ed). New York, NY: Worth Publishers.

Blustein, D. L. (2017). Epilogue. In *Psychology of career adaptability, employability and resilience* (pp. 449–450). doi:10.1007/978-3-319-66954-0

Bolden, R. (2014). Ubuntu. In D. Coghlan & M. Brydon-Miller (Eds.), *The SAGE encyclopedia of action research* (pp. 799–801). London, UK: SAGE Publications Ltd.

Brabender, V. A., Fallon, A. E., & Smolar, A. I. (2004). *Essentials of group therapy*. Hoboken, NJ: John Wiley & Sons.

Briddick, W. C., & Sensoy-Briddick, H. (2013). The role of audience in life design. In *Psychology of career counseling: New challenges for a new era* (pp. 69–81). New York, NY: Nova Science Publisher's Inc.

Busacca, L. A. (2007). Career construction theory: A practitioner's primer. *Career Planning and Adult Development, 23*(1), 57–67. Retrieved from https://www.questia.com/library/journal/1P3-1453134911/career-construction-theory-a-practitioner-s-primer

Busacca, L. A. (2017). Career counseling in postmodern times: Emergence and narrative conceptions. In *Postmodern career counseling: A handbook of culture, context, and cases* (pp. 23–36). Alexandria, VA: American Counseling Association.

Busacca, L. A., & Rehfuss, M. C. (2017). Postmodern career counseling: A new perspective for the 21st century. In *Postmodern career counseling: A handbook of culture, context, and cases* (pp. 1–19). Alexandria, VA: American Counseling Association.

Callanan, G. A., Perri, D. F., & Tomkowicz, S. M. (2017). Career management in uncertain times: Challenges and opportunities. *The Career Development Quarterly, 65*(4), 353–365. doi:10.1002/cdq.12113

Chireshe, R. (2012). Career guidance and counselling provisions at a South African university: Career advisors' reflections. *The Anthropologist, 14*(4), 305–310. doi:10.1080/09720073.2012.11891251

Clark, A. J. (2013). *Dawn of memories: The meaning of early recollections in life*. Plymouth, UK: Rowman & Littlefield Publishers, Inc.

Corey, G. (2012). *Theory and practice of group counseling* (8th ed.). Belmont, Canada: Brooks/Cole Cengage Learning.

DeCarlo, A., & Hockman, E. (2004). RAP therapy: A group work intervention method for urban adolescents. *Social Work with Groups, 26*(3), 45–59. doi:10.1300/j009v26n03_06

Del Corso, J. (2017). Counselling young adults to become career adaptable and career resilient. In *The psychology of career adaptability, employability and resilience* (pp. 171–188). doi:10.1007/978-3-319-66954-0

Di Fabio, A., & Maree, J. G. (2013). Career construction and life design: Heralding a new beginning to career counseling in the 21st century. In *Psychology of career counseling: New challenges for a new era* (pp. 1–13). New York, NY: Nova Science Publishers, Inc.

Domene, J. F., Landine, J., & Stewart, J. (2015). Emerging adult career transitions. In P. J. Hartung, M. Savickas, & W. B. Walsh (Eds.), *APA Handbook of career intervention volume 2 applications* (pp. 479–494). Washington, DC: American Psychological Association.

Edgar, K. (1978). The epiphany of the self via poetry therapy. In *Poetry in the therapeutic experience* (pp. 24–40). New York, NY: Pergamon Press Inc.

Evans, N. J., Forney, D. S., Guido, F. M., Patton, L. D., & Renn, K. A. (2010). *Student development in college: Theory, research, and practice* (2nd ed). San Francisco, CA: Jossey-Bass.

Frost, R. (n.d.). The road not taken. Retrieved from https://www.eduplace.com/activity/pdf/frost.pdf

Germeijs, V., Verschueren, K., & Soenens, B. (2006). Indecisiveness and high school students' career decision-making process: Longitudinal associations and the mediational role of anxiety. *Journal of Counseling Psychology, 53*(4), 397–410. doi:10.1037/0022-0167.53.4.397

Gold, R. (2014). *Writing with at-risk youth: The Pongo teen writing method*. Plymouth, UK: Rowman & Littlefield Education.

Goldstein, M. (1989). Poetry and therapeutic factors in group therapy. *Journal of Poetry Therapy, 2*(4), 231–241. Retrieved from https://link.springer.com/article/10.1007/BF03391346

Grace, C. M., Smith, K., & Hinchman, K. (2004). Exploring the African American oral tradition: Instructional implications for literacy learning. *Language Arts, 81*(6), 481–489.

Gustavson, C. B. (2006). *In-versing your life: A poetry workbook for self-discovery and healing*. New York, NY: Blooming Twig Books.

Hartung, P. J. (2013). The life-span, life-space theory of careers. In *Career development and counseling: Putting theory and research to work* (2nd ed., pp. 83–113). Hoboken, NJ: John Wiley & Sons.

Heywood, A. (1983). *Senior poetry anthology*. London, UK: Macmillan Publishers.

Holland, J. L. (1997). *Making vocational choices: A theory of vocational personalities and work environments* (3rd ed). Odessa, FL: Psychological Assessment Resources.

Johnson, D. W., & Johnson, F. P. (2014). *Joining together: Group theory and group skills* (11th ed.). Essex, England: Pearson Education Lt.

Jones, L. B. (1996). *The path: Creating your mission statement for work and for life*. New York, NY: Hyperion.

Law, B. (2010). *A career learning theory*. Retrieved from http://www.hihohiho.com/newthinking/crlrnoriginal.pdf

Lengelle, R. (2014). *Career writing: Creative, expressive and reflective approaches to narrative and dialogical career guidance* (Unpublished doctoral dissertation). Tilburg University, Tilburg, The Netherlands.

Lengelle, R., & Meijers, F. (2009). Mystery to mastery: An exploration of what happens in the black box of writing and healing. *Journal of Poetry Therapy, 22*(2), 57–75. doi:10.1080/08893670903072935

Lengelle, R., & Meijers, F. (2018). De effecten van groepswerk door "career writing". *Loopbaan Visie, 3*, 85–90.

Lengelle, R., Meijers, F., & Hughes, D. (2016). Creative writing for life design: Reflexivity, metaphor and change processes through narrative. *Journal of Vocational Behavior, 97*, 60–67. doi:10.1016/j.jvb.2016.07.012

Lengelle, R., Meijers, F., Poell, R., & Post, M. (2014). Career writing: Creative, expressive and reflective approaches to narrative identity formation in students in higher education. *Journal of Vocational Behavior, 85*(1), 75–84. doi:10.1016/j.jvb.2014.05.001

Lent, R. W., & Brown, S. D. (2013). Understanding and facilitating career development in the 21st century. In *Career development and counseling: Putting theory and research to work* (2nd ed., pp. 1–26). Hoboken, NJ: John Wiley & Sons.

Lerner, A. (1978). Introduction. In A. Lerner (Ed.), *Poetry in the therapeutic experience* (pp. xv–xvii). New York, NY: Pergamon Press.

Lerner, A. (1982). Poetry therapy in the group experience. In *The newer therapies: A sourcebook* (pp. 228–247). New York, NY: Van Nostrand Reinhold Company Inc.

Levy, I. (2012). Hip hop and spoken word therapy with urban youth. *Journal of Poetry Therapy, 25*(4), 219–224. doi:10.1080/08893675.2012.736182

Lowenstein, L. (Ed.). (2011). *Assessment and treatment activities for children, adolescents, and families volume three: Practitioners share their most effective techniques*. Toronto, Canada: Champion Press.

Maree, K. (2017). The psychology of career adaptability, career resilience, and employability: A broad overview. In *Psychology of career adaptability, employability and resilience* (pp. 3–11). doi:10.1007/978-3-319-66954-0

Masambia, F. M. (2014). Embracing counseling and psychotherapy in Kenya. *Educational Specialist*, 1–20. Retrieved from http://commons.lib.jmu.edu/edspec201019/63/

Mazza, N. (2017). *Poetry therapy: Theory and practice* (2nd ed.). London, UK: Routledge.

McNally, D. (1990). *Even eagles need a push: Learning to soar in a changing world*. New York, NY: Dell Publishing.

Meijers, F. (2002). Career learning in a changing world: The role of emotions. *International Journal for the Advancement of Counselling, 24*(3), 149–167. Retrieved from https://link-springer-com.tcsedsystem.idm.oclc.org/article/10.1023/A%3A1022970404517

Mkhize, N. (2015). Qualitative career assessment in African contexts. In *Career assessment: Qualitative approaches* (pp. 247–254). Rotterdam, The Netherlands: Sense Publishers.

Mosak, H. H., & Di Pietro, R. (2006). *Early recollections: Interpretative method and application*. New York, NY: Routledge.

NAPT. (n.d.). History of NAPT – National Association for Poetry Therapy. Retrieved from https://poetrytherapy.org/index.php/about-napt/history-of-napt/

Okri, B. (1997). *An African elegy*. London, UK: Vintage.

Olson-McBride, L., & Page, T. F. (2012). Song to self: Promoting a therapeutic dialogue with high-risk youths through poetry and popular music. *Social Work with Groups, 35*(2), 124–137. doi:10.1080/01609513.2011.603117

Oludhe-Macgoye, M. (n.d.). Marjorie Oludhe Macgoye | Badilisha Poetry – Pan-African Poets. Retrieved from http://badilishapoetry.com/marjorie-oludhe-macgoye/

Osoro, B. K., Amundson, N. E., & Borgen, W. A. (2000). Career decision-making of high school students in Kenya. *International Journal for the Advancement of Counselling, 22*(4), 289–300. https://doi.org/10.1023/A:1005661001209.

Pennebaker, J. W., Booth, R. J., Boyd, R. L., & Francis, M. E. (2015). *Operator's manual: Linguistic Inquiry and word count-LIWC2015*. Austin, TX: Pennebaker Conglomerates, Inc.

Pennebaker, J. W., & Seagal, J. D. (1999). Forming a story: The health benefits of narrative. *Journal of Clinical Psychology, 55* (10), 1243–1254. doi:10.1002/(sici)1097-4679(199910)55:10<1243::aid-jclp6>3.0.co;2-n

Pisarik, C. T., Rowell, P. C., & Thompson, L. K. (2017). A phenomenological study of career anxiety among college students. *The Career Development Quarterly, 65*(4), 339–352. doi:10.1002/cdq.12112

Pugh, S. (n.d.). What if this road. Retrieved from www2.open.ac.uk/openlearn/poetryprescription/what-if-this-road.html

Rehfuss, M. C. (2009). The future career autobiography: A narrative measure of career intervention effectiveness. *The Career Development Quarterly, 58*(1), 82–90. doi:10.1002/j.2161-0045.2009.tb00177.x

Rehfuss, M. C. (2013). The role of narratives in career counseling: Career as story. In *Psychology of career counseling: New challenges for a new era* (pp. 61–68). New York, NY: Nova Science Publisher's Inc.

Rehfuss, M. C. (2017). Using the my career story workbook with an African American high school student. In *Postmodern career counseling: A handbook of culture, context, and cases* (pp. 91–103). Alexandria, VA: American Counseling Association.

Rehfuss, M. C., & Di Fabio, A. (2012). Validating the future career autobiography as a measure of narrative change. *Journal of Career Assessment, 20*(4), 452–462. doi:10.1177/1069072712450005

Reiter, S. (2000). *A poetry therapy guidebook for the helping professional: Part I. Poetry therapy; understanding its essence. Part II. A poetry therapy curriculum* (Doctoral dissertation). ProQuest Dissertations and Theses database.

Savickas, M. (2015). *Life-design counseling manual.* Mark L.Savickas.

Savickas, M. L. (2002). Career construction: A developmental theory of vocational behavior. In *Career choice and development* (4th ed., pp. 149–205). San Francisco, CA: John Wiley & Sons, Inc.

Savickas, M. L. (2005). The theory and practice of career construction. In *Career development and counseling: Putting theory and research to work* (pp. 42–70). Hoboken, NJ: John Wiley & Sons.

Savickas, M. L. (2006). Career construction theory. In *Encyclopaedia of career development* (pp. 85–88). Thousand Oaks, CA: Sage Publications.

Savickas, M. L. (2011). *Career counseling*. Washington, DC: American Psychological Association.

Savickas, M. L. (2013). Career construction theory. In *Career development and counseling: Putting theory and research to work* (2nd ed., pp. 147–183). Hoboken, NJ: John Wiley & Sons, Inc.

Savickas, M. L., & Hartung, P. J. (2012). *My career story: An autobiographical workbook for life- career success.* Retrieved from http://www.vocopher.com/CSI/CCI_workbook.pdf

Schloss, G. A., & Grundy, D. E. (1978). Action techniques in psychopoetry. In *Poetry in the therapeutic experience* (pp. 81–96). New York, NY: Pergamon Press Inc.

Stoll, G., Rieger, S., Lüdtke, O., Nagengast, B., Trautwein, U., & Roberts, B. W. (2017). Vocational interests assessed at the end of high school predict life outcomes assessed 10 years later over and above IQ and Big Five personality traits. *Journal of Personality and Social Psychology, 113*(1), 167–184. doi:10.1037/pspp0000117

Stoltz, K. B. (2017). Early recollections with a paroled African American male: A career-focused group approach. In *Postmodern career counseling: A handbook of culture, context, and cases* (pp. 133–146). Alexandria, VA: American Counseling Association.

Stoltz, K. B., & Barclay, S. R. (2015). *The life design thememapping guide.* Retrieved from http://www.vocopher.com/Susan%20Barclay/THE%20LIFE%20DESIGN%20THEMEMAPPING%20GUIDE_v.3.pdf

Suda, C. (2002). Gender disparities in the Kenyan labour market: Implications for poverty reduction. *Nordic Journal for African Studies, 11*(3), 301–321. Retrieved from http://erepository.uonbi.ac.ke/bitstream/handle/11295/38502/FULL%20TEXT.pdf?sequence=1

Thompson, K. (2006). Warming up and working together. In *Writing works: A resource handbook for therapeutic writing workshops and activities* (pp. 35–55). London, UK: Jessica Kingsley Publishers.

USAID. (2014). *Workforce connections: Kenya youth assessment.* Retrieved from https://www.usaid.gov/sites/default/files/documents/1865/Kenya_Youth_Assessment_Final_Report.pdf

Van Vianen, A. E., De Pater, I. E., & Preenene, P. T. (2009). Adaptable careers: Maximizing less and exploring more. *The Career Development Quarterly, 57*(4), 298–309. doi:10.1002/j.2161-0045.2009.tb00115.x

Watson, M., McMahon, M., Mkhize, N., Schweitzer, R. D., & Mpofu, E. (2011). Career counseling people of African ancestry. In E. Mpofu (Ed.), *Counseling people of African ancestry* (pp. 281–293). New York, NY: Cambridge University Press.

Wendlandt, N. M., & Rochlen, A. B. (2008). Addressing the college-to-work transition. *Journal of Career Development, 35*(2), 151–165. doi:10.1177/0894845308325646.

Whyte, D. (2012). English. Retrieved from http://www.davidwhyte.com/english-poetry#Finisterre

Xerri, D. (2017). Combating voice poverty through spoken word poetry: An interview with Candy Royalle. *Journal of Poetry Therapy, 30*(4), 262–270. doi:10.1080/08893675.2017.1352066

Yalom, I. D., & Leszcz, M. (2005). *The theory and practice of group psychotherapy* (5th ed). New York, NY: Basic Books.

Yücesan, E., & Şendurur, Y. (2018). Effects of music therapy, poetry therapy, and creative drama applications on self-esteem levels of college students. *Journal of Poetry Therapy, 31*(1), 26–39. doi:10.1080/08893675.2018.1396730

Index

Note: Page numbers followed by "n" denote endnotes.